*"Eat Your Vegetables" and Other Mistakes Parents Make: Redefining Hc Raise Healthy Eaters* 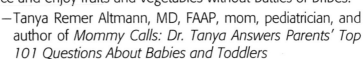 is a pediatrician- and mom-tested guide to help pa and caregivers raise healthy food eaters for life. With many of today's ch being raised on fast food nutrition and couch potato fitness, Dr. Muth parents direction in this step-by-step guide for shaping children's psyches to help them embrace and enjoy fruits and vegetables without battles or bribes.

> —Tanya Remer Altmann, MD, FAAP, mom, pediatrician, and author of *Mommy Calls: Dr. Tanya Answers Parents' Top 101 Questions About Babies and Toddlers*

*"Eat Your Vegetables" and Other Mistakes Parents Make: Redefining How to Raise Healthy Eaters* is an informative guide for parents whose goal is to help their children become healthy eaters. The book impressively integrates developmental psychology and behavioral management techniques with nutritional information, making it easier for parents to help their children make healthy eating choices. It is a voluminous resource, brimming with concrete ideas, suggestions, and recipes. Dr. Muth manages to communicate a great deal of information without "preaching" to parents and with a warm and understanding tone that bridges the perspectives of pediatrician and parent. Thus, her book will not alienate parents who may have initially had difficulty getting their children to eat more healthy foods. I will recommend the book to all of my parent-friends.

> —Kristina L. McDonald, Ph.D., mom and developmental psychologist at The University of Alabama

Natalie Muth has studied the literature and the expert recommendations for infants and toddlers and has written an accessible and easy-to-follow book for parents, grandparents, and pediatricians. This book is destined to be the essential guide for parents on how to feed their young children, helping to create meals that will more likely be healthy, as well as a happy family time.

> —Wendy Slusser, MD, MS, FAAP, mom, assistant clinical professor at UCLA School of Medicine, associate professor at UCLA School of Public Health, and medical director of the UCLA Fit for Healthy Weight Program at Mattel Children's Hospital UCLA

The majority of childhood obesity cases could be avoided or reversed if parents understood and applied the fundamentals of leading a healthy, fit lifestyle based on proper nutrition and regular physical activity. Dr. Muth's book *"Eat Your Vegetables" and Other Mistakes Parents Make: Redefining How to Raise Healthy Eaters* provides a scientifically supported, commonsense approach to improving the overall health and well-being of our nation's youth. She uses her diverse background as a pediatric physician, registered dietitian, and ACE-certified fitness professional to offer parents sensible and practical solutions for addressing their children's nutritional, physical, and emotional needs. This book is a must read for any parent interested in helping their children experience the joys of eating healthy and leading a physically active lifestyle.

> —Cedric X. Bryant, Ph.D., FACSM, dad and chief science officer for the American Council on Exercise

# "Eat Your Vegetables" and Other Mistakes Parents Make

## Redefining How to Raise Healthy Eaters

*Dear Phil + Oksana
I hope that you enjoy!
to happy, healthy mealtimes...
Natalie*

**Natalie Digate Muth, MD, MPH, RD**

With recipes by Mary Saph Tanaka, MD, MS

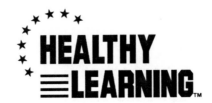

Disclaimer: The content of this book is being offered for education and information purposes only. It should not be used as a substitute for the advice of a child's physician.

ISBN: 978-1-60679-225-4
Library of Congress Control Number: 2012938849
Book layout: Studio J Art & Design
Front cover design: Studio J Art & Design
Front cover images: iStockphoto/Thinkstock
Text photos—Figures 1-3 (toddler and school age), 2-2 (toddler), 4-1 (school age), 5-4 (infant), 7-3 (school age), 11-1 (school age): Jennifer Bonesz
Text photos—recipes: Dig-It Photography

Healthy Learning
P.O. Box 1828
Monterey, CA 93942
www.healthylearning.com

For Tommy, Mariella, and Teddy

# Dedication

# Acknowledgments

When I was a young medical student with a special interest in pediatrics and nutrition, observing child-parent nutrition interactions piqued my interest in the special mealtime struggles that parents face. The initial idea to research and write a book on this topic evolved over the ensuing five years and has finally come together as this book. Along the way, countless individuals have supported me in this process.

First, I'd like to thank my husband, Bob, who encouraged me from the beginning to just do it and who spent hours reviewing ideas, carefully reading through each chapter, congratulating me on those he felt were well done, and politely but bluntly directing me back to the drawing board for those that didn't match the same level of quality. He patiently supported me in spending evenings tied to my computer and did more than his share in helping to keep the house running smoothly as I spent any spare moment writing just one more page or researching just one more article. I'd also like to thank my dad, who has lived with us to help take care of the kids over the past three years while I completed my pediatrics residency and this book and who eagerly supported me throughout the entire process. I can't thank him enough for his commitment to my family and for his patient efforts to apply many of the strategies recommended throughout this book's chapters, even though it would be easier to resort to the old ways of making kids eat healthy rather than teaching them how to do so. The valuable advice and "reality checks" from my mom, who is the inspiration for Chapter 11, played an invaluable role in preparation for what I hope turned out to be a down-to-earth, real-life, realistic, and flexible work. I'd also like to thank her for challenging me and making sure I could defend each statement or assertion. Completing this book would not have been possible without the good humor, flexibility, and charm of my own kids—three-year-old Tommy and one-year-old Mariella—who didn't mind serving as guinea pigs and who highlighted on a very personal basis many of the challenges that parents face in their efforts to raise healthy eaters. I must also thank my great friend and sister, Nikki, and her two kids, Marion and Anneliese, whose mealtime battles served as an inspiration for this book.

To the many moms and dads who contributed their challenges, stories, advice, quotes, and pictures of their kids for the book—thank you! I'd like to especially thank Bridget Jensen, who reviewed every chapter and offered extremely valuable feedback and insights, and Jen Riconosciuto, whose edits and contributions greatly enhanced the book.

Mary Saph Tanaka, an astounding cook, great friend, and fellow pediatrician, enriched this book tremendously with her delicious and healthy recipes. Thank you to my mentor and book reviewer, Wendy Slusser, a phenomenal pediatrician and child health advocate, especially in the areas of nutrition and childhood obesity prevention and treatment. I'm immensely grateful to Dr. Jim Peterson and Angie Perry at Healthy Learning, who believed in my idea and who were willing to take a risk on me as a first-time author, and to editor

Chris Stolle and project manager Kristi Huelsing. Their patience, flexibility, and ongoing support made the process enjoyable. I'd also like to thank Penn State researcher Leann Birch and her lab for the incredible and pioneering work they have done studying child feeding strategies. Their work has served as the scientific basis for much of this book. To the late Dale Fetherling, instructor for the University of California–San Diego extension course on how to write a nonfiction book proposal, thank you for showing me how to transform what was just an idea into what is now my first book—a compilation of all that I have learned over the past five years about how to raise healthy eaters.

# Foreword

Currently, childhood obesity has become a major public health problem, and children's diets are characterized by too many calories from sugar and fat, and too few fruits and vegetables. Dr. Muth provides timely insight on how we create the very unhealthy dietary patterns in our children that we need to prevent—picky eaters who won't eat their vegetables but are eating too much junk food.

*"Eat Your Vegetables" and Other Mistakes Parents Make: Redefining How to Raise Healthy Eaters* gives clear, evidence-based advice to parents on how to help children learn to like and eat "what's good for them" and to support their children in using hunger and fullness cues to decide how much to eat. She also provides clear step-by-step alternative strategies for feeding children, including recipes for healthy foods that should be easy for kids to learn to love. The book includes many clear descriptions and examples of the ways that parents influence what children learn about food and eating, including what, when, and how much they should eat. This perspective provides the basis for helping parents avoid common mistakes. The 10 "Power Ps" summarize her framework for developing patterns of healthy eating and avoiding "food fights." This book is a "must read" for parents (or grandparents)—whether they have an infant, a toddler, or a school-aged child—and a wonderful resource for childcare providers.

—Leann Birch, Ph.D.
   Director, Center for Childhood Obesity Research
   Distinguished Professor, Department of Human Development
      and Family Studies
   College of Health and Human Development
   The Pennsylvania State University

contents

Canned sardines, outdated cereal, and TV dinners comprised my typical diet as a child. My family owned a small independent grocery store, and we were the proud recipients of the food that could no longer be sold: the expired, dented, overstocked, and undersold—but, as my dad said, all perfectly edible. Like many of us, my mom was an ambitious working woman stressed for time and trying to balance the demands of a budding professional career and raising young kids. As such, she would commonly roll through the grocery store about once a month and left with two or three carts full of food. So, we did get fresh vegetables—it just happened to be around the first week of most months.

These fine eating habits and my love of fast food, fried food, and sugar food led me on my way to being known by my peers as "Natalie Fatalie." Like nine million children today, I was an obese kid.[1] But luckily, against the odds, I lost the extra weight and entered adulthood at a healthy weight with healthy habits, including a love of fruits and vegetables and a commitment to a physically active lifestyle. Unfortunately, about half of obese kids aren't so lucky. And many of them develop diseases that used to be seen only in adults, such as type 2 diabetes, high blood pressure, high cholesterol, fatty liver disease, orthopedic injury, and more.[2] In fact, many experts now predict that this generation of children will be the first to have a shorter life span than their parents. The problem, though, isn't just confined to the kids that are already overweight—after all, one in three kids is overweight or obese[3], but two out of three adults are carrying too much weight.[4] Do the math and you've got a lot of normal weight kids becoming overweight adults. All this bad news compelled First Lady Michelle Obama to start the "Let's Move!" campaign to stamp out childhood obesity within a generation. But it's about more than weight—a diet high in fruits and vegetables and a physically active lifestyle add a healthy dose of quantity and quality to life.

Surely, no one needs to be convinced that children *should* eat healthy; it's more a matter of making it happen. And we all know that it isn't always easy. But it doesn't have to be a constant battle. My goal in writing this book is to share what works and what doesn't in raising healthy eaters. The content is based a little bit on personal experience with my patients and two young kids and mostly on what I've uncovered from published research, expert opinions, and anecdotes from parents who have "been there and done that." Ultimately, I hope this information will help us raise a healthier generation of children and get us a few steps closer to reversing the childhood obesity epidemic.

In the ensuing chapters, you'll find numerous easy-to-implement, proven-to-work tips and tricks for raising healthy eaters, along with delicious, healthy, easy-to-make, and kid-tested recipe ideas developed by fellow pediatrician and fantastic and creative cook, Mary Saph Tanaka. Perhaps most importantly, you'll also learn the science and psychology behind the tips so that on any given day, in any given situation, you can come up with your own solutions to common and unique food- and activity-based challenges. The book is about more than kids' nutrition; it's about empowering busy, stressed, and had-it-up-to-here parents. Only then will we move America closer to a healthier future—and on a more personal level, your mealtime battles will be an angst of the past.

# Common "Mistakes" Parents Make

Parents share a wealth of concerns about their kids' eating habits. The three biggest are not eating enough fruits and vegetables, picky eating, and eating too much junk food.[5] In response to the distress and anxiety posed by these concerns, parents have historically responded with a variety of tactics aimed to coerce, bribe, convince, guilt, or otherwise induce compliance in unwilling little ones. Of course, parents are acting in the best interest of the child, hoping that one day, the child will agree that fruits and vegetables are healthy and should be consumed at every meal—and, ideally, the child would also be willing to taste from a variety of new and interesting foods. The problem is that many of these tactics backfire, the kids dig in, and the parents are left with an unending headache dealing with food battles at every meal. Intuitively, all of us probably know this already. Think back to your childhood. Chances are you can produce a story or two in a surprising amount of detail of how your parents' or other adults' good intentions turned you off to some of the "good foods" and on to some of the "bad foods." Seventy-two percent of college students asked to a recall a childhood experience of being pressured to eat reported a current dislike of that food, along with anger and memories of conflict.[6]

This book highlights some common "mistakes" parents make, divided into four categories:
- The inherited mistakes—those passed down from generation to generation
- The underrated mistakes—the ones that have a profound effect on the child psyche, leading to a battle of wills, power struggles, and dreaded mealtime "food fights"
- The everyday mistakes—those that happen day in and day out without anyone realizing the counterproductive effect they have on the child's developing nutrition preferences
- The overlooked mistakes—unintentional acts of omission that sideline parents' best efforts to inspire healthy habits

You likely noticed that "mistakes" is presented in quotations. The reason for this is to highlight that "mistake" is probably not the best word to use, as it might incite a sense of blame, guilt, defensiveness, or various other negative feelings that stand opposite to the purpose of this book. I use the word mostly for lack of a better descriptor. But ultimately, the goal here is to put together the latest information on childhood development, behavior, and shaping healthy eating habits in as unbiased a manner as possible. A major part of parenting is making decisions and then evaluating their consequences. Sometimes, kids will surprise us and do exactly what we ask, but more often, they'll repeatedly refuse and push the limits of our patience. Parenting is a work in progress, with many "mistakes"—or learning opportunities—along the way. Here, I just try to compile this information to give you a head start and take some of the headache out of trying to shape childhood behaviors, especially when it has to do with eating and physical activity. Not every tip or strategy will work for every child. Over the course of experimenting with the ideas presented in this book, you'll find what works and what doesn't for your kids. Ultimately, you, of course, are the number one expert on your child. I'm just here to help you broaden and refine your expertise.

The next several pages highlight the major content of each of the book's chapters. This overview will introduce you to the book's major themes and help you focus on those chapters that will be most useful to you (although if the book is taken as a whole, the likelihood of success with the recommended strategies increases substantially).

## The Inherited Mistakes

The following are the mistakes passed from generation to generation.

### Mistake #1—Insisting "Eat Your Vegetables!"

When left to their own devices, kids eat what they like and leave the rest. And most don't like bitter and bland vegetables. A preference for sweet and salty tastes and the rejection of sour and bitter tastes are innate and unlearned. This reality frustrates parents to no end, and as a result, you may find yourself reasoning that intervention is needed—and it's needed immediately—so you insist that your children eat their vegetables. The alternative, you fear, is that your child will be unhealthy, malnourished, and grow up to be a veggie-hating, overweight, heart-attack-prone glutton. The truth is that the more you pressure your child to eat certain foods, the less likely he'll be to develop a taste for them and continue to eat them often as an adult. In fact, as described in Chapter 1, several research studies have shown that encouraging children to consume a particular food increases their dislike for that food. Kids instinctively resist persuasion. If you want to get your kids to eat vegetables and other healthy foods because they *like* them, you'll have to employ different strategies. The research and strategies are discussed in detail in Chapter 1.

### Mistake #2—Using Food as a Reward

We're all guilty. Using food as a reward is such an easy, inexpensive, and overwhelmingly effective tool that it's hard not to use it. But the short-term benefits from using food as a reward come with a hefty price tag. A series of studies conducted in the early 1980s by psychologist Leann Birch and colleagues at Penn State found that the social environment of children's eating is important in shaping their tastes and food preferences. Children learned to dislike foods eaten to obtain rewards ("Eat your vegetables and you can watch TV") and they learned to prefer foods eaten as rewards ("Clean up your toys and you can have some cookies") or paired with positive interactions with an adult (such as visits to the ice cream store with Grandma). The positive association that develops between the foods used as reward and "feeling good" can lead to later emotional and disordered eating. Chapter 2 offers several alternative ideas.

### Mistake #3—Requiring Membership in the "Clean Plate Club"

For generations, parents have guilted their children into eating what's served by sharing heart-wrenching stories of starving children in developing countries.

When that doesn't work (although it often does), parents then move to the next tactic: eat or no dessert; eat or no play time; eat or Mom and Dad will be disappointed, mad, mean—you name it and parents have tried it. While in the short term these tactics may work, in the long run, they set the stage not only for food battles and power struggles at most meals but worse—they can cause a diminished ability to regulate hunger. In other words, requiring membership in the "Clean Plate Club" teaches children to use external cues (how much food remains on the plate) rather than internal cues (feelings of hunger) to determine how much to eat. Chapter 3 highlights how we can disband the Clean Plate Club once and for all.

## The Underrated Mistakes

The underrated mistakes are those mistakes that have a profound effect on the child psyche, leading to a battle of wills, power struggles, and dreaded mealtime "food fights."

*Mistake #4—Forbidding Potato Chips and Ice Cream*

In one study, children who were tempted with a clear jar of cookies on the table but told they could not eat them for 10 minutes, ate three times more cookies than kids who had free access to the cookies.[7] The results of this and other studies show that kids whose food is highly restricted are more likely to overindulge when they have access to forbidden foods. Regardless of how much you try to protect your children from candy, sweets, and other junk food, they will eat it—if not in your home, then at school, friends' houses, with the grandparents, and so on. If you leave it in your house, they will find it —especially if you've "hidden it" and added the allure of it being "forbidden." The best way to counter the allure of junk food is to make it less enticing. Chapter 4 shows you how.

*Mistake #5—Dismissing "Packaging"*

How many of these can you answer?

1. "Lucky Charms®—they're _____!"
2. Who is the cartoon mascot for Cheetos®? _____
3. Toucan Sam is a fan of what cereal? _____
4. Complete this soft drink slogan: "Do the _____."
5. At McDonald's®, they "love to see you _____."
6. Who is always trying to steal Fred's Cocoa Pebbles? _____
7. What drink is advertised by a big pitcher that says "Oh, yeah!"? _____
8. Name the Rice Krispies® triplets: _____.
9. Complete this cereal slogan: "Silly rabbit, _____ are for kids!"
10. What kind of animal is pizza parlor mascot Chuck E. Cheese? _____

How'd you do?* The fact that you still remember most of this even after all these years exemplifies the harsh reality that manufacturers are experts

*Answers: 1. Magically delicious. 2. Chester Cheetah. 3. Froot Loops®. 4. Dew. 5. Smile. 6. Barney Rubble. 7. Kool-Aid®. 8. Snap, Crackle, Pop. 9. Trix®. 10. Mouse.

in influencing our tastes and desires. Parents who underestimate this power miss an opportunity to intervene in the unhealthy and unproductive mind manipulation of the manufacturers. They also miss the chance to use some very successful packaging strategies in healthy and productive ways—namely, inspiring kids to eat the healthy foods we want them to eat. Chapter 5 gives you the tools you need to use "packaging" to your and your child's advantage.

*Mistake #6—Failing to "Live It"*

Hands down, "living it" will be the most challenging and yet most powerful change that you will make to help your kids adopt a lifetime of healthy habits. If you're not already, now is the time for you to commit to healthy eating and regular physical activity. Ask yourself: Are the foods and beverages available in my home healthful and served in reasonable proportions? Is physical activity a family priority? Do I have rules in place limiting screen time? Don't underestimate your influence—programs that specifically target parents as the exclusive agent of change have demonstrated superior outcomes in improving children's eating and exercise habits.[8] Chapter 6 helps you to "live it." (Note: An unexpected consequence may be a drastic improvement in your own health, quality of life, and body weight.)

## The Everyday Mistakes

The everyday mistakes happen day in and day out without anyone ever realizing their counterproductive effects on a child's nutrition and physical activity.

*Mistake #7—Catering to Picky Eaters*

Go out to any restaurant that at least gives the pretense of being family friendly and you will find that, regardless of whether you're at a fast-food restaurant or a five-star establishment, with rare exception (although a movement is under way to change this), the children's menu offers pretty much the same choices: some version of breaded chicken, macaroni and cheese, peanut butter and jelly, and cheese pizza or a hot dog. Infrequently, you'll find any vegetables other than French fries (which really shouldn't be counted as a vegetable) and maybe you'll come across an applesauce side—if you're lucky. Restaurants offer children these standards because that's what kids want. The kids are happy. The parents are happy because the kids will eat something and be pleasant. Everybody wins. Or not.

While in the short term choosing from children's menus and preparing separate meals (the home-cooked version of the children's menu) to appease picky eaters is the easier and more harmonious choice to make, in the long run, it teaches kids to more strongly prefer the "just for kids" foods, which are almost uniformly high fat, high sodium, high calories, and low in everything else (such as fiber, vitamins, and minerals). To help you get out of this rut and still keep the peace at home, Chapter 7 helps you get a child to accept your previously rejected meals. It also offers some tips and strategies to help you eat out with your kids without blowing your efforts to feed your children healthy foods.

*Mistake #8—Sacrificing Taste*

Can you think of a bad food experience that totally turned you off to ever trying that type of food again? Such as eating spoiled fish or some kind of vegetable soufflé gone very wrong? Taste is the most important factor in determining whether a child will accept a food. It doesn't have to be true that the most delicious foods are "heart attacks on a platter"; likewise, a very healthy meal needn't taste bland. Chapter 8 helps you maximize taste and nutritional density while minimizing extra sugar and calories.

*Mistake #9—Enabling the Couch Potato*

Let's be honest—it's much more convenient to plop a six-year-old in front of the television than to provide the child with seemingly endless entertainment in an attempt to hold his attention half as well. While this offers short-term peace and respite, in the long run, enabling the couch potato leads to overweight, inactive kids and a plethora of missed opportunities. But a little nudge from parents can contribute to a surprising turnaround. You can get your sedentary kid active and having a blast now with some help from the tips outlined in Chapter 9.

**The Overlooked Mistakes**

These are the unintentional acts of omission that sideline parents' best efforts to inspire healthy habits.

*Mistake #10—Remaining Speechless at Doctor's Visits*

How many times have you taken your kids to a doctor's appointment and discussed their weight or physical activity habits or diet? Did your pediatrician plot their weight for length (if younger than two years old) or BMI (if older than two years old) on the growth chart and explain to you what this means? Did he offer you any nutrition, fitness, or health information you internalized and acted on? If your child's doctor is one of the 80 percent of pediatricians who think they lack the tools to effectively help overweight kids change course,[9] parents of overweight and obese kids (which, by the way, is about a third of the population) or parents of kids with less-than-ideal eating and activity habits (which is almost everyone) may not get the help they need—unless they speak up. While parents can't control their pediatrician's behavior, they *can* steer the appointment in the right direction *if* they come to the clinic well informed and prepared. Figure out how to make the most of doctor's visits in Chapter 10.

*Mistake #11—Mishandling Grandparent Sabotage*

Well-intentioned grandparents and other child care providers can wreak havoc on a parent's perfectly planned eating strategy. In fact, one study found that children cared for by their grandparents had a 34 percent higher risk of being overweight than children primarily cared for by parents or an unrelated nanny or babysitter.[10] But let's face it—a large percentage of parents are working full time and have to leave many of the day-to-day decisions to other caretakers—many of whom are unpaid grandparents who sacrifice a lot to help us out.

While it may be easier to "let bygones be bygones," grandparent sabotage can wreak havoc on parents' other nutrition successes. In Chapter 11, parents learn how to speak up without offending and annoying Grandma and Grandpa, who, as we all recognize, are mighty and powerful influences.

*Mistake #12—Missing Opportunities*

Despite its accompanying demands, stresses, mistakes, and disappointments, parenting is supposed to be fun. You have the incredible opportunity to teach your children about the wonders and amazement that the world has to offer. While this role extends far beyond shaping your kids' health habits, you can make learning about healthy nutrition and physical activity fun and educational. Chapter 12 will show you how.

# The Fundamentals

This book is written so you'll get comprehensive answers to your questions compiled into a simple-to-read and organized fashion you can't find anywhere else. While helpful in getting fresh information out to readers, that strategy leaves out a lot of the basic information all parents should know. I've addressed that limitation by including a short recap of the fundamentals here in the introduction. This foundational information is expanded on in each chapter.

## Nutrition Basics

Americans are notoriously lousy eaters, but that's not necessarily due to lack of knowledge. We all know that fruits and vegetables are healthy and that French fries and hot dogs aren't. However, translating knowing into doing is a whole different story—especially when trying to control the behavior of spunky little beings with minds of their own. Research confirms that a wide gap exists between nutrition recommendations for children and what children actually eat. Compared to the recent past, children and adolescents eat breakfast less often, away from home more often, a greater proportion of calories from snacks, more fried and nutrient-poor foods, greater portion sizes, fewer fruits and vegetables, excess sodium, more sweetened beverages, and fewer dairy products.[11,12] As a result, children and especially adolescents eat smaller amounts of many nutrients, such as calcium and potassium, than the recommended values. So, here we start with the "shoulds" and ideals of what would be nice for your kids to eat; throughout the course of the ensuing chapters, I'll help you to actually get your kids to want to eat these foods.

In early 2011, the U.S government released the Dietary Guidelines for Americans, a detailed government document outlining best nutrition practices. Later in the year, the MyPyramid guidelines were replaced with MyPlate, which emphasizes a diet rich in fruits and vegetables by way of an icon of a dinner plate which is half full with fruits and vegetables, one-quarter lean protein, one-quarter whole grain, and a side of dairy (see Figure 1). The Dietary Guidelines for kids were closely aligned with the American Heart Association (AHA) and the American Academy of Pediatrics (AAP) dietary guidelines for children and adolescents aged 2 to 18 years.[13] Both sets of recommendations emphasize a diet rich in fruits, vegetables, whole grains, low-fat and nonfat dairy products, beans, fish, and lean meat. A table of the Dietary Guidelines as they apply to kids is included in Figure 2. Note that the calorie amounts are based on the needs of a sedentary child. If your children are active, they will need more calories.

In short, the AHA/AAP recommendations and the Dietary Guidelines recommend that you pick:

- Mostly whole grains as opposed to refined sugars. When you're deciding on carbohydrates, choose brown—brown bread*, brown rice, brown pasta. Look for cereal that's high in fiber and low in sugar. At first, your kids might abhor the change. Ease them into it by using half whole grain/half white at first and then slowly transition to whole grain only.

- Ample nutrient-dense dark green and orange vegetables, such as broccoli and carrots, rather than disproportionate amounts of starchy vegetables, such as white potatoes and corn, which contain fewer vitamins and minerals. A general rule of thumb is, the more colorful the vegetable, the more nutrients it contains. While potatoes are Americans' favorite vegetable, their health value is limited.

- A variety of fruits, preferably from the whole food sources, as opposed to fruit juices. While the Dietary Guidelines still count 100

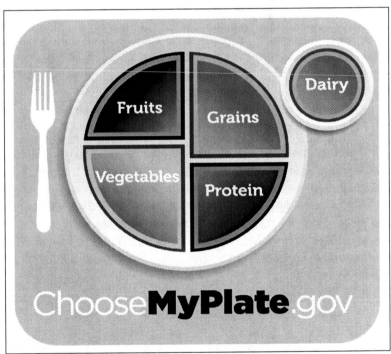

Figure 1. MyPlate, the federal government's nutrition guidance for Americans that replaced the short-lived MyPyramid

*Make sure it says "*whole* grain"—food manufacturers are savvy, and many times, they want you to think something is healthier that it really is. So, watch out for "seven grain," "honey wheat," and the like. They aren't whole grain.

| Daily Estimated Calories and Recommended Servings for Grains, Fruits, Vegetables, and Milk/Dairy by Age and Gender | | | | |
|---|---|---|---|---|
| | 1-3 Years | 4-8 Years | 9-13 Years | 14-18 Years |
| Calories | | | | |
| Female | 900-1000 | 1200 | 1400-1600 | 1800 |
| Male | 900-1200 | 1200-1400 | 1600-2000 | 2000-2400 |
| Milk/dairy | | | | |
| Female | 2 cups | 2.5 cups | 3 cups | 3 cups |
| Male | 2 cups | 2.5 cups | 3 cups | 3 cups |
| Lean meat/beans/nuts/eggs | | | | |
| Female | 2 oz | 3 oz | 5 oz | 5 oz |
| Male | 3 oz | 4 oz | 6 oz | 6 oz |
| Fruits | | | | |
| Female | 1 cup | 1.5 cups | 1.5 cups | 1.5 cups |
| Male | 1 cup | 1.5 cups | 1.5 cups | 2 cups |
| Vegetables | | | | |
| Female | 1 cup | 1.5 cups | 2 cups | 2.5 cups |
| Male | 1.5 cups | 1.5 cups | 2.5 cups | 3 cups |
| Grains | | | | |
| Female | 3 oz | 4 oz | 5 oz | 6 oz |
| Male | 3 oz | 5 oz | 6 oz | 7 oz |

Estimated calorie needs are based on a sedentary lifestyle. Increased physical activity will require additional calories: 0-200 kcal/d if moderately physically active; and 200-400 kcal/d if very physically active.

Table adapted from Appendix 6, Appendix 7, and Appendix 8 of the *Dietary Guidelines for Americans* (2010); http://www.healthierus.gov/dietaryguidelines

Figure 2. Daily estimated calories and recommended servings for grains, fruits, vegetables, and milk/dairy by age and gender

percent juice as a serving of fruit, all that sugar in juice outweighs the benefit from the fruit. (Even though the sugar in 100 percent juice is fructose—a natural fruit sugar—it takes about three apples to make an 8-ounce glass of juice. That's more apple than you would typically eat in a day and you've removed all the fiber contained in the skin.) It's always better to get fruit servings from the whole fruit. Try to limit juice to no more than 4 ounces per day. An easy way to start weaning your juice-addicted kids is to dilute the juice with water.

• Oils in moderation, with an emphasis on mono- or polyunsaturated fats instead of trans or saturated fats. Fat used to be the evil word. And while fats are calorie dense (nine calories per gram versus four calories per gram of carbohydrate or protein), some fats have been shown to be heart healthy, particularly the omega-3 fatty acids contained in salmon, tuna, walnuts, and a variety of fortified products (such as milk and eggs) and other foods. The omega-3s help with brain development and are especially important for children. In fact, some studies suggest that infants and children who consume a variety of omega-3-containing foods have increased attention span and higher IQs.

- Low- or no-fat milk products in contrast to regular whole milk products. Starting at the age of two (and the age of one for kids already overweight), all children should consume 2%, 1%, or, preferably, skim milk. The higher-fat milk contains a lot more calories, saturated fat, and no additional nutritional value.
- Lean meat and bean products instead of higher-fat meats, such as regular (75 to 80 percent lean) ground beef or chicken with the skin. Help your kids choose healthy, low-fat proteins, such as the white meat from chicken (breast and wings) and the leanest red meats (typically round or loin).

Even when consuming the healthiest foods, you should pay attention to serving sizes. In making recommendations, the Dietary Guidelines use measurable terms, such as cups and ounces, to help people control their portion sizes and thus consume fewer extra calories. And while you probably don't intend to measure out your kids' food intake, the ability to "guesstimate" will help you and your family avoid overeating (see Figure 3). More on this in Chapter 3.

In addition to the best foods to eat, the Dietary Guidelines and the AAP emphasize the importance of staying physically active. Children should get at least 60 minutes of physical activity every day.

---

**What does one serving look like? Consult this list for physical examples.**

**Grain Products**

1 cup of cereal flakes = fist

1 pancake = compact disc

1/2 cup of cooked rice, pasta, or potato = 1/2 baseball

 1 slice of bread = cassette tape

1 piece of cornbread = bar of soap

**Dairy and Cheese**

1-1/2 oz. cheese = 4 stacked dice

1/2 cup of ice cream = 1/2 baseball

**Fats**

1 tsp. margarine or spreads = 1 die

**Vegetables and Fruits**

1 cup of salad greens = baseball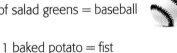

 1 baked potato = fist

1 medium fruit = baseball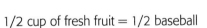

1/2 cup of fresh fruit = 1/2 baseball

 1/4 cup of raisins = large egg

**Meat and Alternatives**

3 oz. meat, fish, and poultry = deck of cards

3 oz. grilled/baked fish = checkbook

2 Tbsp. peanut butter = Ping-Pong® ball

Images: iStockphoto/Thinkstock

Figure 3. Estimating portion sizes

*A Recommended Meal Plan*

If you're up for it, sit down with your child and see how yesterday's food choices stack up against the recommendations or assess your intake online (go to choosemyplate.gov and click "SuperTracker"). Use this information as a starting point, and working with your child, aim to set a goal each week that will help bring you closer to the guidelines. For example, if your son ate no vegetables yesterday, perhaps a good goal for the week would be to eat one vegetable a day. That, of course, is easier said than done. And you may want to wait until you've made it through the rest of the book before you move forward tackling that goal because, as you know, if you push and pressure your kids to eat vegetables, they often resent your efforts and insist even more adamantly that they hate vegetables and refuse to eat them. Not to worry. The average child, of course, doesn't eat as healthy as the guidelines recommend, and as you'll see over the course of the book, that's okay. The objective is to aim for these ideals (without instigating a mealtime food fight) so your kids will eat better than they did before you started. As esteemed pediatrician T. Berry Brazelton said in a *New York Times* piece: "When a young child struggles with you over food, you won't win." He goes on to add: "You can cover them with a multivitamin during this temporary period—usually between 2 and 3 years old—when any battle over food will backfire into even worse nutrition."[14] The goal of this book, of course, is to help you transform mealtimes from potential battle zones into harmonious family time in which your children actually choose to eat the good food. On the way, though, will be a few bumps, in which case a multivitamin is great insurance.

## Developmental Considerations

When attempting to influence a child's food and activity preferences, it's essential to target your strategies to your child's developmental level. Children pass through several predictable developmental phases. One strategy may fail miserably for a two-year-old but work wonders for a five-year-old. Each chapter of this book includes developmentally appropriate suggestions to help you maximize your chances for success in shaping your child's behaviors.

*First Tastes*

In the first few years of a child's life, parents have a unique opportunity to shape future food preferences. Moms-to-be who consume a wide variety of foods during pregnancy have babies who are likely to accept those flavors later. The breastfed infant gets exposure to myriad food tastes from mother's milk and is subsequently more willing to try various foods once solids are introduced. A typical pretoddler loves dirt and anything else that can go from hand to mouth; this is the critical period—a golden opportunity—to shape his food preferences.

Most parents recognize they play an important role in their kids' food choices. It's just that our best efforts sometimes backfire. Time and again, research studies have shown that child-feeding strategies that pressure a child to consume a particular food increase the child's dislike for that food and set the stage for future eating challenges. The Feeding Infants and Toddlers Study (FITS), a study of the eating patterns of children during the first two years of life (four months to two years), found that while most toddlers consume adequate energy, vitamins, and minerals for healthy growth and development, undesirable eating patterns begin to emerge early.[12] As a child transitions from breast milk or formula to an array of solid foods and then to the same table foods that the rest of the family consumes, eating habits slowly erode. In fact, on average, a person's healthiest diet ever is attained at the age of one year. It's all downhill after that for most people.

While infants have a remarkable innate ability to self-regulate caloric intake in response to feelings of hunger and fullness, this ability begins to deteriorate around age two, and by preschool, children's food choices are heavily influenced by such external cues as taste, routine, and social factors. This leads to trouble later, as food preferences are established early in life and tend to predict future eating habits. Genetics and evolution are at least partly to blame. For most of human history, children grew up in times of food scarcity and shortage. It was evolutionarily advantageous to consume calorie-dense foods. An innate preference for sweet tastes and dislike of bitter tastes may have evolved to encourage ingestion of calorie-dense foods and prevent consumption of toxic substances. The most effective parent feeding strategies in times of limited resources assured that children received adequate calories by consuming as much food as was attainable. These parenting strategies have been passed down through the ages, but we must now redefine the best way to raise healthy children. In the current environment of overabundance, the old tools just don't work anymore. Many parents wonder, "But what other option is there?" The alternative, it often seems, to pressuring a child to eat is malnutrition, a 100 percent junk food diet, poor school performance, decreased athletic ability—the list of parental fears around food go on and on. You can now stop worrying, as this book will help put your mind at ease and offer you new tools and strategies to avert the food fights and raise healthy, balanced children.

If you have a kid whose eating and exercise habits are out of control; who is overweight or underweight; who eats everything or nothing; who won't get off the couch to exercise or who exercises too much; or who, like the adult counterpart, struggles to maintain a healthy weight through healthy nutrition and physical activity choices—don't despair. This book will show you how, as a savvy parent, you can "retrain their brains" and reset the course for a healthy future.

### Applying the Techniques to Children of Varying Ages

This book is written for parents of 0- to 10-year-olds. Of course, the techniques will need to be modified and delivered differently for children of different ages and different developmental stages. Each chapter includes a developmental chart you can use with practical suggestions to practice the major principles depending on the age and developmental stage of your child.

## A Little Bit of Psychology Goes a Long Way

Parents and their children have long engaged in a battle of wills, starting from a very young age. Parents desperate to get their kids to eat healthy have tried many tricks and strategies. For example, consider this scenario: Sophia, a rambunctious two-year-old, refuses to eat the crisp peas her mother has carefully placed on her high chair tray. Three minutes of begging and pleading pass. Mom insists: "Sophia, please eat your peas. They're so good. Yummy." Sophia refuses. Mom, an expert two-year-old-mind-manipulator, continues: "Oh, Sophia, I'm so glad you didn't eat your peas because if you're not going to eat them, I will!" Mom slowly brings pea-filled spoon to her mouth. Sophia cries out and opens her mouth wide. Peas in. Mission accomplished.

Mom has mastered the well-known trick of "reverse psychology"—in Sophia's mind, if Mom wants to eat my peas, then they must be good! Many parents around the world play this food game with their toddlers, but then, soon—too soon—the child either catches on to the game or simply outgrows it. After that, getting young kids to eat vegetables often turns into a food fight. But it doesn't have to be that way. By understanding and applying a few principles from the world of child psychology, you can help your kids actually like eating healthy food.

Throughout the book, the application of how children learn to develop certain food preferences will draw on three subdisciplines of learning psychology: classical and operant conditioning, modeling, and information processing or "applying knowledge."

*Classical and Operant Conditioning*

If you took an introductory psychology class as a high school student or while in college, you were probably introduced to classical conditioning and Pavlov's dog. In this experiment, researcher Ivan Pavlov conditioned a dog to salivate at the ring of a bell by continually pairing food (which triggers an unlearned response to salivate) with the sound of a bell. Eventually, he could get the dog to salivate simply by ringing the bell, with no food in sight. This experiment showed that dogs can learn to respond to an unfamiliar stimulus in the same way they respond to a familiar stimulus. Later experiments also confirmed the same type of response in humans. For example, a major contributor to obesity is emotional eating, which is typically a behavior learned in childhood. When an upset child is soothed by a mother's touch paired with food, the child learns to rely on this "comfort food" to feel better. This is known as *classical conditioning*.

With *operant conditioning*, behaviors are learned through rewards and punishments. Examples of operant conditioning include rewarding a toddler who uses the potty with M&M's® and punishing a child who is misbehaving in school by forcing him to run extra laps. While the intended consequences may be to increase use of the potty and decrease unruly behavior (through operant conditioning), the unintended consequences could be a child who learns to rely on candy to feel good (since that reward was inevitably tied with parental praise) and a child who comes to associate exercise and physical activity with negative feelings (through classical conditioning). Classical and operant conditioning both play important roles in shaping children's behaviors. Throughout the book, I'll discuss how to extinguish some of these conditioned responses and also how to use this method of learning to help create healthful behaviors.

## *Modeling*

Social cognitive learning theory says that children learn not only through classical and operant conditioning but also by observing and imitating others. Albert Bandura conducted several studies that showed that children who watched an adult or child behave aggressively were likely to imitate that behavior. Likewise, children who see their parents and friends eating healthy are more likely to eat healthy. But children don't automatically imitate behaviors. This theory also includes a cognitive component in which children select specific behaviors and then the extent of imitation depends on how they process the information. Bandura identified five cognitive processes that must be present for a child to learn a new behavior through observation:

- Notice a particular behavior.
- Retain the observed behaviors in memory.
- Have the physical and intellectual capacity to reproduce the observed behavior.
- Be motivated to want to reproduce the behavior.
- Believe in one's own capability to reproduce the behavior.[15]

Several strategies you can use to maximize your child's positive modeling and minimize the negative modeling are detailed in the text, especially in Chapter 6.

## *Information Processing*

The information processing approach treats the child's mind similar to a computer system. A child hears some information, which is then registered, organized, stored, and finally acted upon. For example, a child may learn at school the health benefits of apples. Then, at some point in the future—and perhaps out of the blue—he may ask his mother to buy apples when she goes to the grocery store. Using this approach as a model, we'll discuss how to effectively use information to best inspire healthy changes in your children.

# **Getting Started**

Now that you've been introduced to the basics and the theoretical and factual underpinnings of this book, let's get started helping your children develop healthier eating habits and eliminating your family mealtime food battles and dietary stressors.

## References

1. Lobstein, T., L. Baur, and R. Uauy. (2004). Obesity in children and young people: A crisis in public health. *Obes Rev.* 5 Suppl 1: p. 4-104.

2. Whitaker, R.C., J.A. Wright, M.S. Pepe, K.D. Seidel, and W.H. Dietz. (1997). Predicting obesity in young adulthood from childhood and parental obesity. *N Engl J Med.* Sep 25 1997; *337*(13): p. 869-73.

3. Ogden, C.L., M.D. Carroll, B.K. Kit, and K.M. Flegal. (2012). Prevalence of obesity and trends in body mass index among US children and adolescents, 1999-2010. *JAMA. 307*(5): p. 483-90.

4. Flegal, K.M., M.D. Carroll, B.K. Kit, and C.L. Ogden. (2012). Prevalence of obesity and trends in the distribution of body mass index among US adults, 1999-2010. *JAMA. 307*(5): p. 491-97.

5. American Dietetic Association. (2006). What's a mom to do? Healthy eating tips for families. *Nutrition Fact Sheet.* Chicago, IL: American Dietetic Association.

6. Batsell, W.R. Jr., A.S. Brown, M.E. Ansfield, and G.Y. Paschall. (2002). "You will eat all of that!": A retrospective analysis of forced consumption episodes. *Appetite. 38*(3): p. 211-19.

7. Fisher, J.O., and L.L. Birch. (1999). Restricting access to palatable foods affects children's behavioral response, food selection, and intake. *Am J Clin Nutr. 69*(6): p. 1264-72.

8. Golan, M., and S. Crow. (2004). Targeting parents exclusively in the treatment of childhood obesity: long-term results. *Obes Res. 12*(2): p. 357-61.

9. Jelalian, E., J. Boergers, C.S. Alday, and R. Frank. (2003). Survey of physician attitudes and practices related to pediatric obesity. *Clin Pediatr (Phila). 42*(3): p. 235-45.

10. Pearce, A., L. Li, J. Abbas, B. Ferguson, H. Graham, and C. Law. (2010). Is childcare associated with the risk of overweight and obesity in the early years? Findings from the UK Millennium Cohort Study. *Int J Obes (Lond). 34*(7): p. 1160-8.

11. French, S.A., M. Story, and R.W. Jeffery. (2001). Environmental influences on eating and physical activity. *Annu Rev Public Health. 22*: p. 309-35.

12. Dwyer, J.T., N.F. Butte, D.M. Deming, A.M. Siega-Riz, and K.C. Reidy. (2010). Feeding Infants and Toddlers Study 2008: Progress, continuing concerns, and implications. *J Am Diet Assoc. 110*(12 Suppl): p. S60-7.

13. Gidding, S.S., B.A. Dennison, L.L. Birch, S.R. Daniels, M.W. Gilman, A.H. Lichtenstein, K.T. Rattay, J. Steinberger, N. Stettler, and L. Van Horn. (2005). Dietary recommendations for children and adolescents: a guide for practitioners: consensus statement from the American Heart Association. *Circulation. 112*(13): p. 2061-75.

14. Parker-Pope, T. (2008). Dr. T. Berry Brazelton's advice on childhood nutrition. *New York Times*'s Well blog. Available at http://well.blogs.nytimes.com/2008/09/16/dr-brazeltons-advice-on-childhood-nutrition.

15. Bandura, A (2001). Social cognitive theory: An agentic perspective. *Annu Rev Psychol. 52*: p. 1-26.

# THE INHERITED MISTAKES

iStockphoto/Thinkstock

## Part One

# 1

# Mistake #1—Insisting "Eat Your Vegetables!"

*"Vegetables! I hated them as a child—and I still hate them. My younger brother hated them more. As I watched my mother hover over him for hours trying to shovel vegetables into him, while completely ignoring me, I began to hate my brother even more than vegetables. Now you know why I became a pediatrician—to stamp out vegetables, and to overcome my guilt at wanting to kill my brother!"*

—Esteemed pediatrician T. Berry Brazelton in response to a reader's question on the *New York Times*'s Wellblog (September 16, 2008)[1]

Nine-month-old Owen amazes his mom as he eagerly chomps down her homemade baby purees, regardless of what she offers. His repertoire includes a scrumptious (Owen thinks) lentil-veggie concoction; cauliflower and tomatoes; spinach, peas, and broccoli; chicken with sweet potatoes and apple; and even a baked salmon special. Mom is pleased. She wonders if it will always be this easy to get Owen to eat healthy foods. Fast-forward two years. Owen balks at anything green on his plate, is reluctant to taste anything unfamiliar, and, if left to his own devices, would eat macaroni and cheese or peanut butter and jelly for his full weekly sustenance. Given these eating habits, Owen's mom is very tempted to insist that Owen "eat his vegetables!" But she resists this temptation. And day after day, she continues to introduce and reintroduce Owen to an array of vegetables in hopes that one day he'll come to love them. And as he approaches his third birthday, he actually does (most of the time)!

## Why "Eat Your Vegetables!" Doesn't Work

The current state of nutrition among children in the United States and worldwide is discouraging. The dietary recommendations advocate a diet high in fruits, vegetables, and whole grains and low in added fat, sugar, and salt. Despite an emphasis on consumption of at least five servings of fruits and vegetables per day, actual intake for kids and adults is much lower. In fact, a study of 1,797 second- and fifth-grade children found that 40 percent of the children ate zero vegetables on the days studied.[2] Surveys of eating habits have shown that only about one in four children and adolescents consume the recommended amount of fruits and vegetables and that one-fourth of those "vegetables" are French fries; none of the top five vegetables consumed by toddlers were dark green, and a significant amount of "fruit" comes in the form of fruit juice.[3] Dietary practices are typically at their best around age one,[4] however, about 30 percent of 12- to 15-month-olds eat no vegetables and 25 percent eat no fruits on any given day.[5] Eating habits tend to worsen after about a year, with an increasing consumption of nutrient-poor snacks, sweets, soda, and sugar-sweetened beverages.[4] By the time a kid starts school, overall fruit and vegetable consumption is pretty lousy. School-aged kids eat about 1.5 cups of fruits and vegetables per day. That's half of the recommended amount.[6] Clearly, a blatant disconnect exists between what's recommended as the healthiest diet for our children and what our children actually eat. In response, parents quite understandably aim to fix that problem by demanding "Eat your vegetables!" After all, vegetables are some of the healthiest foods on the planet. (Refer to the sidebars "What's So Great About Fruits and Vegetables Anyway?" and "Do Vegetables and Fruits Have to Be Fresh to Get the Nutritional Benefit?")

The problem with this strategy is that kids, much like the rest of us, have minds of their own, and they only want to eat what tastes good to them. In a study that looked at many psychological, social, and demographic factors that affect a child's fruits and vegetables intake, researchers found that only one factor predicted fruit and vegetable consumption. It wasn't parents' insistence or an appreciation of all the health benefits fruits and vegetables provide in maintaining health or staving off disease. It was simple: the kids ate the fruits and the vegetables that tasted good.[7] When left to their own devices, kids eat what they like and leave the rest. Not surprisingly, the most familiar and preferred foods in childhood tend to combine sugar and fat. It's not that surprising, then, that among kids as young as 9 to 12 months old, about half eat a dessert or candy on any given day.[5] The number bumps to 75 percent for 19 to 24 month olds.[5] The preference for sweet and salty tastes and the rejection of sour and bitter tastes are innate and unlearned. When is the last time you had to convince a child to eat ice cream?

This reality frustrates parents to no end, and as a result, they may find themselves reasoning that intervention is needed—and needed immediately—so they insist that their children eat their vegetables. But the more adults pressure children to eat certain foods, the less likely they'll be to develop a taste for them and continue to eat them often as adults. Kids instinctively resist persuasion. If you really want your kids to eat vegetables and other healthy foods because they *like* them, you'll have to employ different strategies.

# Parent Feeding Styles Predict Fruit and Vegetable Consumption

Most of us have never taken a parenting class or graduated from a how-to course on achieving our full parenting potential. We tend to learn as we go. Maybe we do things the same way our parents did raising us or maybe we purposefully do the opposite. We pick tips up along the way from our friends, neighbors, television shows, strangers (generally unsolicited), magazines, and books like this one. In any case, you may not have thought about how your parenting style influences how your kids eat (and, alternatively, how your kids eat might influence your parenting style). But it turns out that researchers have studied this and described how the four major categories of parenting styles compare to our parent feeding styles.

In the early 1970s, a researcher named Diana Baumrind did an extensive study on how parents exercise their authority in raising children.[8] In the study, she described four types of parenting styles: authoritarian, authoritative, permissive, and neglectful. The parenting characterizations were based on a parent's responsiveness versus unresponsiveness and tendency to be demanding versus undemanding. Modern-day psychologists use the terms "warmth" (in lieu of "responsiveness") and "control" (in lieu of "demanding") (Figure 1-1). Following is a description of the four parenting styles:

- *Authoritarian* (low warmth, high control) parents set rules and guidelines for their children and tolerate very little flexibility. They emphasize obedience and often withhold love and warmth. An authoritarian parent may restrict junk food completely and not allow for an occasional sweet or unhealthy deviance.

- *Authoritative* (high warmth, high control) parents set structures and guidelines for their children but leave room for flexibility and negotiation. Children experience certain freedoms within well-described rules. They show their children love and warmth. An authoritative parent may generally avoid sweets and other unhealthy foods but will occasionally allow them for her children while acknowledging that they're tasty but not necessarily healthy for children's growing bodies.

- *Permissive* (high warmth, low control) parents have few or no rules for their children and make very few demands of their kids. They tend to shower their children with love and warmth. A permissive parent may allow unlimited snacking and access to unhealthy foods, with no limitation on intake or explanation of the risks of eating too much of it.

|              | High Warmth    | Low Warmth    |
|--------------|----------------|---------------|
| **High Control** | Authoritative | Authoritarian |
| **Low Control**  | Permissive    | Neglectful    |

Figure 1-1. Parenting styles

---

## What's So Great About Fruits and Vegetables Anyway?

Once your kids get the message that fruits and vegetables are great for their health, they might ask you what's so great about fruits and vegetables anyway? What follows are a few talking points to help answer that question. (It's a good idea to avoid "Because I said so" or "They just are.") Information is persuasive and in some cases may convince a skeptical seven-year-old to—on his own—decide to try just a bite of a hated vegetable.

Specific types of vegetables are especially important because they contain high levels of nutrients known to be lacking in the diets of young children. These include leafy dark green vegetables, such as broccoli and spinach, and deep yellow vegetables, such as carrots and sweet potatoes. The following table highlights some of the most important nutrients for children and the vegetables and fruits that contain large amounts of these nutrients. A diet high in fruits and vegetables may cut a child's risk of heart disease and ward off clogged arteries later in life,[21] protect against many childhood illnesses,[22] and help set the stage for a child to have healthier eating habits later in life when the consequences of a lousy diet are most pronounced.

Fruits and vegetables are low in calories and fat, so you can eat more of them and not have to worry so much about gaining unwanted weight or eating too many calories. In fact, a diet rich in fruits and vegetables can a play a very important role in managing weight for an overweight or obese child.

For more information, visit www.fruitsandveggiesmatter.gov/benefits/nutrient_guide.html.

- *Neglectful* (low warmth, low control) parents have few or no rules for their children and make very few demands of their kids. They tend to withhold love and warmth. A neglectful parent won't limit or necessarily even be aware of a child's junk food intake. The neglectful parent will not be discussed further.

Baumrind's work and the work of others have found that, in general, authoritative parents have children who are more independent and socially responsible. Specifically:

- The most influential models are parents perceived by their children as having a high social status and who are most strongly involved with the child (high warmth).
- When parents positively reinforce good behavior and negatively reinforce deviant behavior, their kids are more likely to be socially responsible (high control).
- Parents who use reason to explain their decisions to their children are more potent models and reinforcing agents than parents who disallow children from questioning a parent's decision or who frequently answer "because I said so" in explaining their decisions (high control and high warmth versus high control and low warmth).

| FIBER | |
|---|---|
| Diets rich in dietary fiber have been shown to have a number of beneficial effects, including decreased risk of coronary artery disease. Fiber also helps food move through the digestive tract, and that makes going to the bathroom easier. | **Good fruit and vegetable sources:** navy beans, kidney beans, black beans, pinto beans, lima beans, white beans, soybeans, split peas, chick peas, black-eyed peas, lentils, artichokes, dates, raspberries, pears, and apples<br><br>A rough estimate of how much fiber (in grams) your child needs per day is his age (years) + 5 (for example, a four-year-old needs about 9 grams of fiber). |

| POTASSIUM | |
|---|---|
| Diets rich in potassium may help to maintain a healthy blood pressure. | **Good fruit and vegetable sources:** sweet potatoes, tomato paste, tomato puree, beet greens, white potatoes, white beans, lima beans, cooked greens, carrot juice, and prune juice |

| VITAMIN A | |
|---|---|
| Vitamin A keeps eyes and skin healthy and helps to protect against infections. | **Good fruit and vegetable sources:** sweet potatoes, pumpkin, carrots, spinach, turnip greens, mustard greens, kale, collard greens, winter squash, cantaloupe, red peppers, and Chinese cabbage |

| VITAMIN C | |
|---|---|
| Vitamin C helps heal cuts and scrapes and keeps gums and teeth healthy. | **Good fruit and vegetable sources:** red and green peppers, kiwi, strawberries, sweet potatoes, kale, cantaloupe, broccoli, pineapple, Brussels sprouts, oranges, mangoes, tomato juice, and cauliflower |

| IRON | |
|---|---|
| Iron is very important for a child's developing brain, and it also helps the body use energy. Many children are iron-deficient (anemic) due to poor intake of iron-rich foods. Also, iron is poorly absorbed, but absorption can be greatly increased by pairing an iron-rich food with a food high in vitamin C. | **Good fruit and vegetable sources:** spinach and other leafy dark green vegetables, beans, peas, and dried apricots<br><br>Other sources: fortified cereals and breads, lean beef, and eggs<br><br>The average child needs about 10 mg of iron per day. |

| CALCIUM | |
|---|---|
| Calcium is important for strong bones and teeth. Childhood and young adulthood offer the only opportunities for us to build bone strength. After that, the goal is to prevent bones from weakening. | **Good vegetable sources:** broccoli, kale, and other leafy dark green vegetables, soybeans, and tofu<br><br>Other sources: milk, yogurt, cheese, sardines, and frozen yogurt<br><br>Kids need 500 to 800 mg of calcium per day depending on their age. |

- Children exposed to a stimulating environment (as orchestrated by highly invested parents) are more independent (high control).
- Parents who value individuality and self-expression have more independent children, provided that the parent isn't unwilling to make demands on the child (high warmth and high control).
- Firm parental control is associated with a child's independence as long as the control isn't restrictive of the child's opportunities to experiment and make decisions within defined limits (high warmth and high control).

## Do Vegetables and Fruits Have to Be Fresh to Get the Nutritional Benefit?

We always hear that one of the best ways to take care of our health is to eat a wide variety of fresh fruits and vegetables. But what if you can't always purchase fresh food—whether due to cost, taste preferences, spoilage risk, or any other of several possible reasons to choose frozen or canned over fresh? You can stop worrying about it. Most of the evidence suggests that frozen fruits and vegetables are just as good for you (if not better in some cases) than fresh food.

Unless you're choosing fresh produce from a farmers' market or your own backyard, chances are good that your produce was picked at least several days ago—likely not at its peak ripeness (otherwise, it would spoil too quickly en route to the store) and with degradation of some of its nutritional value after picking and during transport. Once fresh fruits and vegetables are harvested, they undergo higher rates of respiration— a physiologic process in which plant starches and sugars are converted into carbon dioxide, water, and other by-products—leading to moisture loss, reduced quality, and susceptibility to microorganism spoilage. Refrigeration during transport helps to slow the deterioration, but still, by the time you eat a fresh vegetable that traveled across a continent to reach your dinner table, a substantial amount of its nutritional value may be lost. You can help maximize nutritional value of your fresh produce by choosing locally grown produce, refrigerating the fruits and veggies to help slow down nutrient losses, and steaming rather than boiling to minimize loss of water-soluble vitamins.

Produce destined for freezing is picked at its maximal ripeness, quickly frozen to a temperature that maximally retains its nutritional value and flavor, and kept frozen until it gets to the freezer in your local store. While some initial nutrient loss occurs with the first steps in the freezing process—washing, peeling, and heat-based blanching (done for vegetables but usually not fruits)—the low temperature of freezing keeps the produce good for up to a year on average. Once you thaw and eat frozen food, you get the majority of the food's original nutritional value. Be assured, if

- Parents who rely on reinforcement techniques but who don't appeal to reason or explain the rationale for their decisions to the child are more likely to see dependent, overly compliant, or passive-aggressive behaviors in their children (low warmth and high control).
- Parental self-assertiveness and self-confidence—demonstrated by a moderate use of power-oriented techniques—is associated with increased independence in the child (high control).

So, what does all this have to do with raising healthy eaters? These parenting styles parallel parent feeding styles. Some parents take a highly controlling authoritarian approach in which mothers (typically) assume total

you love blueberries and all their health benefits, for example, the frozen version is just as good as the fresh. And depending on how you cook or prepare the food, it may taste quite similar to its fresh counterpart.

The process is somewhat different for canned produce, and in some cases, your nutritional value may suffer. Similar to the freezing process, in the canning process, the produce is picked at its maximal ripeness, blanched (this time for longer duration and with somewhat increased nutrient loss for heat-sensitive compounds compared with frozen), and then canned. Oftentimes, sugary syrup or juice is added to canned fruit. Salt is added to many vegetables to help retain flavor and avoid spoilage. These additions can take a very healthy fruit or vegetable and make it much less desirable than its fresh or frozen counterpart. But without these additions, the nutritional value of canned fruits and vegetables is generally similar to fresh and frozen. For fruits, look for canned fruit "in its own juice." For vegetables, check the sodium content on the nutritional label and aim for vegetables with "no added salt" and without added butter or cream sauces. Because the canned produce is maintained in an oxygen-free environment, canned foods can last for years (but be weary of dented or bulging cans).

By the time they're consumed, most fresh, frozen, and canned fruits and vegetables seem to be nutritionally similar. Each has the same fat, carbohydrate, and protein content as the preharvest fruit. While variable loss in water- and fat-soluble vitamins can occur depending on the postharvest processing method, for the most part, you can feel confident that frozen and canned (without additives) fruits and vegetables are just as good for you and your family as fresh food. Ultimately, you might find that choosing a mix of fresh, frozen, and canned fruits and vegetables will help you and your family to more easily, inexpensively, and creatively enjoy the nine or more servings per day of fruits and vegetables recommended by the Dietary Guidelines for Americans without sacrificing nutritional value.

**Resource**

http://www.fruitsandveggiesmatter.gov

control, essentially force-feeding a child. Others are more permissive, believing fully that children instinctively know when, what, and how much to eat. Food is never forced. Others are more authoritative, controlling which foods are offered to the child but allowing the child to choose what and how much to eat. The differences in "control" affect a child's ability to use internal cues of hunger and satiety to determine food intake as opposed to external cues imposed by a parent (e.g., "clean your plate"), which may be part of the reason why children of parents with a high-control authoritarian parenting style have higher rates of obesity, eating disorders, and chronic dieting.[9] The effects of authoritarian parenting on nutrition and health are discussed in detail in Chapter 4.

The ideal parenting approach to raising healthy eaters who actually choose to consume a healthy diet including fruits and vegetables is to adopt an authoritative style. With this strategy, the parent controls the "big picture," but the child is given the flexibility and freedom to make some choices. How does this play out? Caloric intake and the nutritional quality of a child's diet depend on what meals are eaten, how much time passes between each meal (meal timing), how much is eaten at each meal (meal size), and the specific foods that are eaten (food selection). The parent plays an important role in determining meal timing—when meals are served and what food is offered. Children should be allowed to control their meal size (parents frequently overestimate the amount of food children need to eat) and food selection (in the context of the healthy foods you make available). Don't despair. Your veggie-hating picky eater need not go to bed hungry. Several strategies can help you get your kids to actually want to eat the healthy foods you offer.

# Counterstrategy: The Techniques

The following sections offer a few ideas to help translate this information into action.

### Give Them a Little Control

*Children instinctively seek control over their own lives.* In general, kids have very little control over their lives. Their daily schedule is determined by someone else; they're constantly being told what to do by various adult figures; and, ultimately, they have very little opportunity to make their own decisions—except for when it comes to food (and potty training). While parents and other adults can attempt to pressure children to eat in a certain way, no one can ultimately force a child to eat a particular food. While a parent can't control whether a child eats a food, a parent can usually control to what foods a child is exposed. The last thing that you want to do is get into a battle of wills with your toddler. Chances are pretty good you'll lose. It seems counterintuitive, but you're more likely to get your kids to like vegetables and fruits if you let them choose not to eat them.

### Make It Taste Good

Children have an innate preference for sweet and salty foods and a dislike for sour and bitter. Evolutionarily, this may be due to several factors. To start, we're programmed to fulfill physiologic hunger with food. We thus tend to prefer foods that make us feel full. Typically, these are high-calorie, sweet, and fatty foods. This unlearned preference for "bad foods" is matched with an unlearned distaste for sour and bitter. Unfortunately, many of the healthiest vegetables, such as broccoli, taste bitter and therefore tend to be disfavored. However, these innate preferences can be unlearned with training. Think about it—how much do you love your morning coffee, afternoon tea, or evening beer? Each of these readily consumed beverages tastes bitter, but with a little bit of training and exposure, we can come to prefer these tastes.

Researchers and psychologists have described several food-preference learning strategies we can apply to mold our children's taste preferences.[10]

*Taste-Nutrient Learning*

Evolutionarily, we've come to prefer foods that fill us up. This is known as taste-nutrient learning. It can help explain why a hungry child learns to prefer filling high-calorie foods, such as a cheeseburger and French fries. Taste-nutrient learning is an example of operant conditioning in which the stimulus (eating high-calorie foods) is positively reinforced or rewarded by a feeling of fullness. We can help the child unlearn this tendency. One way is to work with the child in an effort to avoid getting to the point of "starving." In this case, less-filling, lower-calorie foods can do the trick of helping the child to feel "full" without becoming "stuffed." You can also make available higher-fiber foods, such as most fruits, vegetables, and whole grains, that contribute to a feeling of fullness without the excess calories.

*Taste-Taste Learning*

A toddler has a natural and unlearned dislike for new flavors; this well-described phenomenon is referred to as *neophobia*. Paul Rozin first speculated that this tendency to reject new flavors and tastes has evolutionary origins.[11] He described it as the "omnivore's dilemma." Back in the days of hunters and gatherers, it was advantageous to avoid potentially poisonous unknown and untried foods. At the same time, the hunters and gatherers had to be sure to consume an adequate diet. They eventually came to consume new foods via "learned safety" in which eating small amounts of the food and suffering no ill effects led to a greater consumption and a liking of the foods. The same approach works with children. (The negative downfall can also occur. A food can come to be permanently rejected if a child experiences ill effects, such as food poisoning or gastrointestinal distress, after eating a particular food.) You can help your child overcome food neophobia, or fear of trying new foods, without the mealtime battles if you understand and capitalize on taste-taste learning.

Taste-taste learning is a form of classical conditioning in which people learn to like unfamiliar foods that taste similar to foods they already know and like. That is, food likes and dislikes extend to foods that are similar. For example, if your child likes green beans, chances are pretty good that he'll also like snow peas. Alternately, if your child dislikes spinach, he probably won't care for kale. Knowing this, parents can start to capitalize. You can help your child to like unfamiliar foods with tastes that your child innately dislikes (sour and bitter) by pairing them with familiar foods that the child innately prefers (sweet and salty). For example, grapefruit (sour) paired with a teaspoon of sugar is more likely to be accepted than the grapefruit alone. A holiday family favorite at our house is fresh cranberries (tart) boiled with a little bit of sugar (sweet). Broccoli (bitter) with cheese sauce (salty) could facilitate broccoli's entrance into your child's list of tolerable foods. Or you could try pairing vegetables with sauces, such as sweet barbeque or salty soy (go with the low-sodium version to retain the salty flavor without loading up on sodium). One mother interviewed for this book said she could get her five-year-old son to eat *anything* if she paired it with A.1.® sauce.

You can also use food bridges to help get a child to extend his liking of a well-known vegetable, such as potatoes, to a similar but much healthier alternative, such as sweet potatoes. When using bridges, keep in mind a food's appearance, taste, and texture. For example, an orange and tangerine look and taste similar. You can expand an orange-loving child's repertoire of fruit by introducing its smaller and slightly tangier cousin. Or you might be able to introduce your child to a new vegetable, such as eggplant, by bridging from chicken parmesan to eggplant parmesan. A child who eats pumpkin pie might like mashed sweet potatoes. From there, he might come to enjoy mashed carrots.

*Taste-Environment Learning*

Taste-environment learning occurs when a person comes to prefer foods or tastes that are associated with a pleasant physical or social environment and to dislike foods associated with an uncomfortable or negative environment. Highly palatable "unhealthy" foods that our kids already prefer are omnipresent when we celebrate joyful, positive experiences, such as ice cream after a baseball game win. It's not to say that we shouldn't have ice cream after a tough game or a decked-out birthday cake at a kid's party. It just helps to balance it out with nonfood celebrations and with healthy foods. Maybe on occasion, instead of ice cream, try smoothies or fresh watermelon? Regularly having a calm and peaceful nutritious family dinner can also become a fond childhood memory and can reinforce taste preferences for those healthy foods. On the other hand, constant food battles in which parents pressure a child to eat his veggies creates an unpleasant experience and, oftentimes, that child's dislike for that pressured food.

You can work with your child's preferences, your time availability, your budget, and your motivation and level of enjoyment for cooking to prepare healthy foods that your children will actually like because they taste good. Check out Chapter 8 for some detailed tips on how to do this.

## Increase Accessibility and Exposure

Children heavily rely on parents and caregivers to provide them with access to food. They aren't typically able to go to a grocery store or a restaurant by themselves and choose whatever meal or snack they would like, although, admittedly, many do have this freedom at school. (We'll discuss how to deal with this in Chapter 7.) In any case, children are only able to eat foods that are readily available. Thus, you as the parent play a tremendous role in determining what foods your children get to eat—at least while they're in your house. You can make your home a much healthier place for your whole family (yourself included) if you only purchase foods you want your children to eat. Then, your kids will have little choice but to eat healthy foods. (The alternative is to be hungry, which most people tend to avoid. While a toddler may attempt this approach, it generally lasts for only a meal or two at most.) The more exposure your kids have to healthy foods, the more likely it is that they'll come to like those foods.

Consider this study. Researchers wanted to figure out the best way to get children to eat a red pepper. They randomly assigned five- to seven-year-old children to either be in the exposure group, the reward group, or the control group. Then, each day, for a period of eight days, children in the exposure group were offered a taste of sweet red pepper and told they could eat as much of it as they would like. Children in the reward group were given a sheet of cartoon stickers and told they could choose whichever one they wanted as long as they first tried the red pepper. The kids in the control group went about their normal routine and were simply asked to eat and record their liking of the red pepper at the beginning and end of the intervention. At the end of the study, children with the increased exposure to the red pepper significantly increased their liking and their consumption of the red pepper compared with the children in the control group. No significant difference was exhibited in either liking or consumption in the reward group compared with the control group or the exposure group.[12] This is just one example of many studies that have shown that increased exposure and accessibility to fruits and vegetables increases both liking and consumption of vegetables.

If you leave fruit and vegetable snacks out and readily available for your children to eat, they're more likely to eat them. With repeated tasting, the child is more likely to begin to like the food and to ultimately prefer it. Fill your household candy bowls with apples, oranges, and bananas. Fill your refrigerator and freezer with in-season and low-cost fruits and vegetables. Include dried fruit and vegetable-based snacks and chips in your pantry. You don't have to say anything or pressure the kids to eat it. If it's there (and the unhealthy alternative isn't), they'll eat it. You can also increase exposure by offering a fruit and a vegetable at every meal (even if they reject it). Involving children in grocery shopping (check out Figure 1-2 for a fun grocery store game to play with your younger kids) and meal preparation, planting a fruit tree or a garden (even if it's an herb garden on your windowsill), and taking kids to a farmers' market are other powerful strategies to increase exposure and help your children enjoy fruits and vegetables. These ideas are further discussed in Chapter 12.

Don't be afraid to try this strategy with all kinds of vegetables and fruits, even those that have already been rejected by your children. If your kid hates spinach, don't write spinach off and conclude that your child will never eat it. Taste preferences aren't fixed. With repeated exposure—about 15 tries is what seems to be the magic number—children can learn to like previously rejected foods. But they have to have actually tasted the food (merely looking at it or smelling it doesn't help).[13] One way you can get your children to taste previously rejected foods without pressuring them to eat them is to use the *food bridges* previously described, and, if all else fails, you can sneak the food into their favorite foods. The best way to get the "rule of 15" to actually work is to expose the child to the food and then wait 3 to 14 days before introducing the food again.

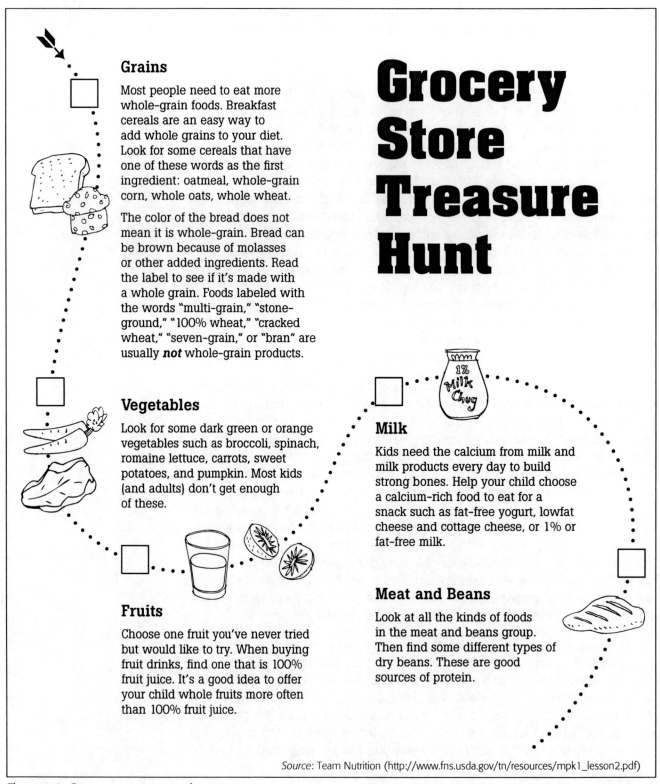

# Grocery Store Treasure Hunt

## Grains

Most people need to eat more whole-grain foods. Breakfast cereals are an easy way to add whole grains to your diet. Look for some cereals that have one of these words as the first ingredient: oatmeal, whole-grain corn, whole oats, whole wheat.

The color of the bread does not mean it is whole-grain. Bread can be brown because of molasses or other added ingredients. Read the label to see if it's made with a whole grain. Foods labeled with the words "multi-grain," "stone-ground," "100% wheat," "cracked wheat," "seven-grain," or "bran" are usually **not** whole-grain products.

## Vegetables

Look for some dark green or orange vegetables such as broccoli, spinach, romaine lettuce, carrots, sweet potatoes, and pumpkin. Most kids (and adults) don't get enough of these.

## Fruits

Choose one fruit you've never tried but would like to try. When buying fruit drinks, find one that is 100% fruit juice. It's a good idea to offer your child whole fruits more often than 100% fruit juice.

## Milk

Kids need the calcium from milk and milk products every day to build strong bones. Help your child choose a calcium-rich food to eat for a snack such as fat-free yogurt, lowfat cheese and cottage cheese, or 1% or fat-free milk.

## Meat and Beans

Look at all the kinds of foods in the meat and beans group. Then find some different types of dry beans. These are good sources of protein.

*Source*: Team Nutrition (http://www.fns.usda.gov/tn/resources/mpk1_lesson2.pdf)

Figure 1-2. Grocery store treasure hunt

This concept of increasing a child's familiarity with healthy foods is the most central and basic principle of how to raise healthy eaters. Kids like what they know.

## Minimize Competition

That brings us to the next point. Yes, you can set the stage to teach your child to like vegetables and fruits. But we can't ignore that kids have an innate, unlearned preference for sweet and salty tastes and an innate, unlearned dislike of sour and bitter tastes. Many vegetables, especially the really-good-for-you ones, such as broccoli, have a bitter taste. Liking broccoli is somewhat of an acquired preference. You don't have to teach a kid to like junk food. Keeping that in mind, if you give a child a choice between potato chips or a raw veggie platter, the child is going to choose the chips every time. If you have junk food snacks in your home that are readily available and accessible to your kids, it might not matter how much fruit you have in the house. Your kids will most likely go for the sweet and salty snacks. Help set your kids up for veggie-loving success by minimizing the competition. That means:

- Make fruits and vegetables readily accessible and junk food snacks very hard to access. That is, keep the junk food out of your house. The extra effort required to actually go to the store to get it will decrease intake of the empty calories. Hiding it is unlikely to work. Your kids will find it, and the allure of the "hard to get" will make it even more desirable. If you've got to get your own junk food fix, try to do it outside of the house and without the knowledge of your kids. Eat it at work. Go for an evening walk and make a stop at the store to get your candy bar. This isn't to say that junk food should be off limits to you or to your kids. It just shouldn't be so available.

- Give your kids a choice between similar foods. A key to authoritative parenting is to create a structured environment for your child so the child has an opportunity to exercise choice. Let your child choose between, say, broccoli or cauliflower for the vegetable that goes with dinner. Remember, if you offer uneven choices, such as a choice of broccoli or French fries, your child will choose the more innately palatable fries. You might also consider planning ahead and letting your child pick any vegetable he'd like for the whole family to eat at a given meal.

- Be creative in how you offer and present food. For example, one study found that by increasing the portion size of carrots at the start of a meal, preschoolers ate twice as much of the veggie.[14] But when increased portions of fruits and vegetables were offered to the kids, fruit—but not vegetable—consumption increased.[15] Kids prefer the sweeter fruit tastes, so if you really want to increase vegetable intake, you have to minimize the competition, even if the competition is fruit. Try it out—offer your hungry kid a bowl of edamame before dinner and see what happens. I was shocked when this worked beautifully with my preschooler. He thought popping the beans out of the pod was a blast. But if he had to choose edamame or grapes, he might have gone with the grapes.

## Model

Children learn to like the taste of foods they see their parents, peers, and other important people in their lives eat. The most powerful models are the people children see as similar to themselves (peers) or as particularly powerful (older peers and siblings and parents). In one study, toddlers put food in their mouths more readily when they were following the example of their mother compared with a stranger.[16] In another study, younger siblings got up the courage to try the generally aversive-tasting chili peppers when they watched older family members eat them.[17] This also works in reverse—children of overweight parents are more likely to be overweight and daughters of dieting mothers are more likely to have problems controlling their eating and are more likely to exhibit a preoccupation with weight.[18] It goes without saying that one of the most powerful strategies you can apply to raise healthy eaters is to model healthy eating for them and to expose them to healthy models (say, the girl next door who loves vegetables). Learn more about modeling and why it works in Chapter 6.

## Vow Not to Say Anything

Just as children are innately programmed to prefer sweet and salty, parents seem to be programmed to persuade children to "Eat your vegetables!" It's just one of those things that get passed down from generation to generation—reinforced by all the other parents out there who do the same thing. Although this tactic does sometimes improve short-term compliance, in the long run, it usually backfires. We'll talk about all the science in upcoming chapters (specifically, Chapters 2 through 4), but the following offers a quick overview as to why it's better to resist the urge to persuade your kids to eat their "yummy vegetables."

To start, children resist persuasion and active encouragement. Remember, children have very little control in their lives, but food is one area where they can dig in, and you can't do much about that. The more they pick up that you really want them to eat something, the more likely they are to recognize that they're in the position of power and can take advantage of that. They'll do this by further refusing to eat. You'll pressure more. They'll refuse more. Then, suddenly, you have yet another battle of the wills. Not to mention the bad rap that those healthy foods you're pushing have just attained. First of all, the child is thinking "How great can this really be if they're selling it so hard?" Second, by pressuring your child to eat the healthy foods (and not pressuring him to eat the less healthy foods), preferences for less-healthy foods are reinforced.

You can avert all this if you make a concerted effort to avoid overt persuasion. Instead, offer your children food opportunities. Use the authoritative parenting strategy of controlling what foods you offer your children and then letting them decide what and how much to eat. Chances are pretty good that if you put a meal of baked salmon, steamed spinach, and Brussels sprouts in front of your picky two-year-old, he's probably going to refuse to eat it. He'll either go to bed hungry or his not eating will stress you out so much that you'll throw this strategy to the wind and prepare him macaroni and cheese or some other favorite. You can meet him halfway. Try some of the following strategies to make mealtime less stressful for everyone and also increase the odds your child will happily eat:

- Keep mealtimes relaxing and enjoyable.
- Choose at least one food the child will like.
- Engage the child in meal preparation.
- Use food bridges.
- Spice it up (see Chapter 8 for some tips on how to do this).
- Offer the previously rejected foods often (eventually the kids will come around).

**Sneak It In**

Entire recipe books are available on how to sneak healthy foods into your child's diet. No need to recreate them here, although a couple of our favorite recipes, which happen to taste great and include such nutrient-dense and oft-rejected vegetables as peppers and spinach, are included at the end of this chapter. Sneaking healthy foods in offers a last-ditch strategy you could employ for those difficult nutrient powerhouses that your kids just won't eat. Unless your kids witness you making these recipes, they won't even know that their most rejected vegetables are included.

The advantages of "sneaking it in" are obvious. You can relax now that you know your kids are getting the nutrients their bodies need to grow and be healthy. But don't forget the potential drawbacks to this strategy. To start, it's deceptive. Second, if your kids can't see or taste the foods that you've snuck in, then they aren't going to gain the benefits of repeated exposure and potential acceptance of the food. This strategy can also backfire. If your kids find out you're sneaking in vegetables, it reinforces that vegetables are "foods that must taste so bad that Mom has to trick us into eating them." Then, your kids aren't likely to willingly try them anytime soon. Use this strategy judiciously, but definitely keep it in your arsenal of counterstrategies.

The sidebar "Counterstrategies in Action: A Recipe for Healthy Eating Without the Mealtime Food Fights" highlights some approaches from parents who have successfully gotten their kids to eat rejected healthy foods without coercion or bribery.

# Developmental Considerations

Although the general rules apply to children of all ages, you'll experience much greater success (and much less frustration) if you understand the normal trajectory of children's eating behaviors and tailor your approach to your child's developmental stage (Figure 1-3).

---

## Counterstrategies in Action:
## A Recipe for Healthy Eating
## Without the Mealtime Food Fights

### Give Them Control

"Letting my daughter eat food off my plate has worked to get her to try new things. I don't suggest that she eat it, but if I sit her on my lap, she will almost always want to try what is on my plate."

—Michelle, mother of three-year-old
Jacob and one-year-old Jessie

### Make It Taste Good

"I have had success getting [my daughter] to eat foods that she previously rejected. For example, she didn't care for raw spinach, but if I sauté it with a little olive oil and garlic, she will inhale it! Also, she didn't care for oatmeal plain, but once I added cinnamon and blueberries, it became her favorite thing to eat in the morning."

—Nina, mother of two-year-old Nora

### Minimize Competition

"With my son, we have been able to get him to eat whole wheat products and avoid juice by just not giving those as options. We started with the whole wheat [instead of white] and milk/water [instead of juice] from the beginning, so that is all that he really knows."

—Rebecca, mother of three-year-old
Alex

---

### Infant (0–1 years)

The diet for the first four to six months of a child's life is simple: breast milk or formula. The American Academy of Pediatrics recommends that all babies be breastfed exclusively without supplementation for the first six months of life. Breastfed babies experience a variety of benefits, including, it seems, a more sophisticated palate. While in one study breastfed and formula-fed infants ate a larger quantity of pureed vegetables after repeated exposure, the breastfed infants ate more overall.[19] It seems that a breastfed baby develops a taste for a

**Model**

"We try to be sure he sees us eating fruits and vegetables even though he's refused for that day."

—Mollie, mother of two-year-old
Charlie and one-year-old Claire

"My daughter definitely saw how frequently I was drinking soda and started to internalize that … grownups could drink as much as they wanted. I cut back for my health (and weight!), but it's certainly had an effect on her assumptions too."

—Caitlin, mother of seven-year-old
Molly

**Engage Them**

"I let him help me 'cook' by standing on a chair, sprinkling in spices or mixing. And I have a toy knife and cutting board that he can cut up really soft canned fruit or veggies while I cook. This also doubles as a healthy snack he can munch on while he 'cooks' if he is really hungry but I don't want him to get too full before a meal. Sometimes, I will also offer 'appetizers' of fruits or veggies to get more of those eaten before I give whatever meat/ grain that I know he eats without issue."

—Amber, mother of two-year-old Xavier

**Sneak It In**

"'Sneaking' fresh spinach into our smoothies is wonderful—I don't hide it from them; they know that's just how we make them. I fill the blender half full of spinach, then add some 100 percent fruit juice (although I know water would be healthier)—blend completely and then add a mix of frozen and fresh fruit. All four of us—and anyone we've had try them—really enjoy it. Especially since the boys get to use straws with them."

—Jen, mother of five-year-old
Jack and two-year-old Nick

wide variety of foods he's exposed to from the maternal diet *if* his mom regularly consumes the food or similar tasting foods.[20] On the other hand, a formula-fed baby tastes only the same formula ingredients at each feeding. If you weren't able to breastfeed your child exclusively for the whole six months, put your guilt aside. For various reasons, only a small minority of babies consume strictly mother's milk for the first half year of life. Any amount of breast milk a baby can get is great, and it may help him to be a healthier eater later on. With that said, a formula-fed baby isn't destined for a lifetime of picky eating.

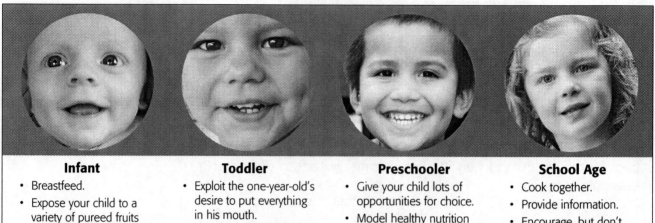

| **Infant** | **Toddler** | **Preschooler** | **School Age** |
|---|---|---|---|
| • Breastfeed.<br>• Expose your child to a variety of pureed fruits and vegetables.<br>• Pair bitter and sweet purees. | • Exploit the one-year-old's desire to put everything in his mouth.<br>• Use chapter strategies to counter neophobia.<br>• Avoid a battle of wills. | • Give your child lots of opportunities for choice.<br>• Model healthy nutrition choices.<br>• Capitalize on peer influences. | • Cook together.<br>• Provide information.<br>• Encourage, but don't pressure your child to try new tastes. |

Figure 1-3. Developmental considerations

The second half of the first year marks the parents' first opportunity to introduce a child to the wonder of vegetables and fruits, although breast milk or formula is still an important part of your child's diet. While no one perfect way exists to transition to solids, the key is to strategically introduce your child to a wide variety of tastes. Babies are accepting of most any flavor at this age, but they're also very smart. Remember, a preference for sweet tastes is innate. Your baby will prefer pears to broccoli and applesauce to your pureed spinach. You can help minimize the competition by introducing your child to vegetables before you add the fruits. The general rule is to start with single-ingredient purees and then introduce a new food every three to four days or so (this is to help to be able to identify food allergies). Expose your baby to as many different vegetables and fruits as possible during this transitional period before your child starts eating the same table food that the rest of the family consumes. After your baby has been exposed to a few different vegetables and fruits, try pairing the more bitter vegetables with the sweet fruit to see if your baby's acceptance of the vegetable increases. If you're still breastfeeding, keep it up and continue to eat as varied of a diet as you can.

You may notice with feedings that your baby makes many different facial expressions in response to various tastes. Although it's reasonable to assume that an expression that seems to indicate dislike is good reason to call a food off limits, use your baby's other signals to decide whether you should keep feeding or stop. For example, is your baby still opening wide and willing to eat the food? If your baby starts to turn his head away, close his mouth, or spit the food out, he's letting you know that he's not so fond of that food for now. These may be signs that he's full and no longer interested in eating or that he doesn't like the particular food you're offering. Don't pressure him to keep eating. Instead, respect that he's telling you he's had enough. At the same time, don't declare that food off limits either. Wait 3 to 14 days to try again.

## Toddler (1–3 years)

The peak healthiness of a typical person's diet is achieved at the ripe age of one. After that, it goes downhill. Your one-year-old is starting to eat table food. That means you have the more challenging job of making sure your meals and snacks are healthy and rich in fruits and vegetables. A typical one-year-old wants to put everything in his mouth. You can exploit this window of opportunity and introduce him to a smorgasbord of new foods. Take advantage of this opportunity because within the next year, neophobia will set in. When it does, remember that it's completely normal and age appropriate for a two-year-old to reject vegetables and fruits. Previously readily accepted foods may now be forcefully rejected. Don't despair. If you stay the course and experiment with the strategies described in this chapter, you'll see that your toddler will start to eat previously rejected vegetables and fruits. But you have to be patient. The toddler years are the time when the food fights begin, and if you're not careful, these fights can persist for years. The investment you make early on in your child's life will pay dividends later. Your child won't starve and become malnourished during this trying time. If you're worried, give your child a multivitamin each day and work with your pediatrician to make sure your child is at a healthy weight.

## Preschooler (3–5 years)

Your preschooler exerts increasing independence and has a decent grasp of the basics; he knows where you keep the food in the cupboard and is resourceful enough to access it (so make sure it's healthy). He loves when he gets to choose. Let him pick what vegetable to have with dinner, take him along when you go grocery shopping, and make it a family project to plant a few seeds (preschoolers generally love to eat what they grow). Modeling also becomes extremely powerful at this age for adult models and peer models. Make sure you (and other adults in the house) have a healthy and positive attitude toward vegetables and fruits. Also, strategize with the parents of your child's closest friends—does your son not eat a vegetable that his best friend loves? Have his best friend's mom offer it up at their next playdate. With time, you might find that food on your child's list of favorites. As an example, one mother interviewed for this book shared the story that her neighbor's kids were over for dinner and she was offering fresh clementine wedges as a side. The neighbor's mom said that one of the children doesn't care for clementines, but the host mom gave him some anyway because three other kids sat at the table with him, happily eating. He ate his portion! (This is also a reminder to parents to try to avoid saying things such as "Oh, you won't like this" or "He won't try that." You might be surprised!)

## School Age (5–10 years)

A school-aged child already has some relatively stable eating preferences. Undoing them takes some effort. While providing information on the health value of an apple may not go far with a three-year-old, it can hold some weight with an eight-year-old. You can offer up some of this information, but don't push it or pressure your child too much. If you're trying to undo unhealthy behaviors, transition slowly. Make sure your child has access to some of the foods he likes, but also encourage—but don't pressure—him to try some new tastes. Include some of his favorites in a dish with an unfamiliar or a previously unliked food. The strategies described earlier in this chapter will still work with this age group, but you have to be sensitive to the fact that just as it's difficult for an adult to break a bad habit, it takes time and patience to undo some of the old preferences and broaden your child's repertoire of acceptable vegetables and fruits.

# Chapter Summary

Now that you're armed with the information you need to set the stage for your kids to eat their vegetables without your having to nag or pressure them, go ahead and give it a try:

- Aim for an authoritative parenting approach in which you control what food is offered and when. Your child controls what food to eat and how much.

- Encourage—but don't pressure—your child to eat his vegetables. Much of this encouragement will be nonverbal in the form of modeling, increasing accessibility and exposure, and making the veggies taste good.

- Be okay with your child refusing some foods at first. Remember, you have a multivitamin as a backup during the uncomfortable period of time it takes for the strategies to work.

- Remember the "rule of 15." It can take 15 to 20 tries for a child to accept a new food. Every 3 to 14 days, reintroduce the rejected food.

- Make fruits and vegetables readily available in your home. Include a fruit and vegetable at every meal. Involve your kids in choosing and preparing meals and consider planting a fruit tree or small garden or even growing something as simple as a couple of herbs on your windowsill.

- Make it taste good. Taste is the number one predictor of whether a child will eat a food. Kids have an innate preference for sweet and salty and an innate distaste for bitter and sour. Pair bitter vegetables with sweet fruits to increase acceptance of the vegetable and up the overall daily intake of produce.

- Use food bridges to help a child accept the new food or come to accept a previously rejected food.

- Be a good role model for your children. In addition to raising healthier eaters, you might experience an unintended benefit of improved health and body composition for yourself.

- Take advantage of opportunities as they present themselves. For example, are your kids *really* hungry? Give them a large amount of a veggie snack. A hungry kid will eat almost anything.

- Tailor your feeding approaches to your child's age and developmental stage.

# Recipes: Yummy Fruits and Vegetables Galore

## Spaghetti and (Spinach) Meatballs

1 pound ground beef, chicken, or turkey

8 ounces of frozen spinach, defrosted

2 carrots, peeled and grated

1 zucchini, grated

1/2 cup of rolled oats

1 jar of tomato sauce

1 16-ounce package of whole wheat spaghetti

2 tablespoons of olive oil

1 teaspoon of salt

2 teaspoons of pepper

To make the pasta: Cook the pasta according to the instructions on the package.

To make the meatballs: Place oats into a blender and blend until roughly chopped. Using your hands or a kitchen towel, squeeze out all the water from the defrosted spinach. Place meat, spinach, and oatmeal in a large mixing bowl. Stir contents to mix well. Add salt and pepper. Take 1 spoonful of the mixture and roll into a meatball. Continue with the rest of the meat/vegetable mix.

Place pot over medium heat on the stove. Put 2 tablespoons of olive oil into the pan. Place meatballs in the pan, approximately 2 inches apart from each other. Cook for approximately 3 minutes and then flip the meatballs onto other side, until lightly browned. Remove the cooked meatballs from the heat and repeat with remaining mixture. Once all meatballs have been pan fried, add the grated carrots and zucchini to pan and cook for 4 to 5 minutes. Add the jar of tomato sauce and cook for 10 minutes.

Place all meatballs back into pan with the sauce. Simmer on low heat for 20 to 30 minutes.

Serve the meatballs and sauce on top of the cooked pasta.

## "Veggieful" Hamburgers

1 pound of lean ground beef or turkey

2 cups of shredded vegetables (carrots, zucchini, peppers)

1/2 cup uncooked oatmeal

1 teaspoon of salt and pepper

Whole wheat hamburger buns

Toppings: Lettuce, tomatoes, onions, mushrooms, cheese

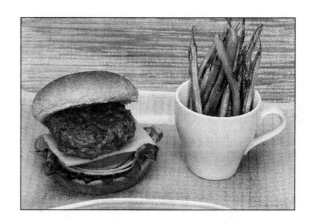

Hamburger patties: Mix vegetables, meat, salt, pepper, and oatmeal in a bowl and stir. Take 2 large spoonfuls of mixture and roll into a ball and then flatten to form a patty.

Place pan on stove at medium heat. Place 1 tablespoon of olive oil in the pan. Place hamburger patty on pan and cook for 5 to 6 minutes. Turn the patty over and cook for another 5 to 6 minutes. Serve on hamburger bun with your favorite toppings!

*Tip*: Serve with Crispy Green Bean "Fries" (see Chapter 7 for recipe).

## Baked Sweet Potato Fries

3 medium-sized sweet potatoes
Olive oil

Preheat oven to 450 degrees. Wash sweet potatoes well. Cut into 1/8-inch round slices and put into a bowl. Drizzle 2 tablespoons of olive oil on top of the potatoes and mix well until potatoes are coated. Place potatoes on a baking sheet in a single layer and then put into oven. Bake for approximately 25 minutes or until crispy and brown.

*Tips:*

- Like pumpkin pie? Try adding cinnamon and nutmeg to the potatoes.
- Like southwestern flavors? Try adding cumin and garlic to the potatoes.

## Choose Your Own Oatmeal

2 cups uncooked oats
3 cups of water
1/2 teaspoon of salt

Bring milk and salt to boil over medium heat. Add oats and stir. Cook for 8 to 10 minutes or until most of the liquid is absorbed.

*Tip*: Spice it up with the following variations:

- "Banana Bread" Oatmeal: Add 1 tablespoon of cinnamon and 1 tablespoon of brown sugar or honey to water and bring to a boil. Peel 2 ripe bananas into a bowl and mash with a fork. After you add the oats to milk, add bananas to oatmeal and stir. Cook for 8 to 10 minutes. Top with chopped toasted walnuts.
- Cinnamon Apple Oatmeal: Dice 2 apples into 1/4-inch pieces and place into pot over medium heat. Add 1 tablespoon of cinnamon and 2 tablespoons of brown sugar or honey to water and pour over apples. Bring the mixture to a boil and then lower heat. Add the oats and stir. Cook for 8 to 10 minutes.
- Strawberries and Cream Oatmeal: Cook basic oatmeal as instructed in the previous variation. Add 1/2 cup of nonfat milk to oatmeal and stir. Add 1/4 cup of strawberry jam/preserves to oatmeal and stir. Cook for 3 to 4 minutes and serve with a dollop of strawberry jam on top.
- Peanut Butter and Jelly Oatmeal: Cook basic oatmeal as instructed in the previous variation. When serving oatmeal, place 1 spoon of jelly and 1 spoon of peanut butter on top of oatmeal.

## Creamy Roasted Red Pepper Tomato Soup With Spinach Grilled Cheese

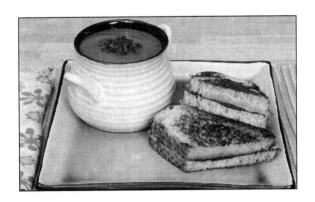

2 15-ounce cans of chopped tomatoes
3 red bell peppers
1 medium yellow onion, diced
2 garlic cloves, chopped
3 tablespoons of tomato paste
1 medium Yukon Gold potato
3 cups of water

Wash and dry all vegetables. To prepare the roasted red peppers, preheat oven to 400 degrees. Place the washed red peppers on a baking sheet and place in oven for approximately 30 minutes. Once skin is blistered or charred, remove peppers from oven and place in a bowl and cover with plastic wrap. Let cool for 15 minutes.

While peppers are roasting, prepare other ingredients for the soup. Dice the medium onion and garlic into small pieces. Wash the potato and scrub the skin. Cut the potato into 1/2-inch chunks. Heat a large pot over medium heat with 2 tablespoons of olive oil. Place onions and garlic into pot and stir. Once onions and garlic are slightly browned, add in the potatoes and tomatoes and stir. Remove peppers from bowl, peel the charred skin, remove seeds, and place into pot. Add water and let simmer for 40 minutes, stirring occasionally. Remove from heat and let cool for 15 minutes. In batches, transfer the soup to a blender and blend until smooth. Serve with spinach grilled cheese.

*Spinach Grilled Cheese*

8 pieces of whole grain bread
2 cups of light cheddar cheese
2 cups of baby spinach
Olive oil

Place the bread on a baking sheet and preheat oven to 375 degrees. Brush both sides of each slice of bread lightly with olive oil. Place cheddar cheese on 4 slices of bread (1/4 cup per slice). Next, place 1/2 cup of baby spinach on top of the cheese and then sprinkle another 1/4 cup of the cheese on top of the spinach. Place the remaining slices of bread on top to make 4 sandwiches. Put the baking sheet into the oven for 10 minutes. Remove the sheet from the oven, and using a spatula, press down each sandwich and then flip each sandwich onto the other side. Place back into the oven for 10 minutes and then remove the sheet from the oven and slice each sandwich diagonally in half.

## References

1. Parker-Pope, T. (2008). Dr. T. Berry Brazelton's advice on childhood nutrition. *New York Times*'s Well blog. Available at http://well.blogs.nytimes.com/2008/09/16/dr-brazeltons-advice-on-childhood-nutrition.

2. Wolfe, W.S., and C.C. Campbell. (1993). Food pattern, diet quality, and related characteristics of schoolchildren in New York state. *J Am Diet Assoc. 93*(11): p. 1280-4.

3. Lorson, B.A., H.R. Melgar-Quinonez, and C.A. Taylor. (2009). Correlates of fruit and vegetable intakes in US children. *J Am Diet Assoc. 109*(3): p. 474-8.

4. Dwyer, J.T., N.F. Butte, D.M. Deming, A.M. Siega-Riz, and K.C. Reidy. (2010). Feeding Infants and Toddlers Study 2008: Progress, continuing concerns, and implications. *J Am Diet Assoc. 110*(12 Suppl): p. S60-7.

5. Siega-Riz, A.M., D.M. Deming, K.C. Reidy, M.K. Fox, E. Condon, and R.R. Briefel (2010). Food consumption patterns of infants and toddlers: Where are we now? *J Am Diet Assoc. 110*(12 Suppl): p. S38-51.

6. Hellmich, N. (2010). We're still too low on fruit, vegetable consumption. *USA Today*. Available at http://www.usatoday.com/yourlife/food/diet-nutrition/2010-11-17-noveggies17_ST_N.htm.

7. Domel, S.B., W.O. Thompson, H.C. Davis, T. Baranowski, S.B. Leonard, and J. Baranowski. (1996). Psychosocial predictors of fruit and vegetable consumption among elementary school children. *Health Education Research. 11*: p. 299-308.

8. Baumrind, D. (1971). Current patterns of parental authority. *Developmental Psychology Monograph. 4*(1, Part 2): p. 1-101.

9. Rhee, K.E., J.C. Lumeng, D.P. Appugliese, N. Kaciroti, and R.H. Bradley. (2006). Parenting styles and overweight status in first grade. *Pediatrics. 117*(6): p. 2047-54.

10. Brug, J., N.I. Tak, S.J. te Velde, E. Bere, and I. de Bourdeaudhuij. (2008). Taste preferences, liking and other factors related to fruit and vegetable intakes among schoolchildren: Results from observational studies. *Br J Nutr.* 99 Suppl 1: p. S7-S14.

11. Rozin, P. (1976). The selection of food by rats, humans and other animals. In R. Rosenblatt, R.A. Hinde, C. Beer, and E. Shaw (eds.), *Advances in the Study of Behavior*. New York: Academic Press.

12. Wardle, J., M.L. Herrera, L. Cooke, and E.L. Gibson. (2003). Modifying children's food preferences: The effects of exposure and reward on acceptance of an unfamiliar vegetable. *Eur J Clin Nutr. 57*(2): p. 341-8.

13. Birch, L.L., L. McPhee, B.C. Shoba, E. Pirok, and L. Steinberg. (1987). What kind of exposure reduces children's food neophobia? Looking vs. tasting. *Appetite. 9*(3): p. 171-8.

14. Spill, M.K., L.L. Birch, L.S. Roe, and B.J. Rolls. (2010). Eating vegetables first: The use of portion size to increase vegetable intake in preschool children. *Am J Clin Nutr. 91*(5): p. 1237-43.

15. Kral, T.V., A.C. Kabay, L.S. Roe, and B.J. Rolls. (2010). Effects of doubling the portion size of fruit and vegetable side dishes on children's intake at a meal. *Obesity (Silver Spring). 18*(3): p. 521-7.

16. Harper, L.V., and K.M. Sanders. (1975). The effect of adults' eating on young children's acceptance of unfamiliar foods. *Journal of Experimental and Child Psychology.* 20: p. 206-14.

17. Rozin, P., and D. Schiller. (1980). The nature of a preference for chili pepper by humans. *Motivation and Emotion.* 4: p. 77-101.

18. Birch, L.L., and J.O. Fisher. (1998). Development of eating behaviors among children and adolescents. *Pediatrics*. *101*(3 Pt 2): p. 539-49.

19. Sullivan, S.A., and L.L. Birch. (1994). Infant dietary experience and acceptance of solid foods. *Pediatrics*. *93*(2): p. 271-7.

20. Forestell, C.A., and J.A. Mennella. (2007). Early determinants of fruit and vegetable acceptance. *Pediatrics*. *120*(6): p. 1247-54.

21. Aatola, H., T. Koivistoinen, N. Hutri-Kahonen N, M. Juonala, V. Mikkila, T. Lehtimaki, J.S. Viikari, O.T. Raitakari, M. Kahonen (2010). Lifetime fruit and vegetable consumption and arterial pulse wave velocity in adulthood: the Cardiovascular Risk in Young Finns Study. *Circulation.* 122(24): p. 2521-8.

22. Knai, C., J. Pomerleau , K. Lock, M. McKee (2006). Getting children to eat more fruit and vegetables: a systematic review. *Prev Med.* 42(2): p. 85-95.

# 2

# Mistake #2—
# Using Food as a Reward

*"Rewarding children with unhealthy foods ...
undermines our efforts to teach them about
good nutrition. It's like teaching children a lesson
on the importance of not smoking, and then
handing out ashtrays and lighters to the kids
who did the best job listening."*

—Marlene Schwartz, Ph.D., co-director,
Rudd Center for Food Policy and
Obesity, Yale University

The online community Momversation.com queried its readers about if and how they used food as a reward to motivate their children. Check out some of these responses, cited exactly as they were written by the mothers. Do any strike a chord?

*"We felt like potty training needed a little nudge in the right direction, so we started offering a piece of candy after every pee-pee. Now the kid tries to make himself go whenever he wants candy, and he barely hops off the toilet seat before he's asking for his candy. Not exactly what we were looking for."*

*"My five-year-old boy got a flu shot yesterday and cried! I felt so bad for him, I immediately whipped out a sucker!"*

*"They are expected to eat a good portion of dinner to be eligible for dessert. ... Have a cookie if you don't like 'my' dessert, but you have to eat like a reasonable human being in order to get to that point."*

# What's Wrong With Using Food as a Reward? After All, It Works.

We're all guilty. Using food as a reward is such an easy, inexpensive, and overwhelmingly effective tool that it's hard not to use it. But the short-term benefits come with a hefty price tag. To start, foods commonly used as rewards (such as candy, cookies, and ice cream) are typically high in fat and sugar and can contribute to various health problems for children, such as obesity, diabetes, hypertension, and cavities. And while children come to prefer nutrient-void, calorie-dense foods, they simultaneously develop a dislike of foods eaten to obtain rewards. This is known as the "discounting principle." A child figures out pretty quickly that those vegetables must be pretty gross if you're going to pay him with delicious desserts and other enticements in exchange for taking a bite. Furthermore, the positive association that develops between the foods used as reward and "feeling good" can lead to later emotional and disordered eating. As one self-reflective mother posted on the Momversation.com blog about rewarding kids with food: "I really try hard not to offer up food as rewards because I struggle with my own weight. … I am an emotional eater. I eat when I'm sad, when I'm upset … hell, even when I'm happy. Birthdays are about the cake, Christmas is about the cookies … Halloween is about the candy."

With this said, the parental tendency to use food as a reward is powerful, especially because it's so effective. The goal of this chapter is to convince you that it's worth the extra effort to forever abandon this strategy and instead apply a few different techniques and offer up other enticing rewards (when appropriate) to encourage your child to comply with your non-food-related requests.

# The Psychology of Rewards

The use of rewards as a motivational strategy seems like an obvious way to shape a child's behavior. After all, this is the essence of operant conditioning—give a child a reward for a job well done and the child will continue to strive to do jobs well. On the other hand, take a reward away or punish a child for a behavior and the behavior will eventually stop. While all this is true, we have to be careful when using rewards that may lead to unanticipated negative consequences, such as when food is used as a reward or when a reward is offered for eating certain foods.

### How Food Rewards Contribute to Worse Nutrition and Health

In our efforts to reward kids for eating healthier, we may actually be contributing to worsened nutrition.

*Preference for Unhealthy (and Highly Palatable) Foods*

Parents of toddlers everywhere struggle to figure out the best way to get their children out of diapers. Ultimately, regardless of strategy employed, kids learn.

But society has an expectation that a child of a certain age should be potty trained. (By the way, the average age is 30 months, but the pressure to get the kid on the toilet starts much sooner for many parents, especially those wanting to get their child into diaper-free daycare and preschools.) Whether out of a sense of desperation or the practical reasoning that rewards work, many parents offer their children incentives for "using the potty," including candy. In fact, even in my own house, we had this argument as our son was nearing the time of starting preschool but still not into the idea of using the toilet. Like a lot of kids, my husband and his siblings were potty trained with M&M's. The older kids still vividly remember the allure of the M&M's for the younger ones as they were learning to use the potty. "It worked!" they all agree. I concur, it does. But there are risks. (By the way, we ended up with stickers as our source of "reward," but no big surprise, it wasn't until he was ready that our son successfully learned to use the potty.) Other than the relatively inconsequential sugar overload a smart child is bound to experience when rewarded with candy for sitting on the potty (after all, once they figure out they get candy, toddlers learn real quick to say that they need to use the potty, whether they actually do or not), the kids also learn to like the reward even more.

To illustrate, consider a study of preschoolers who were given a food reward for accomplishing a non-food-related task. The reward was something the researchers determined to be of relatively neutral liking to the child before the experiment, such as crackers or peanuts. The child was then given that snack and verbal praise from the teacher as a reward for various behaviors, such as responding to a verbal request, performing an activity well, sustaining attention to an activity, and playing cooperatively. Ninety-six percent of the time, the child ate the food immediately. The kids' preference for the snack was then reassessed immediately following the experiment as well as six weeks later. The kids given the food reward liked the previously neutral food more after the experiment. Notably, the effect persisted.[1]

And these foods were relatively healthy. If you take a sweet food like candy which is already innately preferred. and use it as a reward, the child is going to prefer it even more. If you pair the food with verbal praise, the liking increases. Thus, while you might get your kid using the potty (which kids eventually figure out how to do anyway), your kid is also developing more of a sweet tooth (see the sidebar "Sweet Tooth Cycle"). While a few M&M's here and there are unlikely to cause childhood obesity, an increased liking for the stuff is going to lead your child to seek out the sweets, and over time, those extra empty calories add up.

### Dislike of Healthy (but Less Palatable) Foods

"Eat your vegetables or no dessert" is probably the most commonly uttered parent statement at mealtimes now and for the past 100 years. Parents everywhere and over the course of several generations have used this line to get their kids to eat their vegetables. What's the alternative? Let a kid have dessert as his dinner? After all, if he doesn't have to eat anything on his plate and he still gets cake, cookies, and ice cream, then what's to make him eat his veggies? Valid points for sure. But the consequence of this strategy in the

**Sweet Tooth Cycle**

Most of the foods your kids love—cookies, ice cream, candy, juice, and chips—tend to be high-fat, high-calorie, heavily processed foods. Food manufacturers manipulate the ingredients in just the right way to create an addictive food. Without good portion control, it's easy for a child or adult to eat way too many calories and to keep eating long after hunger has subsided. Not only does this set the stage for weight gain, but it also displaces healthier, more nutrient-dense foods and creates a psychological desire for more—whether that "more" comes now or if that "more" comes as a strong desire to eat dessert every night after dinner. A "sweet tooth" is a learned phenomenon. If you go cold turkey for a while, you'll find that you don't need sweets so much anymore. But if you're in the habit of eating them on a regular basis, it becomes very difficult to cut them out, especially if they're readily available. If you rely on dessert to bribe your children into eating their vegetables, you set the stage for dessert on a regular basis, which only reinforces the need for sweets. Furthermore, if those desserts are typical (i.e., high fat, high calorie, highly processed), regularly offering them compromises your child's health. Try to limit how often dessert is available, and when you do offer it, try to go for more natural and healthier sweets. (See this chapter's recipes.)

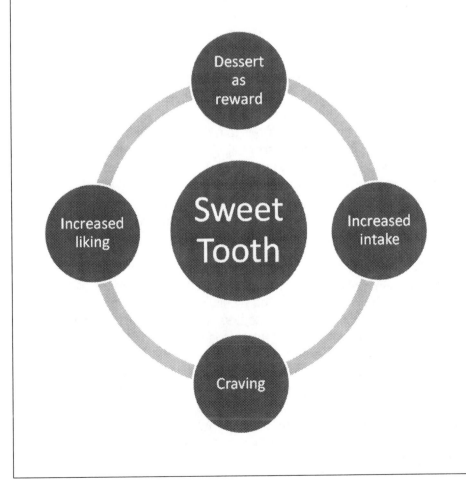

long run is that not only do kids like the dessert more, but when a reward is given to eat certain foods, the kids come to dislike the food they had to eat to get the reward even less (the discounting principle). For example, in one study, children given a reward for drinking a juice they initially rated as "neutral" showed a significant decrease in their preference for the juice when they had to drink it in order to engage in a desirable play activity.[2] A follow-up study showed the same; furthermore, liking decreased even when the reward was verbal praise, such as "You're a really good taster" and "Good job," after a child tried the drink.[3]

*Emotional Eating*

In the study previously discussed in which preschoolers were given snacks as rewards, researchers also assessed how much children liked the previously neutral food when the food was paired with adult attention. The children didn't have to complete any particular task or "earn" the food reward. Rather, at random times, a teacher gave the child individual attention and offered the snack food. At the end of the study, these kids liked the snack foods significantly more than the kids who simply got the snack at snack time or who got the snack in a nonsocial context (the snack left at their locker). But they didn't like it quite as much as the kids who got the snack food as a reward. This arm of the study attempted to quantify the effect of all those social interactions kids have that are paired with food: cake at children's parties, ice cream with Grandma, candy at Halloween, a feast at Thanksgiving, etc.

Essentially, most all the fun stuff in our social lives revolves around or at least includes food—usually, the unhealthy kind. We then become classically conditioned to associate these unhealthy foods with enjoyable social interactions. When times are tough and we long for those enjoyable experiences, we then turn to those unhealthy "comfort" foods to make ourselves feel better and try to recreate the "good times." This emotional eating is prevalent, affecting about a quarter of children aged 5 to 12 years[4]; the rates are higher among adolescents. That's not to say we should completely abandon these enjoyable experiences. Rather, we need to set the stage for our children to help them enjoy sweets in moderation, let hunger be their guide in determining how much and when to eat, and consume an overall healthy, balanced diet.

We also need to be very careful not to use food to make our kids feel better. One study evaluated the relationship between the extent of a mother's use of food to regulate emotions and a child's food intake after being put into a negative mood. Those kids with mothers that used food to make their kids feel better had significantly higher intake than the other kids.[5] In real life, this happens all the time. For example, at one recent family event, one of the kids became upset that one of the other kids took his toy. To help him "feel better," his grandma gave him a hug and asked if he would like a bowl of ice cream. This use of food for emotional regulation reinforces emotional eating and is associated with increased caloric intake. These relationships with food that start so early in life persist to adulthood and have played a role in the current worldwide epidemic of obesity.

We can help minimize the impact and extent of emotional eating for our kids. One way is to cut out the strategy of using food as a reward. Another is to rely less on unhealthy foods to create positive emotional experiences. A child will love going to the bookstore or playground with a special visitor as much as he'll enjoy going out for ice cream. And, finally, we can't rely on unhealthy "comfort foods" to heal a child's pain.

## Extrinsic Rewards Undermine Intrinsic Motivation

A goal of writing this book—and, presumably, a goal of yours in reading it—is to help you raise children who choose of their own will to eat a healthy, balanced diet filled with nutrient-dense fruits and vegetables. Given the innate preference for unhealthy foods and a distaste for vegetables—and as evidenced by the poor dietary habits of American children and adults alike—it's a relatively major undertaking to achieve this goal. My job is to provide you with the information and tools you need so that with careful planning, persistence, and parental savvy, we can achieve our mutual goal. One of our major tasks is to inspire, nurture, and support a child's intrinsic motivation to eat healthy.

Pay careful attention to the "inspire." Kids aren't programmed to love vegetables. Recall the innate preference for sweet and salty and the dislike of sour and bitter. This book describes ways to effectively shape your child's taste preferences and foster a liking for eating healthy. Each of these strategies helps your child to actually *want* to eat these foods. The book also discusses in detail what *not* to do—those well-intentioned but counterproductive tactics that diminish a child's *intrinsic motivation* to choose healthy foods, such as offering food as a reward or offering rewards for eating.

Intrinsic motivation is the desire to engage in some activity out of one's own volition—free of coercion or expectation for some external reward. Play, exploration, and challenge seeking offer a few examples. A child who's intrinsically motivated to eat healthy chooses healthy foods because he likes the taste or because they make him feel energetic or strong. The need for autonomy and competence underlie intrinsic motivation. Instances in which a child is allowed to exert some control and prove his competence will help build his intrinsic motivation. When his autonomy is undermined or he feels a sense of coercion or pressure to do an activity (such as in the case of desiring to receive a reward), his intrinsic motivation is diminished.

Offering up extrinsic rewards to do something, such as eating vegetables, lessens a child's intrinsic motivation to eat these foods. Thus, when you're not looking, he's not going to choose the good stuff. The more you push him, the less he's going to like it. The child is thinking something along the lines of: "*If Dad is going to make me eat my vegetables in order to get dessert, then those vegetables must be pretty gross.*" This is the discounting principle.

One meta-analysis, a type of research paper that evaluates the results of many similar studies, looked at 128 experiments that explored the relationship between extrinsic rewards and intrinsic motivation. Looking at all the studies together, the researchers concluded that the evidence is clear and consistent:

tangible rewards, especially those that are perceived as controlling or coercive (as is often the case in shaping children's behavior), have a negative effect on intrinsic motivation on all kids from preschool children to college (and presumably adults too, although they weren't studied).[6] While rewards may be effective in shaping short-term behavior, in the long run, they're often counterproductive.

However, this isn't to say to never use rewards (although, hopefully, you'll abandon food as a reward). In some cases, we may not care if intrinsic motivation is undermined for the sake of completing a task, such as in the early stages of potty training. In other cases, we can minimize the harmful effects on intrinsic motivation by offering the rewards in a particular way so as to increase the informational value and decrease the perception of controlling. Motivation experts suggest some ways to make rewards more informational:

- Offer a reward spontaneously, when a child isn't expecting it.
- Minimize the use of an authoritarian style and pressuring.
- Provide choices about how to do tasks.
- Acknowledge good performance, but don't use rewards to try to strengthen or control the behavior.
- Emphasize the interesting or challenging aspects of the tasks.[6]

# Counterstrategy: The Techniques

Let's apply these strategies to your mealtime goal of having your children eat a healthy and balanced diet.

### Rewarding Healthy Eating Without Undermining Intrinsic Motivation

We want our children to choose to eat a healthy diet. When left to his own devices, a child is capable of choosing a well-balanced diet, but this isn't the case in the era of food overabundance and access to an overload of calories, processed foods, sugar, and salt. (Read more about this in Chapter 3.) However, with some parental structure and quiet nudging, we can set the stage for our children to be exposed to an array of healthy options and come to prefer these foods. In those cases, when a child has access to primarily healthy choices, his unconscious ability to meet nutritional needs works very well. The difficult task of a parent is to create this healthy environment, which includes structure, guidelines, and rules, while letting the child make some decisions. As soon as your child begins to feel coerced or controlled into doing what you want, he's going to push back. Your prompts and rewards, then, must not be perceived as controlling but rather should be withheld or at least be perceived by the child as informational in nature. The following are a few tips:

- *Don't be so predictable.* Your child is expecting you to pressure him to eat his vegetables. He's waiting for the mealtime power struggle. Refuse to fall into that trap. Instead, try to prepare a healthy meal that includes one healthy food that he likes. (For some parents, it may be difficult to come up with a healthy food that your child likes—how about applesauce or baked sweet potato fries or brown rice?) The rest of the dinner should be healthy too, but recognize before you even serve it to him that he may not eat any of it. Be okay with that. Serve the food, don't worry if he eats it or not, and have an enjoyable meal with the family. After you're done, finish it off with something fun as a family that your child really likes to do, whether that's a board game, a walk around the block, or reading a book. Do something like this spaced out (and unannounced) a few times over the course of the next few weeks or months. Your child will come to unconsciously associate this healthy family meal with fun and pleasure.

- *Practice authoritative parenting techniques.* The quintessential authoritative parent feeding strategy, which was first described by renowned dietitian and therapist Ellyn Satter, is to live by the "division of responsibility" principle. That is, you as a parent control what foods are offered and when and your child chooses which of those foods to eat and how much. This gives your child the satisfaction of choosing, which goes a very long way in helping him enjoy the foods he's chosen to eat. Just make sure the choices you're giving him are between healthy foods and that you're equally happy with whatever choice he makes. Then, if you would like to reward him, make the reward for being such a big kid and making a great choice rather than rewarding him for eating the healthy food.

- *Acknowledge when your child makes a healthy choice, but don't make a big deal out of it and don't use it as an opportunity to control his behavior.* You can acknowledge a healthy choice by saying something along the lines of "That milk you just drank is going to help you have strong bones" rather than "Drink that milk so you can have strong bones." The first statement is informational. The second is controlling. If your child perceives that you're trying to control him into doing the behavior again, he's less likely to be intrinsically motivated to do it again spontaneously. For example, in one of the studies previously discussed, the researchers found that verbal praise for trying a healthy food lessened intrinsic motivation. However, in another study, kids ate more of the healthy food when it was paired with adult attention. The difference is that in the first study, the kids felt controlled or pressured by the praising comments, whereas in the second, the attention had nothing to do with the food; it just happened to occur at the same time.

- *Experiment together.* Challenge your child to make a vegetable taste better. For example, ask him: "What could we do to make this spinach taste good?" By simply acknowledging that the vegetable may not taste good to him, you give him the freedom to not like it. From that alone, he may be willing to see if anything he could add would help him like it. Hey, if he insists on chocolate-covered spinach or sugar-coated broccoli, letting him try it out is a small price to pay. (After all, wouldn't the old you have offered up the sweet stuff in exchange for eating his veggies?) Other ways you might emphasize interesting or challenging aspects could be to take your child with you to the grocery store and give him the task of picking a fruit and vegetable that he would like to eat. If on occasion he happens to want to get a candy bar while you're there, so be it. But don't verbally elevate the candy to being a "reward" for picking the produce.

## Alternative to Rewards

You don't need to offer illustrious rewards, such as chocolate chip cookies or ice cream sandwiches, in exchange for enduring Brussels sprouts or green beans. You *can* get through mealtimes without having to break out this ultimately counterproductive negotiation technique requiring vegetable consumption before dessert. You control what's offered and when and your child controls how much and what to eat. Leave it at that. The concern that many parents express in response to this is that if they don't make their kids eat their vegetables and other healthy items on their plate, then they'll end up not eating anything; then, if you allow them to eat dessert, you're basically rewarding them for not eating anything healthy. First off, you can limit how often dessert is offered. No one needs to eat dessert after every dinner, but so many of us have developed a sweet tooth, which makes the habit hard to break. By limiting how often dessert is offered, you can help reduce your child's reliance on the sweets. Secondly, you can get your kids to eat their vegetables without being coercive. You might just have to get creative. (Refer to the sidebar "Counterstrategies in Action: Raising Healthy Eaters Without Using Food as a Reward" later in this chapter for some ideas.)

Next, practice the strategies that are emphasized throughout this book, such as improving taste, increasing exposure and accessibility, allowing the child to choose between healthy alternatives, and modeling. Remember that it takes time, consistency, and persistence. The strategies aren't going to magically work the first time you employ them, but eventually, you'll see that some of the strategies discussed here and others that you come up with on your own will help your children eat well without the pressure and enticements of extrinsic rewards.

## Rewarding Without Food

Sometimes, you just want to reward your children for a job well done. You may want to shape their future behavior without regard to the effect on intrinsic motivation or you may just need them to behave in a certain way right now and offering up a reward as an enticement is the best way to do it. In the past, you may have used food as the reward. Hopefully, you're adequately convinced that using food in this way is counterproductive in the long term, so you may be trying to think up something else.

This comes down to the art and science of disciplining children, which is based in large part on operant conditioning. (See this book's introduction for a review of the psychology of learning.) Discipline is defined as "teaching the child" and encompasses all the methods parents use to change behavior. It's not the same as punishment; in fact, the use of rewards is a form of discipline when the rewards are offered in an attempt to shape behaviors. Parents need to be very thoughtful and strategic when disciplining children so as to encourage those behaviors that are "good" and discourage those behaviors that are "bad." Typically, this is done through rewards and punishments. Rewards are a form of *positive reinforcement*—something desirable is given to the child and in turn the desired behavior increases. You could also increase the desired behavior by taking away some aversive stimulus (for example, rewarding a child who's behaving well by not making him take out the trash). This is known as *negative reinforcement*. On the other hand, *positive punishment* refers to the scenario in which a behavior is followed by some aversive stimulus (for example, getting yelled at), which leads to a decrease in behavior. *Negative punishment* is when an undesirable behavior is followed by the removal of an enjoyable stimulus (such as taking away a child's toy after he hit his sister). This leads to a decrease in the "bad" behavior (see Figure 2-1). The goal, of course, is to increase the wanted behaviors and decrease the unwanted behaviors.

In order for rewards to be effective in shaping a behavior, they must be:
- Offered continuously to build a new skill (continuous reinforcement) and then intermittently to maintain a skill (variable reinforcement). For example, when a child is first learning to use the potty, he may receive a sticker every time he sits on the toilet. Once he's successful using the potty several times, he's given the stickers only sometimes.
- Tailored to the child's motivators. If your child isn't interested in stickers, then giving him a sticker as a reward isn't going to be very effective. On the other hand, if he's obsessed with Elmo from *Sesame Street*, then giving him an Elmo book for a job well done is going to be highly effective. You have to offer something they *really* want.
- Tied to the desirable action in time. That is, you need to give the reward immediately after the desired behavior so the child clearly understands *why* he was given the reward.

Keeping these principles in mind, the following are a few nonfood strategies you can apply to positively shape your child's behaviors. Each of these strategies was outlined and described in an excellent summary, which appeared in *Pediatric Clinics of North America*.[7]

**Positive reinforcement =** behavior followed by rewarding stimulus, resulting in an increase in that behavior

**Negative reinforcement =** behavior followed by the removal of an aversive stimulus, resulting in increase in that behavior

**Positive punishment =** behavior followed by an aversive stimulus, resulting in a decrease in that behavior

**Negative punishment =** behavior followed by removal of a favorable stimulus, resulting in a decrease in that behavior

| | Something given to the child | Something taken from the child |
|---|---|---|
| Increases the likelihood of repeated behavior | **Positive Reinforcement** | **Negative Reinforcement** |
| Decreases the likelihood of repeated behavior | **Positive Punishment** | **Negative Punishment** |

Figure 2-1. Shaping behaviors

- *Praise.* Praise given to a child after a desirable behavior socially reinforces the behavior. For example, when a child is given a high-five and told "Great job picking up your toys," he'll likely engage in this behavior again in order to receive more praise. To be most effective, praise should be labeled and specific. That is, the child should know exactly why he's being praised rather than just being told "Good job." Parents who give praise sincerely and freely, even for such mundane tasks as saying "please" and "thank you," have children who are overall better behaved. After all, the children are getting ample amounts of positive attention rather than mostly negative attention (such as "No!" and "Don't do that!"). Unfortunately, many children prefer negative attention to no attention at all; thus, they may act out in an effort to get a parent to take notice.

- *Sticker charts (good for kids two to six years).* Identify your child's target behavior(s) and then every time the child does the desirable behavior(s), award him a sticker to put on a chart. The chart can have rows to identify target behaviors and columns listing days of the week. Make sure the chart is in an easily visible place, and review the chart with the child each time he does the desired behavior. At the bottom of the chart, include the number of stickers the child needs to obtain a "reward." Possible rewards could include a toy, a playdate or slumber party, a special outing, a special bedtime story, or a family game night with a game of the child's choice.

- *Token economy systems and a grab bag (best for kids 6 to 12 years).* This method is similar to the sticker charts but is geared toward older kids. When your child does something you like, reward him with tokens that at the end of the day can be exchanged for a "prize." Prizes could be similar to those offered for the sticker charts or perhaps access to a box of special toys, computer games, or art supplies that can only be used on special occasions.

- *Positive practice.* With this strategy, every time a desirable behavior is completed, the child is rewarded with either verbal praise or some tangible item. For example, a child who often forgets to pick up his toys could be given a reward every time he actually remembers. The desired behavior is increased through repetition and reminders. Another variation of this is the removal of annoying repetitive reminders (negative reinforcement). For example, if you tend to nag your child to eat his vegetables, if you stop nagging (removal of an aversive stimulus), then your child may spontaneously increase his vegetable consumption. The use of negative reinforcement to change behavior tends to be more difficult because the aversive stimulus has to be salient enough for the child to care when it's removed.

The sidebar "Counterstrategies in Action: Raising Healthy Eaters Without Using Food as a Reward" offers real-life examples of how parents have gotten their kids to choose healthy behaviors without using food as a reward.

*Mistake #2—Using Food as a Reward*

---

## Counterstrategies in Action: Raising Healthy Eaters Without Using Food as a Reward

### Reward Healthy Eating Without Undermining Intrinsic Motivation

Tali, the mother of six-year-old Averie, four-year-old Sami, and two-year-old Bennett, gets her kids excited about eating fruits and vegetables without even mentioning the idea of a reward. One way she does this is by making eating healthy fun with "make your own taco" night. Together, they make seasoned ground turkey with a variety of toppings for the kids to choose from, including corn, diced tomatoes, shredded spinach leaves, brown rice, avocado, and black beans. The kids at Tali's house also love "make your own pizza" night, when the kids get to use whole wheat pita breads and assemble their own veggie-ful pizzas. These special nights make eating together as a family fun, create lasting memories, and exemplify the perfect application of the "division of responsibility" principle: Mom decides what foods are offered and the kids choose what and how much to eat.

### Use Alternatives to Rewards

How to deal with the problem of letting the kids eat dessert even if they don't eat their vegetables? Try a trick that Jen, mother of six-year-old Jack and three-year-old Nick, uses: make the dessert one of the healthiest parts! The kids' favorite dessert is yogurt—just regular, nonfat, healthy adult yogurt with a few sprinkles on top. The sprinkles don't hurt the healthiness of the dessert much, and the kids think it's quite special. You could spice this idea up a little and pack an even greater nutritional punch with a yogurt and oat flour-based "carbazu" (carrot/banana/zucchini) cupcake. (See the recipes for this chapter.)

### Reward Without Food

While food is the easiest (and arguably a very highly effective) strategy to shape child behaviors, you can get by without using food as a reward, just as these mothers have:

- Christine, mother of three-year-old Olivia, found the perfect trick to inspire good listening and manners. She bought small butterfly wall decals at IKEA. A new one appears on Olivia's wall each morning if she had been a good listener the previous day. Olivia can't wait to wake up to see if a new butterfly appears. (Note that Christine's award is so effective because it's highly motivating for Olivia.)

- Ann put the token economy system/grab bag to perfect use when potty training her kids: three-year-old Patrick and two-and-a-half-year-old William. They made a star chart and decorated a "treasure chest." When the kids filled up a row of stars, they got to pick a racecar (or another $1-or-less toy) from the treasure chest. Ann attributes this token system for keeping the kids' interest in learning to use the potty and getting them out of diapers once and for all.

# Developmental Considerations

The following strategies are most effective when tailored to a child's developmental stage (Figure 2-2).

### Infant (0–1 years)

Classic attachment theory speculated that mother-infant attachment resulted from the mother's reduction of a baby's primary drive of hunger—in essence, a form of classical conditioning in which the mother provides the infant with food and ultimately she herself is associated with the positive feeling of satiety. According to this theory, the ability to satisfy a baby's hunger forms the basis for infant attachment to his mother or other people associated with feeding. However, in a classic experiment, researcher Harry Harlow separated infant monkeys from their biological mothers and raised them by one of two surrogate "mothers." One was made of stiff wire and had a feeding bottle attached to it. The other was made of soft terrycloth and had no bottle. Especially in moments of stress, the monkeys preferred the cloth "mother" even though she did not dispense food. Research on humans has played out a similar point: attachment isn't automatic and the provision of food isn't necessary to comfort infants, especially when their bellies are already full and they aren't hungry.[8] Attempt to understand why your infant is upset rather than automatically assuming hunger with every tearful bout. This becomes even more important for older infants, who can learn to rely on breastfeeding or a bottle for comfort if every time they're upset they're offered food for comforting. You probably know of a child who's almost one year old who wakes up multiple times in the night wanting to be fed. This isn't due to hunger; it's because he's come to rely on the milk for comfort.

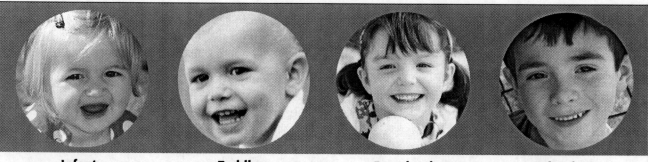

| Infant | Toddler | Preschooler | School Age |
|---|---|---|---|
| • Look for signs of hunger. Remember that not all tears are tears of hunger.<br>• In the second half of the first year, avoid using feeding to comfort. | • Reinforce good behaviors with attention and nonfood rewards.<br>• Avoid using bribes to induce compliance with your dietary requests.<br>• Once you say "No!" don't give in. | • Reinforce good behaviors with sticker charts and other motivating rewards.<br>• Encourage hunger to be the guide; be aware of signs of emotional eating.<br>• Minimize linking junk food with enjoyable social activities. | • Watch for signs of emotional eating.<br>• Provide information about a food's health value.<br>• Use token reward systems to shape behaviors. |

Figure 2-2. Developmental considerations

## Toddler (1–3 years)

A toddler's growing sense of self and all the accompanying opinions, demands, and tantrums that characterize this age set the stage for an overwhelming parental urge to begin to use food as a reward. From buying candy at the store to get a kid to stop crying (in which case, he's unintentionally being awarded for throwing a tantrum) to offering desserts in exchange for eating vegetables, you're dealing with an age at which using food as a reward becomes incredibly tempting. For that reason, this is the critical age in which well thought out and consistently applied parental feeding strategies become extremely important to set the stage for healthy eating down the road.

Mealtime power struggles can be mostly avoided if you create a healthy eating environment without pressuring your toddler to eat in a particular way. Remember, neophobia (reluctance to try new foods) is common and normal at this age. Expose your child to a wide variety of foods, but don't force him to eat and you should avoid offering sweets as an incentive to eat other foods. It's also important to avoid unintentionally rewarding "bad" behaviors. For example, if you're in the grocery store and your child wants candy or some other item, think carefully before you say "No." Once you do say "No," you can't give in— no matter what. Even if your child has an extraordinarily embarrassing temper tantrum, if you give in and buy the desired item, he learns that he just has to escalate enough to get his way. Next time, he'll throw an even bigger tantrum because he's learned that if he's loud and embarrassing enough, he'll get what he wants. Ignoring bad behaviors helps to extinguish them, while sticker charts and a lot of positive attention go a long way in reinforcing good behaviors.

## Preschooler (3–5 years)

Preschool-aged children are highly motivated by rewards. While it's true that overuse of rewards will undermine a child's intrinsic motivation to engage in certain activities, you may often find yourself using a reward system to teach your child appropriate behaviors and to shape his actions so as to make him more pleasant to be around and to make your life function more smoothly. The strategies discussed earlier, such as praise, sticker charts, and positive practice, will help you achieve your goal. Of course, try to avoid using any food items as rewards.

At this age, your child is also learning to associate "good times" with food. From cupcakes to celebrate birthdays at school to further involvement in social activities focused on foods to picking up on the emotional eating that older kids and adults engage in, your child is unconsciously learning to rely on food as a "reward." In fact, it's at age three that children lose their ability to rely on hunger to guide their intake; instead, like the rest of us, they eat (despite not being hungry) when they're sad, tired, bored, or stressed. Chapter 3 discusses how we can help our children use hunger to guide their food intake rather than their emotions.

## School Age (5–10 years)

School-aged children already have a pretty good idea of which foods they like and which foods they don't like, but they also tend to be less neophobic than younger kids. While coercing them to eat their vegetables in exchange for some desirable reward might help to get the veggies down in the short term, it will simply reinforce their dislike in the long term. A better strategy to help shape positive eating behaviors in this age group is to pair information with enjoyable activities. For example, a child may have learned some nutrition lessons at school that taught him about the benefits of healthy foods. Ask him about what he's learning and then try to create such experiences as visiting a farmers' market, planting a garden, or participating in a cultural event to reinforce his learning. Creating rewarding experiences and sharing a little bit about the "why" of healthy eating will help to inspire healthier behaviors, but also remember that it took years for some of the less healthy behaviors to develop; they aren't going to disappear overnight.

Your positive attention, token reward systems, and cash rewards are alternatives to using food incentives to successfully shape behaviors at this age, but also remember that these strategies will dampen a child's intrinsic motivation to do a particular task. While it sometimes doesn't matter (after all, who expects a 10-year-old to be intrinsically motivated to clean the bathroom?), in those cases when it might, remember that information is influential at this age. Instead of answering requests with "Because I said so," try giving your child a compelling explanation. You might find that in some situations, that's all it takes for compliance with your request.

# Chapter Summary

Hopefully, you now feel equipped with strategies you can use to shape healthy behaviors in your children instead of using food as a reward to get children to eat. Let's recap with ways to turn this information into action:

- Vow to never again say "Eat your vegetables or no dessert!" Offering sweets as a reward for eating vegetables increases liking of the sweets and decreases liking of the vegetables.
- Increase your child's healthy food intake without pressuring by using such strategies as including a healthy food he likes and finishing off the meal with a fun nonfood activity; practicing authoritative parenting and the "division of responsibility"; and acknowledging but not making a big deal out of it when your child makes healthy choices.
- Minimize the impact of rewards on a child's intrinsic motivation by making rewards informational in nature rather than coercive.
- Resist the temptation to use food to comfort (e.g., offering ice cream or candy to a child who scraped his knee).
- In an effort to counter all the positive emotions your child will develop with less healthy foods (cake at birthday parties, candy at Halloween, baked goods as holiday gifts), create positive emotional experiences with healthy foods (such as a farmers' market trip, a family garden, etc.) and nonfoods (such as a visit to a bookstore or a museum).
- Decrease how often you offer dessert to once or twice per week or less.
- When a reward is in order, offer nonfood rewards for a job well done.

- Remember that positive attention goes a long way in reinforcing behaviors. Try to create mealtime harmony by praising good behaviors (helping to make dinner, setting the table, etc.) and ignoring less desirable eating behaviors (such as leaving all the vegetables).
- Use the principles of operant conditioning (positive and negative reinforcement, positive and negative punishment) to shape behaviors, but remember that these strategies may dampen intrinsic motivation.
- Tailor your strategies to your child's age and developmental stage.

# Recipes: Sweet but (Relatively) Healthy Recipes for Special Occasions

## Peanut Butter and Honey Crispy Treats

1/2 cup of peanut butter
1/2 cup of honey
1 cup of fiber cereal
2 tablespoons of butter

Mix peanut butter, honey, and butter in a microwaveable bowl. Microwave for 45 seconds or until peanut butter is melted. Mix in cereal. Pour mixture and press into a 9x13 pan. Let rest for 20 minutes and then cut into squares.

## Go Green Smoothie

1 banana
2 cups of baby spinach (washed and dried)
1 cup frozen peaches
1 cup frozen pineapples
2 tablespoons of honey
1 cup of orange juice

Blend all ingredients until well blended and smooth. Divide into 4 glasses and serve.

## Oatmeal Banana Cookies

1 ripe banana
1 cup of rolled oats
1/3 cup of flaxseed meal
2 tablespoons of olive oil
2 tablespoons of maple syrup
1/2 teaspoon of salt
2 teaspoons of vanilla extract
1/3 cup of chocolate chips
1/3 cup of dried cherries

Preheat oven to 350 degrees. Mash banana well with olive oil and vanilla extract. Mix in rolled oats, flaxseed meal, and salt with banana mixture until well combined. Add in 1/3 cup of chocolate chips and 1/3 cup of dried cherries. Drop spoonfuls of cookie dough on baking sheet. Bake for approximately 12 minutes.

Try different combinations, such as dried cranberries and white chocolate or diced dried apples and butterscotch chips.

## Frozen Chocolate Bananas

2 bananas
1/2 cup of chocolate chips
4 wooden skewers or popsicle sticks
1/4 cup chopped nuts (optional)

Peel the bananas. Cut bananas in half. Insert the skewer through the banana. Melt chocolate chips in the microwave and stir until smooth. Dip bananas in chocolate and place on baking sheet lined with foil. Sprinkle bananas with nuts—if desired. Place in freezer at least one hour before serving.

## Quick Graham Cracker Apple Crisp

2 apples (any variety)
1/4 cup of brown sugar
1 tablespoon of cinnamon
1 teaspoon of nutmeg
1 tablespoon of lemon juice
6 graham crackers
1/4 cup of pecans, chopped
2 tablespoons of butter, melted

Core and slice apples in half. Then, slice apple halves horizontally in half, resulting in 4 total pieces. Next, slice apples across into 1/4 inch chunks and place in a large mixing bowl. Add sugar, cinnamon, nutmeg, lemon juice, and half of the melted butter. Mix well and pour into a microwaveable dish.

For the topping, crush graham cracker into crumbs and pour into a bowl. Add pecans and butter to the bowl and stir. Sprinkle graham cracker/pecan topping onto apples and place dish in microwave. Microwave on high for 10 to 12 minutes. Serve with a dollop of low-fat vanilla yogurt.

## CarBaZu Muffins or Cupcakes

1 cup oats
2/3 cup whole wheat flour
1/3 cup all-purpose flour
2 small carrots, peeled and grated

1 small zucchini, grated

1 ripe banana, mashed

2/3 cup buttermilk or plain yogurt

2 eggs

1/3 cup brown sugar

2 tablespoons of unsalted butter, melted and cooled

1 teaspoon baking powder

1 teaspoon baking soda

1/2 teaspoon of salt

2 teaspoons ground cinnamon

1/2 teaspoon ground nutmeg

Preheat oven to 375 degrees. Break eggs into a medium mixing bowl and lightly beat eggs. Add yogurt or buttermilk to eggs and stir. Add cooled butter to wet ingredients and then brown sugar and stir. Squeeze excess water out of grated zucchini. Mix in grated carrots, zucchini, and mashed bananas and then stir.

For the dry ingredients, place oats in a blender and blend until a fine powder. Pour oat flour into a mixing bowl and add the whole wheat and all-purpose flour. Mix in the baking soda, baking powder, and salt. Stir in the cinnamon and nutmeg to the flour mixture.

Pour half of the flour mixture into the wet ingredients and gently stir. Add the remainder of the flour mixture and mix gently until well incorporated. Pour batter into lined muffin tins approximately 2/3 full from the top. Bake for approximately 20 minutes.

Makes approximately 16 muffins.

*Tip:* Transform the muffin into a cupcake with a dollop of honey cream cheese frosting.

*Honey Cream Cheese Frosting*

1 8-ounce package of light cream cheese, room temperature

1/4 cup honey

1 tablespoon of cinnamon

Mix all ingredients together using an electric mixer. Serve on top of muffins to make a cupcake.

## References

1.  Birch, L.L., S.I. Zimmerman, and H. Hind. (1980). The influence of social-affective context on the formation of children's food preferences. *Child Dev. 51*: p. 856-61.
2.  Birch, L.L., D. Birch, D.W. Marlin, and L. Kramer. Effects of instrumental consumption on children's food preference. (1982) *Appetite. 3*(2): p. 125-34.
3.  Birch, L.L., D.W. Marlin, and J. Rotter. (1984). Eating as the "means" activity in a contingency: Effects on young children's food preferences. *Child Development.* 1984;55:431-9.

4.  Carper, J.L., J. Orlet Fisher, and L.L. Birch. (2000). Young girls' emerging dietary restraint and disinhibition are related to parental control in child feeding. *Appetite.* 35(2): p. 121-9.

5.  Blissett, J., E. Haycraft, and C. Farrow. (2010). Inducing preschool children's emotional eating: Relations with parental feeding practices. *Am J Clin Nutr. 92*(2): p. 359-65.

6.  Deci, E.L., R. Koestner, and R.M. Ryan. (1999). A meta-analytic review of experiments examining the effects of extrinsic rewards on intrinsic motivation. *Psychol Bull. 125*(6): p. 627-68; discussion p. 692-700.

7.  Larsen, M.A., and E. Tentis. (2003). The art and science of disciplining children. *Pediatric Clinics of North America. 50*: p. 817-40.

8.  Hetherington, E.M., R.D. Parke, M. Gauvain, and V.O. Locke. (2006). *Child Psychology: A Contemporary Viewpoint* (6th ed.). New York: McGraw Hill.

# 3

# Mistake #3—Requiring Membership in the "Clean Plate Club"

*"I will always remember my mom cooked this
cabbage casserole concoction for dinner, which
was disgusting. My dad insisted that I eat it—and
eat it all. When I refused, my dad calmly placed
the plate in the refrigerator and forced me
to eat it for breakfast the next day before I
could have any real food. It was traumatizing."*
—Steve, 26

To understand the origins of parental insistence on eating everything on our dinner plates even if we don't care so much for the food or if we're already full, we need to take a step back in American history.

In the early 1900s, as World War I escalated and food shortages threatened the health of American troops and European civilians, family mealtimes across the United States underwent a massive overhaul. In 1917, Herbert Hoover, then head of the now-defunct Food Administration, called on all households to demonstrate their patriotism by dramatically decreasing food consumption and eliminating food waste. Citizens were encouraged to grow "victory gardens" in their backyards and participate in "meatless Tuesdays" and "sweetless Saturdays." Posters plastered across towns read "Food Will Win the War. Don't Waste It." Schoolchildren showed their patriotism by signing the pledge: "At table I'll not leave a scrap of food upon my plate. And I'll not eat between meals, but for supper time I'll wait." The "Clean Plate Club" was born.

Then, during the Great Depression and World War II, Americans once again were tasked with the job of demonstrating their patriotism and commitment to the troops and fellow citizens by conserving food. Consider this excerpt from *Time* magazine, published on Monday, May 11, 1942:

*"World War I moppets rallied to the defense of freedom by planting Victory Gardens and licking their platters clean. This year the Jack Spratlike platter came back. In Glencoe, Ill., Margot, 5, and John Chinnock, 7, with their father, formed the Clean Plate Club, pledged themselves always to "finish all the food on my plate and drink all of my milk. ..." Penalty for failure: "I will turn in my button." Club records last week showed only one recalcitrant among 200 members: five-year-old Betsy Brown, who refused to drink her milk. Betsy was dropped for several days, is now a member in good standing."*[1]

## Why the "Clean Plate Club" Needs Disbanding

Who would have thought that a wartime movement initiated almost 100 years ago would so profoundly affect the eating habits of children for generations? Although times have changed, many parent feeding practices haven't. Instead of telling our kids to clean their plate as a patriotic duty in time of war, we paint heart-wrenching images of starving children. Although we should certainly teach our children to be thankful for the food they eat and all of us need to work harder to minimize our food waste, we should also recognize that putting the calories in a child's stomach versus the garbage can doesn't affect the nutritional status of anyone other than the kid who's forced to eat too much.

When we make our children "clean their plates," we teach them to use external cues (such as how much food is left on the plate) rather than internal cues (such as how hungry they feel) to determine how much to eat. This overrides their ability to let hunger be their guide in controlling food intake. The Clean Plate Club, founded in a patriotic effort to conserve food in an era of food scarcity, has contributed to an epidemic of obesity in a time when cheap, heavily processed, high-calorie, and low-nutrient foods are abundant. If we want to help our children develop lifelong healthy eating habits, we must disband the Clean Plate Club once and for all.

## Clean Plate Club Risks of Membership

Many risks exist when pressuring children to eat against their will. Many of the risks, such as decreased liking for the food they're forced to eat and mealtime food battles, are detailed elsewhere in this book. But perhaps the most alarming consequence of this parental feeding strategy is the dysregulation of a child's internal ability to use hunger to guide caloric intake. For some children, this will result in obesity—either during childhood or later in adulthood. For others, it will contribute to emotional eating. For everyone, it makes maintaining a healthy weight with a balanced diet and a healthy relationship with food nearly impossible.

If left to their own devices—free of adult influence and outside pressures— and with access only to a wide variety of healthy foods, children seem to consume a calorically balanced, varied, and healthy diet.[2] Similarly, if a child is taught to rely on his internal feelings of hunger and fullness, he does a pretty good job regulating caloric intake. However, a child's innate ability to choose wisely is quickly eroded in an environment filled with highly palatable, low-nutrient-dense foods and external pressures and triggers to eat. For example, in one study, preschoolers who were taught to rely on internal hunger cues to guide their intake consumed less of an enticing snack of cookies and granola bars after being given a yogurt snack than preschoolers taught to snack at the ring of a bell and who were rewarded for "cleaning their plates." It didn't matter how full the kids were—the ones taught to eat by external cues ate the whole extra snack.[3] A follow-up study in a more natural environment (not many of us eat at the ring of a bell much these days) found that kids who were taught to rely on feelings of hunger and satiety were very good at regulating their intake based on the caloric density of the foods. Those kids encouraged to eat in response to external cues (such as the time of day), the amount of food remaining on their plates, and in order to obtain a reward were not.[4]

Parents are charged with the difficult task of ensuring that their young children—who, by the way, tend to be neophobic, picky, opinionated, and stubborn—consume a diet that will promote optimal health, growth, and development. Concerned that their kids may not be getting enough of the right nutrients, parents use various feeding strategies to encourage their kids to eat. A popular strategy is to provide a child with a relatively balanced mix of foods and to require children to eat all the food on their plates. That way, the parent can be sure that the child is getting enough of the right foods. But parents often overestimate the amount of food that a child needs, and a child can become full long before his plate is clean. It often goes something like this: The parent gives the child a plate of food containing more calories than the child actually needs. The child doesn't eat all the food on his plate. The parent insists. The child refuses. The parent more forcefully insists or employs contingencies and bribes. The child gives in and eats the food.

Consider this real-life example from Bridget, mother of two-year-old Maeve, who still vividly recalls the experience that happened well over two decades ago:

> *"I remember being a child at a babysitter's, and the babysitter was forcing me to finish my meal. I kept telling her I was not hungry anymore, but I still had a lot of food left on my plate. She told me I could not leave the dinner table until I had finished my meal. I finished my meal, and not two minutes later, I threw it all up. I honestly was not hungry anymore and was so full I couldn't hold it in my stomach."*

These type of scenarios, which have been documented in observational studies, suggest that parental demands to eat may serve to override a child's own attempts to use internal signals to control the amount of consumption.[5] If forced to override his feeling of fullness and to continue to eat, not only does he get more calories than his body needs, setting him up for excess weight gain, but with time, he also loses the ability to use feelings of hunger and fullness to control food intake.

# If Only We Could Let Hunger Be Our Guide

The human body is well equipped to tell us when our body needs food for energy and sustenance (hunger) and when we've had enough (satiety). On a simplest level, a grumbling stomach lets us know it's time to eat, but the physiology of hunger and satiety is intricate and complex. The brain is in constant communication with the gastrointestinal system and the body's fat stores to regulate food intake. The two main gut hormones that get the messages of hunger and satiety across are *ghrelin*, also known as the "hunger hormone," and *peptide YY*. When the body is low on energy, the stomach releases ghrelin to signal that it's time to eat. After a meal, ghrelin levels decrease and peptide YY, an appetite suppressant released by the small intestine, increases. The increase in blood sugar that results after a meal triggers the pancreas to secrete insulin, which, among other functions, suppresses appetite. Through this system, the body tries very hard to maintain a healthy weight. But when the system gets overridden, havoc can ensue. A person who ignores the signals of hunger and satiety and continues to eat is bound to gain weight and fat stores. The chronically elevated insulin levels stimulate increased fat storage. This extra fat is metabolically active and also influences intake. When energy stored in fat is depleted, the level of a hormone called *leptin* decreases. The decrease in leptin signals to the brain to eat more (see Figure 3-1). Putting on extra weight in childhood is particularly risky because the fat cells that are accumulated can never be lost. Their size may shrink, but the total number can only increase and never decrease over a lifetime. This makes it even more difficult for an overweight child to lose the weight and keep it off as an adult and is one more reason why preventing obesity in the first place is so important. One way parents can help to do this is by helping a child to retain the innate but easily overridden ability to let hunger guide food intake.

Some research studies suggest that kids as young as preschool can be taught to better trust their bodies. In one experiment, researchers taught preschoolers to pay attention to their own feelings of hunger and fullness by using a doll with a clear glass stomach. The adult showed the children the doll's stomach and then asked them to point to their own stomachs and say if they felt hungry or full. Next, they talked about what it feels like to be hungry and to be full. Then, the children fed the doll a small number of dried beans to show how the stomach fills up with eating and how feelings of hunger would start to change. Afterward, the children were fed a snack and told to eat only until they felt full and then to stop eating. These children were able to regulate their intake based on the amount of calories contained in the food.[4] Another study that elaborated on this methodology also found that children can be taught to rely on their body's signals of hunger and fullness to guide intake.[6]

Parents have the responsibility to provide their children with the food and nutrients a child's body needs to grow and develop optimally. The immediate and salient instinct is to accomplish this task through exertion of power. But if we step back and take a more relaxed approach—focused on empowering a child to make good decisions when we're not looking—we can help our kids

*Leptin*: Produced in the adipose tissue. Acts on the appetite centers in the brain. When body fat levels are high, leptin levels are high and appetite is suppressed. When body fat levels decrease, leptin levels fall and appetite increases.

*PYY:* Released by the small intestines. Acts on the appetite centers in the brain. After meals, PYY levels increase and appetite decreases.

*Ghrelin:* Secreted by the stomach. Acts on the appetite centers in the brain. As mealtimes approach, ghrelin levels increase, triggering feelings of hunger. People who lose weight have high ghrelin levels, which may be one reason why maintaining weight loss is so difficult.

*Insulin:* Secreted by the pancreas. Acts on the brain to suppress appetite, among many other functions, including facilitating the transfer of blood glucose to cells and stimulating fat deposition.

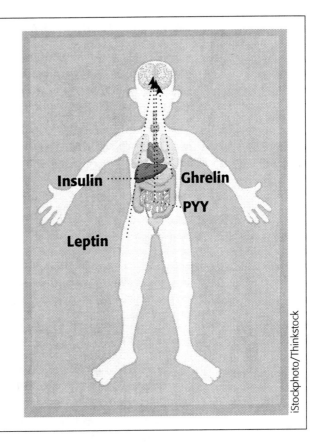

Figure 3-1. Hormonal control of appetite

learn to not only choose healthy foods but to also listen to their bodies when deciding when and how much to eat. With all the environmental and social factors that influence eating, parents have the special opportunity to help their children engage in social cultures and practices without losing this invaluable ability to control intake with hunger. After all, if we all followed this, we wouldn't have to experience feeling guilty after having a decadent dessert or overstuffing ourselves at a dinner party. If we would only eat when we're hungry and stop when we're full, we would eat just the right amount of calories to maintain a healthy weight. But we don't do this—and so many of us can't do this—because we have for so many years ignored our body's signals. Now as adults, we have many struggles with food, weight, and emotional eating. We can best serve our children by helping them avoid this predicament. We'll do more to ensure their optimal growth and development by empowering them to listen to their body's signals, even if that means not eating all their dinner rather than forcing them to eat what we consider an optimal diet.

## Counterstrategies

The good news is that with the application of a few simple strategies, we can permanently ban the Clean Plate Club and help kids use hunger to guide intake.

## Reestablish Internal Cues for Eating

A lot of individual variation occurs in how well children can self-regulate intake. Based on a few research studies, it seems that boys are much better at it than girls. And children whose parents exert the most control over what, when, and how much children eat are worse off. This is especially the case for girls whose mothers are highly restrictive and forbid "junk food." Studies have shown that when the girls have access to those foods in an unrestricted setting, they eat the most—even when they aren't hungry. And mothers who have a high degree of dietary disinhibition—or "out of control" eating—have daughters with dietary disinhibition.[7] This and what to do about it are detailed in Chapter 4, but it's important to mention here that ditching the diet mentality is an essential first step in helping our kids—girls *and* boys—to reestablish internal cues for eating. That doesn't mean loading up the house with an unlimited supply of junk food. It simply means "allowing" all foods in moderation, even though you may choose not to have the less desirable items readily available in your house. It also means making the whole pursuit of healthy eating a family affair in which the adults commit to modeling healthy eating and activity habits for their children.

Strategies to reestablish internal cues for eating should be tailored to a child's age and developmental stage in order to have the greatest impact. Several suggestions for each age group are included in the "Developmental Considerations" section of this chapter. However, you can also make changes in general to help make eating when you're hungry and stopping when you're full the household norm. First, make an effort to track for one day food intake of the whole family. You don't need to be overly detailed or analytic. The idea is to get a gist of how everyone is eating, when, and why. (See the sidebar "How to Keep a Food Log" for a step-by-step guide on how to keep a food log.) Then, identify and eliminate triggers in your physical environment that encourage family members to eat when they aren't hungry. Maybe it's filled candy dishes in the living room and cookie jars in the kitchen. Or perhaps you've always got a juice box or regular soda cold in the refrigerator. Whenever possible, try to plan out each week's meals ahead of time and make a list of needed ingredients. Then, when you go grocery shopping (ideally, right after eating so you have a full stomach), try to limit your purchases to foods on the list and avoid ready-to-eat highly processed foods. Next, identify where in the house will be the "eating" room (typically, this should be a dining room and not in front of the TV or kitchen sink). Encourage family members to do the majority of their eating in that location. Finally, make some systematic changes, such as using smaller dishes, discarding leftovers, removing food from inappropriate storage areas in the house, and storing food out of sight. Plan your approach to holidays and social gatherings ahead of time. For example, teach your kids polite ways to decline food, decide how much dessert you plan to eat, and graciously decline offers to bring home leftovers.

## Portion Control

People need strategies to help manage caloric intake because otherwise, if the food is there, we eat it. It doesn't matter if we're already full or don't really like the food all that much or are consciously trying to restrain ourselves. This unfortunate reality holds true for children and adults alike. In one study, for example, when age-appropriate portions of an entrée were doubled in size, preschoolers increased their intake by 25 to 29 percent. It's not that the kids were still hungry—when given the standard age-appropriate portion, they only ate about two-thirds of it. The kids didn't decrease their intake of other foods to compensate for their increased consumption of the main course. As a result, their overall caloric intake increased 9 to 15 percent.[8] Over time, this can lead to significant unnecessary weight gain.

A big part of the problem is that over the past 20 years, standard portions offered in restaurants and grocery stores have morphed our perspective of how much food is a normal amount. You may recall that this inspired the documentary *Super Size Me*, after which McDonald's and other fast-food restaurant chains eliminated "supersized" meals (though most places still have combos that, based on calories, saturated fat, and sodium, might still be considered "supersized," even if they aren't named that anymore). Overall, portion sizes continue to be out of control. Figure 3-2 includes a few examples prepared by the National Heart Lung and Blood Institute.

To help kids maintain a healthy weight, parents have got to decrease portion sizes. One way to start is to recognize that we're pretty bad at "guesstimating" how much our kids need. Most parents overestimate when doling out serving sizes to their kids. It doesn't help that if after we've given them too much, we then require them to clean their plates. Whenever possible, kids should be encouraged to choose their own portion sizes. Research supports that when given this opportunity, they do a pretty good job of estimating the right amount.[9] If they aren't old enough or you don't quite trust them to do this, then make sure you offer them an age-appropriate amount. A general rule of thumb is that an appropriate serving size is about a tablespoon of food for every year in age. Then, if your child wants more, he'll let you know and should be allowed seconds. One exception exists to this valiant effort to control portion size. You can use the human tendency to eat more when more is put on our plate to your advantage when it comes to serving up foods you want your kids to eat,

| | 20 Years Ago | | Today | |
|---|---|---|---|---|
| | *Portion* | *Calories* | *Portion* | *Calories* |
| **Bagel** | 3-inch diameter | 140 | 6-inch diameter | 350 |
| **Cheeseburger** | 1 | 333 | 1 | 590 |
| **Spaghetti with meatballs** | 1 cup sauce 3 small meatballs | 500 | 2 cups sauce 3 large meatballs | 1020 |
| **Soda** | 6.5 ounces | 82 | 20 ounces | 250 |
| **Blueberry muffin** | 1.5 ounces | 210 | 5 ounces | 500 |
| *Reference*: National Heart, Lung, and Blood Institute (http://hp2010.nhlbihin.net/portion/index.htm) | | | | |

Figure 3-2. Portion distortion

## How to Keep a Food Log

For anyone on a mission to eat better, having a good idea of what your baseline eating habits include is essential. You can simply and effectively figure this out by keeping a food log. By following these five simple steps, you and your kids will have a much better idea of how your eating habits measure up and where you have some room for improvement. To the best of your ability, try to go through this process with each family member. The steps outline what "you" should do for yourself, but you can also follow a similar process for your other family members.

### Step #1: Prepare

The purpose of a food log is threefold: record what you eat and drink and some of the factors that influence when and what you decide to eat; assess the quality of your diet; and evaluate how your diet compares with the recommendations. The first step to keeping a good log is planning ahead as to how you're best going to achieve this purpose. Start by choosing a recording system. Thedailyplate.com or MyPlate SuperTracker (choosemyplate.gov) are two useful websites to help you get started. (You can also access many other equally good websites with a quick Internet search.) In addition to writing down *what* you eat, it's also important to record what *time* of day, *where* you were while eating, what kind of *mood* you were in, and *how hungry* you were on a scale of 1 (ravenous) to 10 (completely full to the point of discomfort). This additional information will help you identify patterns of non-hunger-related eating and other opportunities to cut calories. Finally, have the Dietary Guidelines or MyPlate guidelines (discussed in the Introduction, with more individualized details at choosemyplate.gov) on hand so you can compare your diet to the recommendations.

### Step #2: Record Intake

The best way to get a good idea of your usual intake is to commit to recording everything you eat or drink for two "typical" weekdays and a weekend day. A "typical" day is one that's as close as possible to your usual routine. From the moment you wake up to the moment you go to sleep, commit to recording everything you eat—down to the cups and ounces if possible. Yes, this is an extremely tedious process, and you'll likely find yourself choosing not to eat a snack or that extra serving during a meal just so you don't have to write it down. It's also difficult to do for your preschool and school-aged kids, who spend a good part of the day at school. But just do the best you can. The more detailed and specific, the more useful your food log will be. For example, if you eat a bowl of cereal with milk and a banana for breakfast, actually measure out the amount of cereal and milk you use. Is the banana small, medium, or large? What kind of cereal? Did you add any sugar? How much? When you input your food intake into a database, such as dailyplate.com, you'll find that the program will have nutrition information for a lot of foods but not everything. For best results for your food log, try to approximate your intake to a food available on the database as best you can. Recognize that no matter how diligent you are, the analysis isn't going to be 100 percent accurate. That's okay. Your goal is to try to get as close of an idea to your usual eating habits as possible, realizing that some fluctuation from day to day and from the inherent error of using a food log is inevitable.

## Step #3: Assess the Quality of Your Diet

Once you input your three days of food intake into an online database, you'll get a summary of your eating habits, including calories, grams of fat, and other information, such as the number of servings from various food groups. Once you get the results from your analysis, you might suffer from information overload. Think about what parts of your diet are most important to you and pay special attention to those results. Also, review your log to see if you can identify patterns. For example, do you find yourself eating a large number of calories around 8 p.m. when your mood is "bored" and your hunger rating is "8" (not hungry)? Did you skip breakfast and then eat a 1,000-calorie lunch, whereas you might otherwise eat a 300-calorie breakfast and a 500-calorie lunch, thus saving about 200 calories (equivalent to running about two miles)?

## Step #4: Compare Your Intake to Your "Ideal Diet"

Now compare how your results stack up to the MyPlate guidelines and how your kids' measure up to the Dietary Guidelines recommendations for kids.

## Step #5: Set SMART Goals

Finally, you're set to use the information from your food log to set goals. Think about exactly what you'd like to achieve. Do you want to lose weight? Be healthier overall? Eat more fruits and vegetables? Eat fewer sweets? Now try to clearly articulate a SMART (specific, measurable, achievable, results-driven, and time-bound) goal. For example, your eight-year-old's goal to increase fruit and vegetable intake might be to eat at least three servings of fruits and vegetables per day, which he'll do by eating a fruit at breakfast and as a snack when he gets home from school and at least one vegetable at dinner every night for the next three weeks. Whatever the goals, write each family member's goal down and post it someplace you can see every day. Remember, the key here is to set goals you can and will achieve and then to celebrate once you've met them.

such as fruits and vegetables. The studies suggest this phenomenon holds true even for vegetables—if you give kids more, they'll eat more.[10] This, of course, is provided that the kids are actually willing to try the food in the first place. Your best bet is to give them large servings of the fruits and vegetables you know they'll eat. For those that you're less optimistic they'll even try, you're better off giving them a small amount initially. This will help to avoid too much food waste.

Eating meals together as a family gives you an opportunity to model healthy eating for your children and a chance to develop portion control skills. For example, you can help the whole family practice portion control at dinner if you use small plates, avoid serving food family style, and follow the MyPlate eating plan. That is, aim for half of the plate to be filled with vegetables and fruits, one-fourth whole grains, and one-fourth with a protein source, such as meat or fish. Also, aim for a calcium-rich food or beverage at each meal. Encourage your family to be mindful of the body's cues of hunger and fullness and to eat slowly. Let the kids get up for seconds if they're still hungry, but remember, it takes about 20 minutes to feel full. If you think they've already eaten a lot and may be eating more for reasons other than hunger, encourage them to wait 20 minutes before getting more.

And more importantly, enjoy the time together as a family. Socialize during your meals and festivities. You can't eat and talk at the same time—so the more conversation, the less you'll eat. This may seem wonderful in theory, but as a busy parent, you might feel overwhelmed by the idea of having to cook every night or having to coordinate everyone's schedules to eat together. While it's ideal to have a wholesome family meal together nightly, everyone knows that's near impossible. Chapter 7 describes ideas for how to simplify dinnertime and offers tips on how to get the health benefits of a family meal with limited time and scheduling challenges.

Without a plan, snacking can become a portion control nightmare. Too often, kids will get home from school, grab a bag of chips, and sit in front of the TV or computer and mindlessly eat until the bag is gone. Maybe they or you looked at the calorie content on the back of the bag first and figured it's not so bad (refer to Figure 3-3). But did you look and see what the "serving size" is on the nutrition label and how many "servings per container" the bag has? Even items that seem like they should be one serving may have a nutrition label showing the nutritional content for only a fraction of the food. For example, a 20-ounce soda has 2.5 servings. A three-ounce bag of chips contains three servings. You can make portion control easier by purchasing snack foods that are inherently portion controlled (that is, one serving per package), such as string cheese sticks, prepackaged one-ounce bags of mixed nuts, or a small box of raisins. Many packaged convenience foods, such as crackers and chips, also come in single-serving packages. Or you can do it yourself by portioning out multiserving snack foods into single-serving baggies or eating them only after putting them into a small snacking bowl. However you choose to do it, portion control is a very important tool in helping your children rely on cues of hunger and satiety to determine how much to eat rather than the amount of food that's sitting in front of them.

**Serving Size**
Is your serving the same size as the one on the label? If you eat double the serving size listed, you need to double the nutrient and calorie values.

**Calories**
Are you overweight? Cut back a little on calories!

**Total Carbohydrate**
Carbohydrates are in foods like bread, potatoes, fruits, and vegetables.

**Dietary Fiber**
Fruits, vegetables, whole-grain foods, beans, and peas are all good sources and can help reduce the risk of heart disease and cancer.

**Protein**
Most Americans get more than they need. Where there is animal protein, there is also fat and cholesterol.

**Vitamins and Minerals**
Your goal here is 100% of each for the day. Don't count on one food to do it all.

### Nutrition Facts

Serving Size ½ cup (114g)
Servings Per Container 4

**Amount Per Serving**

**Calories** 90 — Calories from Fat 30

% Daily Value*

| | |
|---|---|
| **Total Fat** 3g | 5% |
| Saturated Fat 0g | 0% |
| Trans Fat 0g | 0% |
| **Cholesterol** 0mg | 0% |
| **Sodium** 300mg | 13% |
| **Total Carbohydrate** 13g | 4% |
| Dietary Fiber 3g | 12% |
| Sugars 3g | |
| **Protein** 3g | |

| | | | |
|---|---|---|---|
| Vitamin A | 80% | Vitamin C | 60% |
| Calcium | 4% | Iron | 4% |

*Percent Daily Values are based on a 2,000 calorie diet. Your daily values may be higher or lower depending on your calorie needs:

| | | Calories | 2,000 | 2,500 |
|---|---|---|---|---|
| Total Fat | Less than | | 65g | 80g |
| Sat Fat | Less than | | 20g | 25g |
| Cholesterol | Less than | | 300mg | 300mg |
| Sodium | Less than | | 2,400mg | 2,400mg |
| Total Carbohydrate | | | 300g | 375g |
| Fiber | | | 25g | 30g |

Calories per gram:
Fat 9  •  Carbohydrate 4  •  Protein 4

*(More nutrients may be listed on some labels)*

mg = milligrams (1,000 mg = 1 g)
g = grams (about 28 g = 1 ounce)

**Total Fat**
Aim low: Most people need to cut back on fat! Too much fat may contribute to heart disease and cancer.

**Saturated Fat**
Saturated fat is listed separately because it is the key player in raising blood cholesterol and your risk of heart disease.

**Trans Fat**
Trans fat works a lot like saturated fat, except it is worse.

**Cholesterol**
Too much cholesterol—a second cousin to fat—can lead to heart disease.

**Sodium**
You call it "salt," the label calls it "sodium." Either way, it may add up to high blood pressure in some people.

**Daily Value**
Daily Values are listed for people who eat 2,000 or 2,500 calories each day. If you eat more, your personal daily value may be higher than what's listed on the label. If you eat less, your personal daily value may be lower.

Reprinted with permission from the American Council on Exercise. (2007). *ACE Lifestyle & Weight Management Consultant Manual: The Ultimate Resource for Fitness Professionals* (Second Edition). San Diego, CA: American Council on Exercise

Figure 3-3. Nutrition label

It's worth mentioning that you can also use a child's tendency toward "mindless eating" in a good way. One mother quietly placed a whole plate of julienned red pepper in front of her sons one day when they were playing the Wii™. When she checked on them a few minutes later, the plate was empty. This may be a not-so-sneaky way to sneak the low-calorie, high-nutrient-dense vegetables into a child's diet.

## Minimize Food Waste (Without Cleaning Your Plate)

The whole "clean your plate" mentality started with an admirable and socially responsible desire to reduce food waste. Luckily, you can have it both ways—that is, reduce food waste without overriding internal hunger and satiety cues. The following list offers a few tips:

• Eat at home more often so you have better control over portion sizes and can freeze any leftovers for another day when you don't have time to cook.

- Don't go to the grocery store on a whim. Instead, check what you already have in your refrigerator and pantry, and when shopping, ensure you have your shopping list in hand. This will help you avoid overbuying. Also, go to the store more frequently. You're less likely to accumulate rotting produce this way.

- It seems obvious, but only buy food that you're actually going to eat. And then actually eat it. If time gets away from you and you've got some rotting produce in the refrigerator, think of creative ways to use it—how about tomatoes to make a pasta sauce or ripe fruit for a smoothie? You can still eat those past-their-prime vegetables. Just remove the parts with blemishes.

- Check packages and perishable items for expiration dates and try to pick the latest one possible. (These are usually kept in the back of the shelf because the grocer is trying to unload the stuff that will go bad first by displaying it more prominently.) Generally, "use by" is a good indicator of when a food is going to go bad. The "sell by" or "best before" notations are for stock control and are best estimates of when the taste worsens.

- Teach your children the value of a food budget. Take them shopping with you and teach them to use price, actual need, nutritional value, and portion size to determine buying decisions.

- Donate your excess nonperishable food to your local food pantry.

Follow this advice and you're bound to not only save a lot of food that might otherwise be wasted, but you can also feel a lot less guilty when you have to throw out the small amount of food your child refused to eat.

# Developmental Considerations

The most effective way to get your child eating in response to cues of hunger and satiety is to adapt your approach to your child's developmental stage. Some background information and strategies are detailed here (and summarized in Figure 3-4).

### Infant (0–1 years)

Supporting your child's instinct to let hunger be his guide starts in infancy.

*Breastfed vs. Formula Fed*

Breastfed babies have a lower lifetime risk of obesity compared with formula-fed infants. In the excellent book *Eating Behaviors of the Young Child* (2008) edited by Leann Birch and William Dietz, researcher Kathryn Dewey describes the research evidence supporting several hypotheses to answer the question "Why?"[11] It seems to boil down to three potential mechanisms:

- *Learned self-regulation.* A breastfed baby gets to determine how much to eat, without anyone hovering over him measuring ounces and nudging him

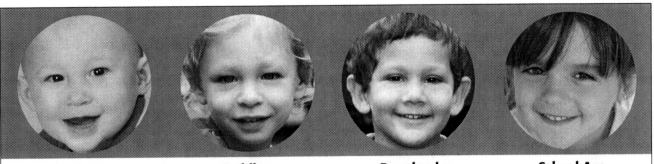

| Infant | Toddler | Preschooler | School Age |
|---|---|---|---|
| • Breastfeed if possible.<br>• Tune in to signs of hunger.<br>• Introduce solids at four to six months but still try to feed "on demand" (versus a schedule) in the first year. | • Regularly offer a variety of healthful options.<br>• Give your child a choice between healthy alternatives.<br>• Let your child feed himself as often as he'd like.<br>• Offer "neutral" prompts to eat, not coercive ones. | • Portion out snack amounts.<br>• Ask "Is your stomach full?" and "Are you hungry?" to help your child develop the ability to use internal cues to eat. | • Fill out a food log together.<br>• Encourage your child to slow down at mealtimes.<br>• Help your child be mindful while eating.<br>• Try to eat family dinners as often as possible. |

Figure 3-4. Developmental considerations

to eat more. Caretakers with a preset idea of how much the baby should eat or who don't want to waste formula or who believe that extra-full babies sleep better are especially prone to overriding the infant's internal hunger and satiety signals.

• *Metabolic programming.* Metabolic programming describes how foods consumed early in life affect a person's metabolism later in life. Some research suggests that formula-fed babies have persistently higher levels of insulin.[8] Higher insulin levels stimulate increased fat deposition and have been associated with increased weight gain and obesity. Formula-fed babies also tend to gain weight more rapidly in the early months. Rapid weight gain in infancy and higher infant fat mass are associated with a decreased sensitivity to leptin later in life, such that the body doesn't respond as well to the hormone. You'll recall that leptin is the hormone that's supposed to tell us to stop eating.

• *Parent feeding practices.* Some research suggests that mothers who breastfed for at least 12 months use less controlling feeding practices than those who didn't breastfeed or who breastfed for shorter periods of time. As we've described, more controlling parenting practices interfere with a child's ability to self-regulate intake.

Regardless of whether your infant is breastfed, try to use your baby's hunger cues rather than the amount of formula in the bottle or length of feeding to determine when he's hungry or full. This will allow him to self-regulate intake and also prevent him from gaining too much weight too fast. Try to adopt an authoritative parenting style in general. And look for formula that mimics breast milk as closely as possible.

*Signs of Hunger*

Whether you're breastfeeding or formula feeding, one of the most important skills you can acquire in feeding your young infant is to use your baby's signals of hunger (and not a specified amount of formula or a specific amount of time for the feeding) in determining when and how much to feed him. When given the chance, a healthy baby skillfully adjusts caloric intake to meet his nutritional needs. Some common signs of hunger include whimpering or smacking his lips, waking and looking alert, putting hands toward his mouth, making sucking motions, and becoming more active. If your baby becomes fussy with feeding, slows down sucking, falls asleep, or spits out or refuses the nipples, chances are good he's trying to tell you he's full.

*Introducing Solids*

Between four and six months, a child experiences his first tastes of solid food. Even though you're starting to give him food that more closely resembles what the rest of the family is eating—and family mealtimes no doubt are important for everyone—it's important to continue to feed your baby on demand during the first year of life. A baby still has an innate ability to listen to internal hunger and satiety cues to guide intake—if you let him. You can still create structure in your baby's life. At family mealtimes and snack times feed your baby however much solid food he would like. Then, at other times during the day when he indicates hunger, give him breast milk, formula, water, or no more than four ounces per day of juice.

## Toddler (1–3 years)

As your toddler develops into his own person with his own thoughts and ideas of how he would like to do things, you play a very important role in helping him develop healthy eating habits and also retain his ability to self-regulate intake. Resist the temptation to overly control mealtimes. The goal is to offer your child a variety of healthy food choices and let him determine what and how much of it he'll eat. Your child wants to exert independence and show you his competence. Let him feed himself as much as he would like. Sure, it's messier than if you do it, but it helps him develop his fine motor skills and a better sense of control over what and how much he eats. Let him decide how much or little he wants to eat. No bribes. No persuasion. Let your child use his internal cues of hunger and satiety to control his intake. Let him refuse food. If your toddler doesn't want to try a new food, let it be okay. Don't make a big deal out of it or force him to taste it. Neutral prompts such as "Don't forget to eat your applesauce" are more effective at encouraging intake (if he's still hungry) than coercive ones such as "I told you to eat the applesauce." On occasion, strategies like "airplane" (where you pretend that the food is an airplane flying into his mouth) may help a hungry toddler to try a new food. If you use this strategy, use it for all kinds of new foods and not just "healthy" ones that he's likely to reject initially. Avoid it as a way to get a full child to ignore his feeling of fullness and instead eat more food.

## Preschooler (3–5 years)

The preschool years are the critical time when, for most kids, the ability to use innate cues to regulate food intake begins to fade and becomes overpowered by external forces. This unfortunate but not inevitable phenomenon is demonstrated in a simple experiment by Penn State nutrition researcher Barbara Rolls. Children three-and-a-half and five years old were given a heaping serving of macaroni and cheese versus a standard portion. The younger kids ate the same amount regardless of how much food was presented to them. But for the five-year-olds, the bigger the portion, the more they ate.[12]

The good news is that you can "retrain their brains." Help your child (and the rest of the family) practice mindful eating so hunger and satiety guide food intake. Talk to your child about the sensations of hunger and feeling full (Figure 3-5). Teach your child to ask himself before eating "Am I hungry?" Before getting seconds, he should ask himself "Am I full?" Strategies to make mindful eating easier include:

- *Eat family meals.* It takes about 20 minutes to feel full. The time spent socializing allows your child the opportunity to feel full rather than mindlessly eating in front of the television. Family meals also tend to be healthier and provide an opportunity for parents to model healthy eating.

- *Encourage portion control.* For example, make it the norm to portion out snacks (versus sitting in front of the TV with the whole bag) and let your child dole out his own portions at mealtimes.

- *Encourage physical activity.* Not only will your child be out there burning off energy and having fun, but it also means he's not inside eating.

- *Set a good example.* When you're bored, angry, tired, or stressed, turn to such alternatives as a quick walk, music, a bath, or a phone call with a friend rather than food.

- *Get rid of the "clean plate" mentality.* If your child refuses to eat, ask him "Is your stomach full?" or "Are you still hungry?" This will help him connect feelings of hunger and satiety with his decisions to eat or not.

| 0 | Starving to the point of feeling sick |
|---|---|
| 1 | Ravenous and feeling dizzy and weak |
| 2 | Really hungry, irritable, and distracted |
| 3 | Hungry with a grumbling stomach |
| 4 | Getting hungry and thinking of food |
| 5 | Comfortable and not hungry |
| 6 | Satisfied |
| 7 | Full and slightly uncomfortable |
| 8 | Overfull and feeling a little bloated |
| 9 | Stuffed and very uncomfortable |
| 10 | Sick and miserable and extremely uncomfortable |

Figure 3-5. The hunger scale

### School Age (5–10 years)

As your child ventures off into elementary school, the parental influence and control over eating choices lessen. Peers and the school environment play a more salient role in his life. If he's a typical school-aged child, his eating habits are fairly well established and he may not do that great of a job regulating caloric intake based on hunger and satiety. This occurs at a time when dietary restraint and disordered eating habits first present.

Many of the strategies for preschoolers can be adapted to help school-aged children listen to their internal cues of hunger and satiety to guide intake. They should be encouraged to consume a balanced diet that *can* include, on occasion, calorie-dense and nutrient-poor foods (but don't make a big deal out of it when they eat these foods). Teaching portion control is very important. Children at this age are also receptive to teaching and responsive to behavior modification strategies to help them better listen to their bodies. For example, overweight school-aged children tend to eat faster and take bigger bites. After an intervention that included education, modeling, and practice, obese kids learned to chew more thoroughly and set food down between bites.[13] The following behavioral modification strategies are useful not only for school-aged kids but also adolescents and adults:

- *Monitor intake.* Get online together and fill out the dietary record at choosemyplate.gov. For older kids, both of you could put in what you've eaten for a 24-hour period to see whose diet stacks up better next to the MyPlate recommendations. Not only does this give you a chance to spend some quality time together, but the information your child gets from an unbiased source might inspire him to eat a little bit better. And by putting your own dietary habits on the line, you're opening up an opportunity for you and your child to set goals together so you can optimize your eating habits.
- *Slow down.* Specifically, take one small bite at a time. Put the fork down between mouthfuls. Chew thoroughly before swallowing.
- *Leave some food on the plate.* Yes, this is the anti–clean plate strategy.
- *Control snacks.* Keep low-calorie snacks, such as baby carrots, apple slices, and yogurt, on hand for snacking. Slow down to eat the snacks. That is, set them on a plate and sit down.
- *Be mindful while eating.* In other words, don't do anything else, such as reading, homework, watching television, texting, or surfing the Internet, while eating.

The sidebar "Counterstrategies in Action: Disbanding the 'Clean Plate Club'" highlights how families can let hunger be their guide.

# Chapter Summary

Ultimately, you can do a lot to help your children adopt healthy eating habits by ditching the "clean plate" mentality and instead focusing on listening to one's body to guide intake. The following summarizes ways to help transfer this chapter's recommendations into reality:

---

## Counterstrategies in Action:
## Disbanding the "Clean Plate Club"

### Reestablish Internal Cues of Hunger and Satiety

At mealtimes, Jessica and Matt make an extra effort to help their kids—six-year-old Alexis, four-year-old Sophie, two-year-old Ben—use their feelings of hunger and fullness to guide how much they eat. The parents are careful not to comment on how much the kids eat or whether they leave food on their plates. If the kids ask Jessica or Matt how much they need to eat, the parents always reply "You're the only one who knows the answer to that. You should eat until your tummy is happy."

### Control Portion Sizes

Gail, mother of now-grown kids, used a six-muffin tin to help with portion control. On hot days, she would fill the tins with a mix of fruits and vegetables. For example, one cup had a handful of frozen peas, another had frozen corn, another had frozen blueberries, and so on, to fill the six tins. When the kids were hot and hungry, they would grab a handful and go back to playing. To promote portion control, you could vary this idea with other snacks, such as Cheerios®, crackers, nuts, and dried fruit.

### Minimize Food Waste

To minimize food waste and promote adherence to the government's MyPlate recommendations that half of eaten foods are fruits and vegetables, Susanna, mother of seven-year-old Daisy and nine-year-old Max, decided to give the refrigerator a makeover. Instead of stuffing the fruits and vegetables in the bottom drawer of the refrigerator, where they tended to rot and mold, she prominently displayed them on the top shelf of the refrigerator—in perfect view every time anyone opened the refrigerator. Not only did her kids eat more fruits and vegetables, but she cut the amount of wasted food in half.

- Don't require your children to eat everything on their plates during mealtimes.
- Don't pressure children who say they're not hungry to eat by using clever strategies, such as "stealing" their food, cooing how "yummy" the food is, or playing "airplane" or various other games. (Although these strategies may be useful at times to help a child *try* a new food, they're counterproductive when trying to get a child to keep eating.)
- Teach your kids to rely on internal cues of hunger and satiety to guide their intake.
- Make the pursuit of healthy eating a *family* affair. Try to eat meals together as often as possible and make sure everyone is on board to improve their eating habits.

- Make it hard to overeat and hard to engage in emotional eating by eliminating triggers, planning ahead, and systematically changing the way you eat.
- Let children choose their own portion sizes whenever possible. If you're choosing their portions, make sure you give an age-appropriate amount.
- Read the nutrition label—especially look at "number of servings" and "serving size." Teach your children to do the same.
- Breastfeed your baby for as long as possible—ideally, at least to one year. If you formula feed, don't require consumption of a certain amount.
- Try to reduce food waste in ways other than "cleaning your plate."
- Try to use less controlling feeding practices in general.

# Recipes: Inherently Portion-Controlled Recipes

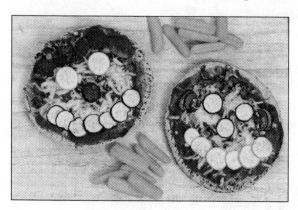

### Smiling Faces Whole Wheat Pita Pizzas

4 whole wheat pita breads
1 cup of tomato sauce
2 cups of assorted chopped vegetables (mushrooms, spinach, onions, peppers, broccoli)
1 cup of shredded mozzarella cheese

Preheat oven to 400 degrees. Place 1 to 2 tablespoons of tomato sauce on each pita bread and spread evenly. Top with vegetables and/or meat of your choice. (Encourage your kids to make a smiling face out of the toppings!) Sprinkle 2 tablespoons of cheese on top of vegetables. Place on baking sheet and bake for 10 to 15 minutes, until cheese is melted.

*Tip:* Make dessert pita pizzas! Slice 1/2 banana over pita bread and sprinkle with 1 teaspoon of cinnamon. Put in oven for 5 to 10 minutes. Remove from oven and drizzle 1 tablespoon of honey over pita.

### Frittata Muffins

4 eggs
1 cup of assorted vegetables, chopped into small pieces
Muffin tin and cupcake liners
1/4 cup of nonfat milk
2 teaspoons of salt
2 teaspoons of black pepper

Preheat oven to 375 degrees. Crack eggs into a medium-sized bowl and beat lightly. Add milk into eggs and stir. Add vegetables into bowl and stir gently. Sprinkle in salt and pepper.

Spray muffin tin with nonstick cooking spray. Line muffin tin with cupcake liners. Pour egg mixture into each muffin tin, until approximately three-fourths full. Bake in oven for approximately 15 minutes. Makes approximately 10 to 12 muffins.

*Tips*:

- For breakfast: Cut one muffin into slices and put in between 2 pieces of toast for a healthy breakfast sandwich.
- For lunch: Serve a frittata with a green salad for a balanced lunch.

## Chicken Chili Baked Potatoes

4 baking potatoes, washed
1 medium onion, chopped
2 celery ribs, chopped
2 carrots, peeled and chopped
1 green bell pepper, diced
2 cups of broccoli, cut into small florets
2 medium zucchinis, cut into 1/4-inch slices
4 links of chicken andouille sausage, chopped into 1/4 inch slices
1 can of kidney beans, drained
2 15-ounce cans of chopped tomatoes
2 cups of water

Cook potatoes: Scrub the outside of the potato well. Using a fork, poke the potato in a few places. For microwaves: Place each potato in the microwave, cook for 10 minutes, flip the potato onto its other side, then cook for an additional 10 minutes (or until a fork can easily pierce the potato). For oven: Preheat to 400 degrees. Place potatoes on baking pan and cook for 45 minutes or until a fork can easily pierce the potatoes.

To prepare the chili: Heat a large pot with 2 tablespoons of olive oil over medium heat. Place onions into oil and cook for approximately 5 minutes. Add celery, carrots, and bell pepper and cook until vegetables have softened. Next, add the chicken sausage and cook for 5 minutes. Add in the broccoli, zucchini, kidney beans, tomatoes, and water. Bring to boil and then turn heat down to low and let simmer for approximately 20 minutes.

For toppings: Cut zucchini lengthwise in half. Lay flat and then cut across into 1/2-inch pieces. Bring pot of water to boil over medium-high heat. Add broccoli and zucchini and cook for 1 minute. Drain water and place vegetables in bowl.

Remove potatoes from oven. Cut potatoes in half. Serve with broccoli/zucchini, chili, cheese, and salsa on top.

*Tip:* Like sour cream in your baked potato? Try nonfat or low-fat plain yogurt instead.

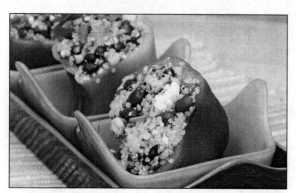

## Mexican Fiesta Stuffed Peppers

4 bell peppers (any color)
1 cup of crumbled feta
1 can of black beans, drained
1/4 cup of cilantro, chopped
1 cup of corn
2 cups of cooked quinoa
1 tablespoon of olive oil

Preheat oven to 375 degrees. Cut tops off of bell pepper and remove seeds from inside. Combine remainder of ingredients in a bowl and mix well. Divide quinoa mixture evenly and stuff into peppers. Place peppers in the oven in a proof pan and bake for 25 minutes. Serve with a side salad.

## Rosemary Apricot Pork Sliders With Apple Cabbage Slaw

1 pork tenderloin, cut into 1/2-inch round slices
8 mini burger buns or dinner rolls
1/4 cup of apricot preserves
2 teaspoons of Dijon mustard
2 tablespoons of fresh rosemary, chopped
Salt and pepper

*Apple Cabbage Slaw*

1 apple (any variety)
1/2 head of green or red cabbage
2 carrots, peeled and grated
2 stalks of green onions
1/2 cup of plain Greek yogurt
1 tablespoon of mayonnaise
Salt and pepper

To prepare the sliders: Place the pork tenderloin slices in a medium bowl with the rosemary, mustard, and 2 tablespoons of the apricot preserves. Mix gently until the pork is covered by the rosemary and preserves. Sprinkle 1 teaspoon of salt and pepper over pork. Let marinate for 15 to 20 minutes in the refrigerator.

To prepare the slaw: Wash cabbage and discard outer leaves. Chop cabbage into thin slices and place in a mixing bowl. Wash and peel carrots and then grate carrots and place into bowl. Wash the apple and then quarter the apple and cut out the core. Slice each quarter into thin slices and then cut each slice into julienne strips and place in bowl. Wash green onions and cut off ends and then slice thinly across the entire length of the onion. Add the yogurt and mayonnaise to the bowl and mix. Add 1 teaspoon of salt and pepper to slaw and then mix well.

Mix remaining apricot preserves with 1 tablespoon of water in a small bowl. Remove the pork from the refrigerator. Heat a pan over medium heat. Place 2 tablespoons of olive oil in the pan. Once oil is heated, place the pork slices on the pan spacing approximately 2 inches apart. Let cook for 7 minutes and flip over. Brush the top of each slice with the remaining apricot preserves. Cook pork slices for another 7 minutes and then remove from heat.

Assemble sliders by placing the slaw on one side of each bun, then top with pork and the remaining half of the bun. Serve with apple cabbage slaw on the side.

## References

1.  Clean plate club. (1942). *Time.* Retrieved from http://www.time.com/time/magazine/article/0,9171,790403,00.html on September 13, 2011.

2.  Davis, C. (1928). Self selection of diet by newly weaned infants. *American Journal of Diseases of Children. 36*: p. 651-79.

3.  Birch, L.L., and M. Deysher. (1986). Caloric compensation and sensory specific satiety: Evidence for self regulation of food intake by young children. *Appetite. 7*(4): p. 323-31.

4.  Birch, L.L., L. McPhee, B.C. Shoba, L. Steinberg, and R. Krehbiel. (1987). "Clean up your plate": Effects of child feeding practices on the conditioning of meal size. *Learning and Motivation. 18*: p. 301-17.

5.  Klesges, R.C., T.J. Coates, G., Brown, J. Sturgeon-Tillisch, L.M. Moldenhauer-Klesges, B. Holzer, J. Woolfrey, and J. Vollmer. (1983). Parental influences on children's eating behavior and relative weight. *J Appl Behav Anal. 16*(4): p. 371-8.

6.  Johnson, S.L. (2000). Improving preschoolers' self-regulation of energy intake. *Pediatrics. 106*(6): p. 1429-35.

7.  Birch, L.L. (1998). Psychological influences on the childhood diet. *J Nutr. 128*(2 Suppl): 407S-10S.

8.  Fisher, J.O., and L.L. Birch. (2008). Feeding children in an environment of plenty: Lessons from the laboratory. In L. Birch and W. Dietz (eds.), *Eating Behaviors of the Young Child: Prenatal and Postnatal Influences on Healthy Eating.* Elk Grove Village, IL: American Academy of Pediatrics.

9.  Orlet Fisher, J., B.J. Rolls, and L.L. Birch. (2003). Children's bite size and intake of an entree are greater with large portions than with age-appropriate or self-selected portions. *Am J Clin Nutr. 77*(5): 1164-70.

10. Spill, M.K., L.L. Birch, L.S. Roe, and B.J. Rolls. (2010). Eating vegetables first: The use of portion size to increase vegetable intake in preschool children. *Am J Clin Nutr. 91*(5): 1237-43.

11. Dewey, K.G. (2008). Breastfeeding and other infant feeding practices that may influence child obesity. In L. Birch and W. Dietz W (eds.), *Eating Behaviors of the Young Child: Prenatal and Postnatal Influences on Healthy Eating.* Elk Grove Village, IL: American Academy of Pediatrics.

12. Rolls, B.J., D. Engell, and L.L. Birch. (2000). Serving portion size influences 5-year-old but not 3-year-old children's food intakes. *J Am Diet Assoc. 100*(2): p. 232-4.

13. Tanofsky-Kraff, M., A.F. Haynos, L.A. Kotler, S.Z. Yanovski, and J.A. Yanovski. (2007). Laboratory-based studies of eating among children and adolescents. *Curr Nutr Food Sci. 3*(1): p. 55-74.

# THE UNDERRATED MISTAKES

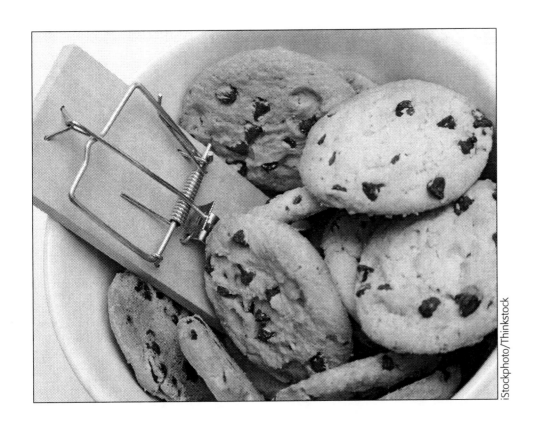

iStockphoto/Thinkstock

# Part Two

# 4

# Mistake #4—Forbidding Potato Chips and Ice Cream

*"The more things are forbidden,*
*the more popular they become."*
—Mark Twain

Among the best anecdotes describing the problem of aggressively forbidding certain unhealthy foods is an essay published in the *New York Times* by writer Joshua Yaffa.[1] In the essay, Yaffa describes his experience as a 10-year-old at school and sleepovers, safely outside the realm of his if-it's-not-good-for-you-you-can't-eat-it mother:

> *"Bargains were struck in the lunchroom. Want a look at my worksheet from math class? Sure. Just make sure your mom throws an extra stash of Pringles in your lunch tomorrow. Sleepovers took on the kind of salivatory anticipation that most children reserve for Halloween. Other kids aimed straight for the Nintendo. … I headed for the kitchen cabinet. After sucking down a few cans of Coke and burying my face in chocolate wrappers, I would streak through the house with a bleary-eyed zeal of an enraptured Pentecostal. 'Perhaps we should call his folks,' I could hear my friend's parents whispering as I collapsed on the kitchen floor."*

## Why Restriction Doesn't Lead to Healthy Eaters

Research plays out the binge phenomenon that Yaffa details. For example, in one study, children who were tempted with a clear jar of cookies on the table but told they couldn't eat them for 10 minutes ate three times more cookies than kids who had free access to the cookies.[2] It turns out that the more restrictive the parent, the more the child eats in an unrestricted setting.[3] In another study, four- to six-year-old girls who reported that their parents restricted snack foods were more likely than the girls of nonrestrictive parents to eat the snack foods immediately after a meal *even though* they said that they weren't hungry. After eating the snacks, half reported they'd eaten too much and nearly half said they felt bad about it.[4] Other studies have also shown that a high level of parental restriction is associated with a decreased ability to regulate energy intake and increased rates of childhood obesity.[5]

In sum, these studies suggest that restriction may contribute to:

• Bingeing
• Decreased ability to use hunger and fullness to guide intake
• Guilt following eating an unhealthy food (which may contribute later to dieting; this tends to emerge around middle childhood)
• Childhood overweight and obesity

In the rest of his essay, Yaffa describes his mom as a highly controlling force that the rest of the family dealt with by sneaking junk foods when she wasn't looking. He details how his now-grown 30-plus-year-old sister takes satisfaction from eating Cool Whip® out of the container at family get-togethers. Yaffa's mom took the approach that so many other parents concerned about their children's health take: if kids aren't allowed to eat unhealthy food, then by default, they'll eat a healthy diet. Thus, the parents restrict. They keep certain foods out of a child's reach or permit them in limited quantities; require consumption of a healthier food first (eat your vegetables and *then* you can have a cookie); and allow them only on special occasions as a "treat." And as long as a parent is there watching, this kind of restriction may inspire healthier eating habits. It's kind of like how people slow down on the freeway when a police officer is in sight, but as soon as that police car exits, traffic returns to its speeding-fast-enough-to-get-a-ticket rate. Kids do tend to choose healthier foods when they know they're being monitored,[6] but if you really want to raise healthy eaters who make smart choices *even when you aren't there*, then restriction may not be the way to go.

Back in the mid-1980s, researchers Philip Costanzo and Erik Woody[7] speculated that parents are most likely to restrict their child's food when they have problems regulating their own food intake, perceive the child is at risk of becoming overweight, or think the child is unable to regulate intake on his own. It's a two-way street: not only may highly restrictive practices inspire kids to binge on unhealthy foods when they finally get access to them, but overweight kids who have an insatiable appetite for junk foods might trigger a parent to limit access to those foods. This parental reaction seems reasonable. After all, haven't we been talking about how to make the home a healthier place by only having healthy food available to the kids?

It's a fine line. The line between not having dessert available in the house and not allowing the child to eat ice cream when he's out with friends. The line between giving out Play-Doh® or a healthy snack at Halloween and disallowing a child from trick-or-treating. The line between not frequenting fast-food restaurants and having a meltdown when Grandma picks up the little one from school and buys him Chicken McNuggets® for dinner. It's the line between authoritative parenting in which the parent sets up structure and guidelines (such as only having healthy food in the house) but leaves room for flexibility and negotiation (such as letting the child choose what he would like off of the menu when going out to eat) and authoritarian parenting in which the parent highly controls the child's life with little room for flexibility.

# Why the Deviance?

It'd be nice if kids would accept that unhealthy foods are restricted because they can contribute to unwanted health problems. But something about human nature pushes us to desire that which we can't have. This applies to adults as much as kids—how many people adopt a restrictive diet and lose a ton of weight, only to gain it all back and then some? This phenomenon has been studied extensively in adults. It seems that unlike unrestrained eaters who tend to regulate their intake in response to bodily cues of hunger and fullness, restrained eaters constantly battle two incompatible goals—the goal of eating enjoyment they get from the good-tasting "forbidden foods" and the goal of eating control. Even a small taste of the "forbidden food" triggers pervasive thoughts about the food and the pleasure of eating. Soon, the "dieter" craves the forbidden food and eats the food (oftentimes in excess).[8] The cycle then repeats itself. While in adults the restriction is self-imposed, the end result of excess intake of the forbidden food seems to be the same for children with parentally imposed restriction.[9]

Even given the staggering obesity rates in the United States, 40 percent of women and 30 percent of men are on a diet at any given time.[10] It's not such a paradox: dietary restriction in adults contributes to bingeing and chronic dieting. Strict parental dietary restriction poses the same two serious risks to children, and both may manifest in the same child. The first is the rebellious instinct to eat the restricted foods at any opportunity. This may contribute to overweight and obesity. The second is the adoption of the parental restrictive practices, possibly to an unreasonable extreme. This may lead to chronic dieting and disordered eating, among other negative consequences. For example, studies have shown that adolescent girls with restrained eating not only tended to be overweight but also had high levels of worthlessness, body dissatisfaction, fear of gaining weight, depression, and social anxiety.[11, 12] Although a parent's goal is to raise a child with a love of healthy foods, the unanticipated consequence of restricting unhealthy food is often a child who develops an unhealthy relationship with food. This seems to be especially true for girls of highly restrictive mothers.

## Dieting Mothers Raise Dieting Daughters

The results of a large body of research looking at food attitudes and behaviors suggest that dieting mothers raise dieting daughters.

*Evaluating the Role of Parental Restriction, Disinhibition, and Child Eating Patterns*

The results of a notable parent-feeding study of 70 three- to six-year-olds are at the same time intriguing and disturbing.[9] The study examined the relationship between parental restriction and child eating practices. The study methods and the results illustrate why highly restrictive feeding practices are detrimental—especially to girls.

*Maternal restriction and disinhibition.* To evaluate levels of maternal restriction, mothers answered nine questions about each of 10 snack foods (popcorn, potato chips, pretzels, nuts, fig bars, chocolate chip cookies, fruit-chew candy, chocolate bars, ice cream, and frozen yogurt). To get at the extent of maternal restriction, for each of the snacks, the questions assessed how often the mother:

- Limited availability of food to special occasions
- Got upset if the child obtained the food without asking
- Monitored the child's consumption of the food
- Generally limited the amount consumed
- Specifically limited the portion size
- Specifically limited when the food was available
- Kept the food out of reach
- Limited how often the food was in the home
- Generally limited opportunities to consume the food

Next, mothers and fathers answered several questions about their own eating habits, such as how often they stop eating when they're not really full in an effort to limit the amount they eat (a measure of restriction) and if they ever keep eating because a food tastes so good even when they're no longer hungry (a measure of disinhibition). Parents also provided self-reported height and weight.

*Child's perception of restriction.* Researchers assessed the children's perception of parental restriction by asking them three questions about each of the 10 snack foods: "Do Mommy or Daddy let you have these foods?"; "Would your parents be upset if you didn't ask before you got these foods?"; and "Are you allowed to eat as much of these foods as you want?" Researchers then measured the children's height and weight.

*The experiment.* Finally, right after the kids ate lunch to the point of feeling full, each went alone to a room stocked with toys and nearly unlimited quantities of each of the 10 snacks. The kids were allowed to play and eat as much as they wanted for 10 minutes. Then, the child answered how much his parents typically restricted access to each of the foods.

*Results.* The researchers found that the average kid ate 215 calories in snacks, even though all had reported they were no longer hungry after eating their lunch. That's a sizable increase in calories when you consider that the average child at this age needs only about 1,800 calories a day. Although girls *and* boys reported about the same overall level of parental restriction, only the girls ate more when parental restriction was higher. Those girls with the least restrictive mothers ate an average of 127 calories from the snack foods. The girls with the most restrictive mothers ate 303 calories. The boys ate about 215 calories, regardless of the extent of maternal restriction.

Girls, but not boys, who perceived the highest maternal restriction ate more of the snack foods when given the chance. The mothers were most restrictive with the kids who weighed the most. And mothers with the most restrained eating habits themselves were most restrictive with their daughters. Put this together and you have overweight girls developing even more dysregulated eating behaviors in response to their mothers' own struggles with food and eating. Not exactly what a well-intentioned mother desperate to prevent her daughter from developing the same destructive issues with food had in mind.

*The Alarming Beginning of a Long-Term Struggle*

The results of this study and others should trigger all mothers of daughters to stop and take a good look at their own eating attitudes and habits. Although dieting practices don't typically emerge until middle childhood, it's not uncommon to find a seven-year-old trying to lose weight. A study of *five-year-olds* found that the girls with mothers who were current or recent dieters knew an awful lot of about dieting and had developed their own opinions about whether it was a good thing to do.[13] Another study showed that a whopping 75 percent of middle- and upper-middle class, white, five-year-old girls ate for reasons other than hunger; 25 percent exhibited emotional eating; and one-third showed dietary restraint[14]—early precursors to long-standing struggles with food.

This is a whole lot of data that adds up to an epidemic problem. Societal pressures to be thin in the context of an environment that promotes overconsumption with few outlets for vigorous physical activity are overwhelming to even the most put-together teenager. A young girl who faces this environment looks to her mom for guidance. When a mom is dieting, bingeing, making negative comments about her own body or that of her daughter, restricting "bad" foods, and encouraging her daughter to diet, the young girl is bound to develop maladaptive eating attitudes and practices. *Forty percent* of women are dieting at any given time.[10] What impact does that have on their daughters?

# Reversing Course

A major facet of getting kids to choose a healthy balanced diet *even when their parents aren't looking* is to grow up in an environment where healthy foods are readily available and where the adult figures have a healthy relationship with food. If this doesn't describe you at present, don't sweat it. Now is the perfect opportunity to change course.

## Say "No" to Dieting

This is a book about getting kids to eat better. In many cases, the most powerful impetus for healthier behaviors in kids is healthier behaviors in influential adults. This especially holds true when it comes to dieting. You can dramatically decrease the likelihood that your daughters will turn to dieting to control their weight if you refuse to diet. (See the sidebar "Diet-Free Ways to Help an Overweight Child.") The following is a list of tips to help you permanently give up on diets and adopt eating behaviors that will not only set you up for optimal health and a healthy weight but will also set a positive example for your kids:

- *Refuse to diet.* Resist the temptation to adopt the newest and latest promise of instantaneous weight loss. Many diets are overly restrictive and nutritionally inadequate, which can lead to preoccupation with food, binge eating, fatigue, depression, and other harmful health consequences. Plus, much of the rapid weight loss from diets comes from water losses and muscle. The decrease in muscle mass slows metabolism, which just makes it easier to gain all the weight back—and then some—when the diet ends.

- *Allow all foods.* Yes, that's right—you and your kids can even eat potato chips and ice cream sometimes. Try to get out of the "good" food versus "bad" food mentality and think in terms of an overall healthy eating plan. Even the MyPlate recommendations and Dietary Guidelines for Americans leave room for "empty calories" (described as "solid fats and added sugars" or "SoFAS" in the 2010 Guidelines). These are the calories that come from foods that contain little nutritional value but taste really good. In moderation, these foods can have a place in a healthy diet.

- *Remember that food is fuel.* Food contains calories from carbohydrates, protein, and fat. These calories provide the energy and fuel for all the body's activities—from creating body heat to competing in a marathon. Think of food as fuel, not a fattening vice to be avoided or a friend to turn to for comfort. With that, actually use the food for its intended purpose and get moving! Commit to at least one hour of physical activity every day (more on this in Chapter 9).

- *Focus on health and fitness.* While the scale is an easy way to measure your weight, your overall health and fitness are much more important. Focus on improvements in energy, strength, endurance, flexibility, heart rate, attitude, and lean body mass more than a number on a scale.

- *Be mindful.* Eat when you're hungry and stop when you're full. It seems simple, but too often, we eat for a lot of other reasons (for example, when we're bored, stressed, sad, and tired). Before you eat, ask yourself: "Am I hungry?" Emotional eating can wreak havoc on a well-planned weight management program.

- *Lose weight slowly and steadily.* If you need to lose weight, aim to lose no more than one to two pounds per week through healthy lifestyle changes. A realistic weight loss goal for someone who's overweight is to aim to lose 7 to 10 percent of your starting weight over a six-month to one-year period and then to keep the weight off for at least six months before trying to lose more. It may feel like it's taking forever to get to your goal weight, but when you lose it slowly, you're more likely to keep it off.

- *Keep perspective!* A major problem with dieting is that it encourages people to think in black and white. This food is okay; that food isn't. When you "break the diet," it opens up a thought process similar to this: "Oh, well, I just screwed that up. Now that I'm off the diet, I might as well eat whatever I want." Then comes the binge, a return to the old way of eating, or some other less desirable eating behavior. Don't worry about if you ate well beyond the point of feeling full one day or if you didn't get in all the recommended amount of fruits and vegetables on another day. Weight and health are affected by an overall way of eating over a longer period of time.

## Diet-Free Ways to Help an Overweight Child

If you have an overweight child, you might feel that restricting the foods your child eats is the only way to help him achieve a healthy weight. After all, for many overweight children, an inability to effectively regulate intake is part of the reason the child became overweight in the first place. That's partly true. A person who eats when hungry and stops when full could probably maintain a healthy weight (although maybe not healthy arteries) from a fast-food-only diet. The problem is that many children lose the ability to use internal cues of hunger and fullness to guide intake from a very young age. Because of this, a lot of children eat more calories than their bodies need. The natural adult action in this situation is to put together a weight loss plan. However, the best weight loss plan for most overweight children is not to lose weight at all. Rather, it's to grow into their weight—that is, to not gain weight while they continue to grow taller. The best way to do this is to adopt a healthy lifestyle plan that includes a healthy overall eating plan and ample physical activity of at least 30 to 60 minutes most days of the week.[16–18]

In fact, a study of 169 moderately obese five- to nine-year-olds found that kids who underwent a healthy lifestyle intervention and whose parents received skills training lost about 10 percent of their weight and kept it off for two years.[19] While for most kids the goal is to not gain weight rather than to actively lose weight, the results from this study are promising. The parents learned some basic parenting skills that weren't specific to weight management. For example, they learned about setting goals, building self-esteem, and developing child behavior modification techniques, including how to encourage desirable behaviors and discourage undesirable behaviors. This is essentially the application of operant conditioning techniques, which are described in the Introduction and Chapter 2. In the healthy lifestyle component of the class, they learned basic nutrition principles, including food groups and serving sizes, how to read a nutrition label, healthy snack ideas, and recipe modifications to make healthier meals. They also learned about the importance of physical activity and some techniques to promote activity in their kids. The program was a success, lending credence to the assertion that the most effective weight management programs for children are ones that focus on parents. You can teach your child *how* to eat for optimal health—and you don't need diets.

## Say "Yes" to Lifestyle Changes

Just because you're giving up on dieting doesn't mean you should abandon any and all weight loss goals. If you're of a healthy weight, then a priority is to maintain that healthy weight (and teach your children to do the same) through a balanced, healthy eating plan and physical activity. If you're a healthy weight but still find yourself obsessed with losing weight, then for your sake and that of your children who are paying close attention to your attitude about eating and exercise, please seek help from a registered dietitian or another health professional to better understand your thought processes. The reality is that many people are overweight and can improve their overall health and quality of life by losing a few pounds. There is a healthy way to do this.

First, take a good look at the way you eat and the way that you think about food. Try to identify any major roadblocks that have gotten in your way in the past to successfully lose weight without going on a diet. It helps to complete a food log (see Chapter 3) to really see what you're doing right and what could be improved. Next, make sure you understand nutrition basics. The Dietary Guidelines for Americans and MyPlate.gov are good places to start. One of the most important principles to understand is that of energy balance. To lose weight, you must consume fewer calories than you expend. You can do this by eating less and exercising more. It takes about a 3,500-calorie deficit to lose one pound, so if you eat 350 fewer calories each day and burn 150 calories more each day, you'll lose about a pound per week. Third, put your knowledge into practice by adopting a healthy eating and exercise program you can stick with *long term*. A program you can still live with is one that includes all foods in moderation—those you eat because they're healthy for you and those you love but aren't healthy. Try to ban the diet mentality (see previous section) and instead get back your ability to let feelings of hunger and fullness guide your food intake.

### Practice Authoritative Parenting

Serving as healthy role models and fostering healthy eating preferences in kids challenge the fortitude of even the most disciplined and patient parents. The task of ensuring children grow up into healthy and productive members of society weighs heavily on many parents' shoulders. Not to mention all the pressure that society places on parents to make sure their children are well behaved, well mannered, and well educated; they must also be well fed. That means they eagerly eat the good food, don't care so much for the bad food, weigh just the right amount, and are immune to societal pressures to look a certain way. In their best effort to get started, many of the most committed parents spend a lot of time and energy learning about *what* to feed the kids. But much less time is spent learning about *how* to feed them. As a result, we push the good food. When kids refuse it, society and all the other people out there judging parents' techniques tell us that we need to force them to eat it. When kids are picky eaters, we push the food even more. When they have a voracious appetite and perhaps eat too much, we restrict. It all makes sense—if you remove the human elements. But when you remember that kids have minds of their own, it shouldn't be so surprising that pushing a food on a kid who doesn't want to eat it will increase refusal. And telling a child he can't have a food brightens its allure. So, what do you do?

## The Counterstrategies

A key strategy is to learn *how* to feed your children using authoritative parenting techniques. Authoritative parents set structures and guidelines for their children but leave room for flexibility and negotiation. Children experience certain freedoms within well-described rules. An authoritative parent sets the stage for healthy eating by focusing on the big picture and the *how* of eating. She gives the child choices and some control over the *what* of eating. She exerts her own control in a more covert way, which goes undetected by the child and virtually eliminates mealtime food battles. See the sidebar "Counterstrategies in Action: Authoritative Parenting" for some specific examples.

The best way to understand what an authoritative parent would do is to contrast it with what an authoritarian (restrictive) parent or a permissive parent would do. Let's look at some of the hallmarks of restrictive parenting (as laid out in the study described earlier in the chapter) and offer alternative *authoritative* parenting methods to achieve the same objective (guiding the kids toward eating the healthier, more balanced options) without being so restrictive.

---

## Counterstrategies in Action: Authoritative Parenting

Many parents struggle with the idea of the authoritative technique of "covert restriction" (such as only having healthy food in the house) versus the more overtly restrictive authoritarian approach (not allowing or severely limiting access to less healthy food). The following are a few examples from parents who have navigated that fine line:

- Amber, mother of three-year-old Xavier, practices one of the most important principles in shaping children's eating preferences: she gives Xavier a sense of control but still helps guide him to healthy choices. She says: "I try to let him have some control. If he requests a snack spontaneously that's healthy, such as fruit or cheese, for example, I will give him what he asked for. If he asks for a not-so-healthy food, I'll try to redirect to a couple better choices and let him choose between the two. I do take him shopping and let him choose which fruit pieces and put them in the bag. Also, he helps stirring and putting in spices for meals."

- Sarah, mom of four-year-old Lucas, has no problem with him eating desserts, but she's careful to make sure they aren't always available: "I don't mind if Lucas eats dessert, but I don't have desserts in our house. If we go to a party or friend's house and dessert is available, then I just let him eat however much of it he wants. And usually, that's not very much. He tells me that his tummy will hurt if he eats too much."

- The "Go, Slow, and Whoa" approach is in use at Alex's house. Alex and his wife Jess help their elementary school–aged kids understand that healthy foods, such as fruits and vegetables, help to make strong bodies, while less healthy foods, such as ice cream and cake, taste good but don't do much to help make strong bodies: Alex says: "The kids are really motivated by the idea that some foods help make them big and strong. They know that other foods aren't really that good for them and so they try really hard to only eat those foods sometimes. It turns out we don't really have to say that much more about it."

- An *authoritarian* parent limits the availability of less healthy* foods to special occasions. The problems with this are detailed in Chapter 2, but most concerning is that the sugar-laden, highly palatable food becomes associated with good times. Later in life, the child may turn to those foods for comfort in a psychological effort to reproduce the positive feelings associated with childhood memories. A *permissive* parent doesn't worry about what foods are in the house, and healthy and unhealthy foods may be readily available. An *authoritative* parent generally doesn't have the less healthy food around (thus covertly "restricting" access to unhealthy foods), but if a child requests a less healthy food while out, a parent doesn't mind buying it on occasion and doesn't make a big deal about it. By creating an environment in which healthy foods are in abundance and readily available (and less healthy foods aren't), an authoritative parent shows her children how to satisfy hunger with wholesome foods. The increased exposure and accessibility to the foods helps the children learn to like the healthy foods. The authoritative parent doesn't mind, then, if a child sometimes chooses less healthy fare—whether it's for a special occasion or not.

- An *authoritarian* parent gets upset if the child obtains a less healthy food without asking. By getting upset, the parent is showing her cards. The child learns that if he wants to push Mom or Dad's buttons, all he needs to do is eat a whole lot of the "bad food." A *permissive* parent doesn't take much interest in what the kids are eating and allows her children to eat whatever food is available. An *authoritative* parent creates an environment where the children are welcome to eat whatever is available in the refrigerator or pantry because only healthy foods that she would like her children to eat are readily available. The parent pays attention and asks the child about his food intake for purposes of information but not regulation. By showing an interest in what her children are eating but not being coercive, she has the opportunity to better understand what foods they really like and use the bridging principle (see Chapter 1) to further expand their repertoire of acceptable foods.

- An *authoritarian* parent monitors the child's consumption of less healthy foods. While being aware of whether what a child is eating is good, keeping too close of a tab on how much a child is eating of a particular "forbidden food" just encourages the child to sneak the food and otherwise try to hide what he's eating. As a result, the parent knows even less about what the child is eating and the situation of sneaking food creates an emotional relationship between the child and the food. A *permissive* parent doesn't pay much attention to what the kids are eating. An *authoritative* parent pays attention to what her children are eating but doesn't set strict limits on how much of a food a child can eat. Instead, she sets him up for success by teaching him how to control portions and use internal signals of hunger and fullness to guide intake.

- An *authoritarian* parent limits the amount consumed of less healthy foods. Intuitively, it makes sense. A child should eat a balanced diet and he needs

*For the purposes of this section, "less healthy" refers to foods with a moderate to high amount of sugar and/or saturated fat.

some adult guidance—eat a little less of this; eat a little more of that—to do so. But overtly setting strict limits can lead to many of the problems detailed earlier in this chapter. On the other hand, *permissive* parenting in which a child is left to his own devices to choose what and how much to eat in an environment that encourages overconsumption sets a child up for weight struggles. An *authoritative* parent guides a child into deciding for himself when he's had enough. She teaches him how all foods can fit in moderation and how some foods are better for our bodies than others. She models this in the way she eats and with her healthy relationship with food.

- An *authoritarian* parent specifically limits the portion size of less healthy foods. When a parent provides the portion control—rather than helping the child learn how to control portions himself—the child doesn't learn for himself how to moderate intake of the unhealthy foods. A *permissive* parent doesn't worry about how much of the unhealthy food a child eats. An *authoritative* parent teaches her children portion control strategies and then lets them practice by choosing their own portion sizes.

- An *authoritarian* parent specifically limits when unhealthy foods are available. For example, dessert is only allowed after dinner (or in exchange for eating vegetables); pizza is only allowed on certain Fridays. The problem with this strategy is that the limitations on when certain foods are allowed make them more appealing. A *permissive* parent allows unhealthy foods whenever the child requests. An *authoritative* parent makes sure a child is frequently exposed to many healthy foods and allows a child to eat less healthy foods on occasion. Her children understand that all foods fit in moderation and that foods aren't "good" or "bad." A way of eating is best judged over the course of days to weeks, not from food to food.

- An *authoritarian* parent keeps the "forbidden foods" out of a child's reach. Research on children's ability to delay gratification shows that children have less self-control when they can see but can't physically access a desired food compared with when the food is out of sight.[15] The old cliché "out of sight; out of mind" holds true. A *permissive* parent lets a child choose however much of unhealthy foods he would like to eat. An *authoritative* parent doesn't even store junk food, dessert, or other foods that are "off limits." Desserts are purchased fresh and served on the same day; leftover desserts are tossed. Children appreciate that all foods can fit into a healthy eating plan but also learn that it's better to reduce temptations to eat when not hungry by not having highly palatable, less healthy foods too readily available.

- An *authoritarian* parent limits opportunities to consume less healthy foods. While a measure of restriction, this is actually one area where restrictive and authoritative parents agree. The research on child feeding practices suggests that if children are given a choice between healthy options, they're able to choose a fairly well-balanced diet. However, if the more innately preferable sweet and salty foods are readily available, then children are going to go for what tastes better (as is the case in homes of *permissive* parents, where unhealthy foods are available without limitation). One way to ensure family meal- and snack-time harmony is to offer a child a choice between healthy alternatives and minimize (but not eliminate) opportunities to consume less healthy foods. Thus, an *authoritative* parent minimizes (but doesn't eliminate) opportunities to consume less healthy foods.

# Developmental Considerations

The best approach to minimizing restrictions while optimizing nutrition varies based on a child's age and developmental stage. The old saying "An ounce of prevention is worth a pound of cure" definitely applies here. Parents of one-year-olds who haven't had much opportunity yet to develop issues with food will have a much easier time implementing some of the strategies detailed in this chapter than parents of 10-year-olds who may have developed some unhealthy eating behaviors, including bingeing or dieting. Still, whether you're starting fresh or if you have to "retrain their brains," the investment you make now will pay dividends as your child grows up into a healthy adult (Figure 4-1).

## Infant (0–1 years)

Parents don't have to worry too much about restrictions in the first four to six months of a child's life—the period of time when an infant's diet consists exclusively of breast milk or formula to be fed on demand. When solids are introduced, it's best to choose healthy baby food options that optimize nutrition. (If you can make your own baby purees, that's great, but if not, try to choose fruits, vegetables, meats, and grains without any extra added sugars or salt.) Capitalize on the opportunity to expose your infant to as many different and varied flavors as possible to help foster a taste for healthy foods, but try to avoid

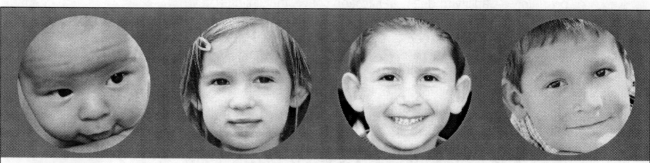

| **Infant** | **Toddler** | **Preschooler** | **School Age** |
|---|---|---|---|
| • Tune in to signs of hunger.<br>• Introduce solids at four to six months but still try to feed "on demand" (versus a schedule) in the first year.<br>• Expose your infant to a wide variety of healthy foods. | • Give your child a choice between healthy alternatives.<br>• Let your child eat less healthy foods sometimes. | • Teach your child the "Go," "Slow," and "Whoa" categorizations of food.<br>• Ask "Is your stomach full?" and "Are you hungry?" to help your child develop the ability to use internal cues to eat. | • Find out your child's attitudes about dieting.<br>• Teach your child about the importance of a balanced diet and how all foods can fit in moderation. |

Figure 4-1. Developmental considerations

juice and less healthy finger foods. If you offer up too much sugar and sweet stuff early on, it will be much more difficult to get your child to accept the less exciting bitter taste of vegetables and other healthy foods later. And at this age, your child isn't sophisticated enough to understand that you're withholding the sugary snacks.

## Toddler (1–3 years)

Toddlerhood is the period in a child's development when he really learns to find his voice—literally as the child's vocabulary multiplies exponentially and figuratively as the child becomes very adept at stating his wants and preferences. Blatant efforts to control him lead to tantrums, downright refusal, and a cunning desire to do the opposite of what you request. This is when mealtime food battles are born. Fortunately, you can avoid most of this by creating a pleasant mealtime environment in which a child is given the opportunity to choose what to eat and how much from the foods you've offered him. While in general it's best to have an array of nutritionally dense foods, everything fits in moderation. A family can enjoy an occasional dessert, pizza night, or the consumption of other nutrient-poor but good-tasting foods. In fact, it's even better if your kids do have access to these foods on occasion so they don't go overboard when given the opportunity to eat them, such as at a friend's house or with Grandma. But do remember that children are most neophobic at this age, and if you allow them to dictate meals based on their preferences for sweet and salty foods, you're going to end up with a child who refuses all the healthy foods and makes unreasonable demands (such as preparing a separate meal at dinner—more on this in Chapter 7).

## Preschooler (3–5 years)

At this age, children are developing an intrigue about the world and an increased desire to learn. Now is a great time to teach your preschooler about the benefits of the healthy foods you're offering and why he still can eat the less healthy foods, but that it's important to do so in moderation. Preschoolers are at the perfect developmental stage to learn about the U.S. government's WE CAN (Ways to Enhance Children's Activity and Nutrition) approach to healthy eating. This technique uses the "Go," "Slow," and "Whoa" categorizations of foods in which a child stops to think about what he's eating. The "Go" foods are nutrient dense and a great snack at almost any time. The "Slow" foods are a bit higher in calories and fat and are good to eat on occasion. The "Whoa" foods are the least nutrient dense and are good to eat just once in a while (see Figure 4-2). If you teach your child this way of categorizing foods, you put the power in his hands to decide what he'd like to eat and why. This gives your child a sense of control and sets the path for healthy eating in the future when you aren't always looking over his shoulder.

## School Age (5–10 years)

Around the time of middle childhood, adult-like issues with food and body image begin to emerge, including dieting, poor self-esteem, and eating

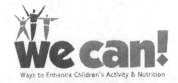
Ways to Enhance Children's Activity & Nutrition

## *We Can!* GO, SLOW, and WHOA Foods

Use this chart as a guide to help you and your family make smart food choices.
Post it on your refrigerator at home or take it with you to the store when you shop.
Refer to the *Estimated Calorie Requirements* to determine how much of these foods
to eat to maintain energy balance.

- GO Foods—Eat almost anytime.
- SLOW Foods—Eat sometimes, or less often.
- WHOA Foods—Eat only once in a while or on special occasions.

| Food Group | GO (Almost Anytime Foods) Nutrient-Dense | SLOW (Sometimes Foods) | WHOA (Once in a While Foods) Calorie-Dense |
|---|---|---|---|
| **Vegetables** | Almost all fresh, frozen, and canned vegetables without added fat and sauces | All vegetables with added fat and sauces; oven-baked French fries; avocado | Fried potatoes, like French fries or hash browns; other deep-fried vegetables |
| **Fruits** | All fresh, frozen, canned in juice | 100 percent fruit juice; fruits canned in light syrup; dried fruits | Fruits canned in heavy syrup |
| **Breads and Cereals** | Whole-grain breads, including pita bread; tortillas and whole-grain pasta; brown rice; hot and cold unsweetened whole-grain breakfast cereals | White refined flour bread, rice, and pasta. French toast; taco shells; cornbread; biscuits; granola; waffles and pancakes | Croissants; muffins; doughnuts; sweet rolls; crackers made with *trans* fats; sweetened breakfast cereals |
| **Milk and Milk Products** | Fat-free or 1 percent low-fat milk; fat-free or low-fat yogurt; part-skim, reduced fat, and fat-free cheese; low-fat or fat-free cottage cheese | 2 percent low-fat milk; processed cheese spread | Whole milk; full-fat American, cheddar, Colby, Swiss, cream cheese; whole-milk yogurt |
| **Meats, Poultry, Fish, Eggs, Beans, and Nuts** | Trimmed beef and pork; extra lean ground beef; chicken and turkey without skin; tuna canned in water; baked, broiled, steamed, grilled fish and shellfish; beans, split peas, lentils, tofu; egg whites and egg substitutes | Lean ground beef, broiled hamburgers; ham, Canadian bacon; chicken and turkey with skin; low-fat hot dogs; tuna canned in oil; peanut butter; nuts; whole eggs cooked without added fat | Untrimmed beef and pork; regular ground beef; fried hamburgers; ribs; bacon; fried chicken, chicken nuggets; hot dogs, lunch meats, pepperoni, sausage; fried fish and shellfish; whole eggs cooked with fat |
| **Sweets and Snacks*** | | Ice milk bars; frozen fruit juice bars; low-fat or fat-free frozen yogurt and ice cream; fig bars, ginger snaps, baked chips; low-fat microwave popcorn; pretzels | Cookies and cakes; pies; cheese cake; ice cream; chocolate; candy; chips; buttered microwave popcorn |
| **Fats/Condiments** | Vinegar; ketchup; mustard; fat-free creamy salad dressing; fat-free mayonnaise; fat-free sour cream | Vegetable oil, olive oil, and oil-based salad dressing; soft margarine; low-fat creamy salad dressing; low-fat mayonnaise; low-fat sour cream** | Butter, stick margarine; lard; salt pork; gravy; regular creamy salad dressing; mayonnaise; tartar sauce; sour cream; cheese sauce; cream sauce; cream cheese dips |
| **Beverages** | Water, fat-free milk, or 1 percent low-fat milk; diet soda; unsweetened ice tea or diet iced tea and lemonade | 2 percent low-fat milk; 100 percent fruit juice; sports drinks | Whole milk; regular soda; calorically sweetened iced teas and lemonade; fruit drinks with less than 100 percent fruit juice |

*Though some of the foods in this row are lower in fat and calories, all sweets and snacks need to be limited so as not to exceed one's daily calorie requirements.
**Vegetable and olive oils contain no saturated or *trans* fats and can be consumed daily, but in limited portions, to meet daily calorie needs (See Sample USDA Food Guide and DASH Eating Plan at the 2,000-calorie level handout)

**Source:** Adapted from CATCH: Coordinated Approach to Child Health, 4th Grade Curriculum, University of California and Flaghouse, Inc., 2002.

*Source:* National Heart Lung and Blood Institute, National Institutes of Health, Department of Health and Human Services. Available at http://www.nhlbi.nih.gov/health/public/heart/obesity/wecan/downloads/go-slow-whoa.pdf

Figure 4-2. Go, Slow, and Whoa Foods

disorders. Girls are particularly susceptible to these issues, which, for some, will persist into and throughout adulthood. This is a good age to find out your child's attitudes about dieting and get an idea for her relationship with food. Teach your child about the importance of a balanced diet but also that all foods can fit in moderation. If you notice any early signs of disordered eating, seek out a local health professional who can provide resources and information to help your child get back on track and avoid an enduring struggle.

School-aged kids also tend to have fairly well-established eating patterns, which for many may include eating for emotional reasons or out of boredom, disliking healthy foods, and having a preference for nutrient-poor foods. You might have difficulty trying to implement the recommendations in this chapter if you have an overweight or obese child or a child who refuses healthy foods and insists on the less healthy foods. Even though excessive restriction is discouraged, this chapter doesn't advocate a laissez-faire approach to your child's eating, especially for those kids who are already struggling with their weight. But remember, the goal is to teach them *how* to eat and focus a little less on restricting *what* they eat. With that, kids need structure and discipline. See the sidebar "How to Provide Structure With Minimal Restriction" for tips on how to provide your children the eating structure and guidelines they need without being overly restrictive. If you're concerned that these steps aren't enough and that your child really needs help with his eating, talk with your child's doctor (more on how to be most effective in doing this in Chapter 10).

# Chapter Summary

Hopefully, you feel like you've got the tools you need to set your children up for eating success without micromanaging their food intake or highly restricting nutrient-poor foods. To help turn the knowledge into action, the following points complement the information in this chapter:

- Test your assumptions about what does or doesn't work in raising healthy eaters. Examine your own parenting style. Do you tend to be more authoritarian, authoritative, or permissive?
- Think about your biggest worry regarding your child's health. Does this worry influence your feeding strategies? Specifically, if you tend to be highly restrictive, is it because you've struggled with weight and eating or that your child is overweight or that you feel that your child isn't very good at regulating his own intake?
- Refuse to diet and don't encourage your children to diet—even if they're overweight. Instead, teach your child *how* to develop healthier habits, including becoming more physically active and reestablishing internal cues for eating.
- Assess your kids' attitudes about dieting and weight control.
- Reframe your thinking from "good foods" and "bad foods" to healthy eating plans and less healthy eating plans. Healthy plans include a majority of nutrient-dense foods but allow for less healthy foods in moderation.
- Allow your kids to eat junk food sometimes. But try not to keep them in your house.

## How to Provide Structure With Minimal Restriction

Kids need structure and discipline. While suggesting you avoid being too restrictive in what your child is allowed to eat may sound like advice to let your kid run haywire, it's actually the opposite. The goal is to provide your children with the structure and discipline to help them learn *how* to eat rather than focusing so much on individual food items. The following are a few household rules you could implement to set them up for eating success:

- Eat meals at home as frequently as possible. Restaurant and fast-food offerings are often loaded with hidden calories.
- Try to eat meals together as a family—at the table with the TV off. Require the kids to stay seated at the table until everyone is done eating.
- Encourage regularly eating a healthy, balanced breakfast.
- Don't allow children to eat meals in front of the television. If you make exceptions to this rule for special occasions (such as Super Bowl Sunday), make the kids put their snacks into small bowls (versus bringing out the whole large bag). This will help with portion control.
- Designate an area in the home (kitchen, dining room, etc.) where most all eating should take place. Eating in one area encourages mindfulness.
- Make a rule that disallows snacks within an hour of mealtimes. This way, the kids will be hungry for dinner and more likely to consume the balanced meal you serve.
- Offer kids water first when they're thirsty. Water quenches thirst and is calorie free. Very little reason exists for most people to "drink calories," such as juice and regular soda. With that, keep only calorie-free beverages in your refrigerator.
- If your child eats too much of a particular healthy snack (for example, granola bars or crackers), tell him that you're only going to buy one box per week (or however much over whatever period of time that you see fit). Once it's gone, he has to wait until next week to get more. Although this is a form of restriction, it helps to teach him about eating foods in moderation and encourages him to add a little variety to his diet.

- Focus your efforts to raise healthy eaters more on *how* your kids eat and not as much on *what* they eat.
- Train your kids to ask themselves "Am I hungry?" before eating.
- Teach your kids the "Go, Slow, and Whoa" approach to deciding whether to eat a particular food.
- Access local resources to help if you have a child who's overweight or who's showing signs of restriction or disordered eating.

# Recipes: Healthy Snacks

## Creamy White Bean Hummus Cucumber Bites

1 can of white beans (also known as cannellini beans)
2 tablespoons of olive oil
2 tablespoons of water
1 garlic clove
Juice of half lemon
1 English cucumber

Place beans, olive oil, water, garlic, and lemon juice in a blender until smooth. Cut cucumber into 1/2-inch slices. Top each cucumber slice with a dollop of hummus and serve.

*Tip:* Try adding different ingredients to the basic bean spread for new flavors:

- Rosemary and sun-dried tomato dip: To previous ingredients, add 1 tablespoon of fresh rosemary and 5 to 6 sun-dried tomatoes.
- Green onion and olive: To previous ingredients, add 1/4 cup of chopped olives (seeds removed) and 1 bunch of green onions.

## Baked Garlic Basil Pita Chips

4 whole wheat pita breads
Olive oil
1 teaspoon of garlic powder
1 teaspoon of onion powder
2 teaspoons of dried basil
1 teaspoon of salt

Preheat oven to 400 degrees. Mix cayenne pepper, garlic powder, onion powder, basil, and salt with 3 tablespoons of olive oil in a bowl. Cut each pita bread into 4 pieces. Place pita breads on baking sheet and drizzle with the spiced olive oil. Bake for 15 to 20 minutes, until pita is crisp.

Serve with hummus or as croutons for a salad.

*Tip:* Want a sweet twist? Instead of the noted spices, mix 1 tablespoon of cinnamon and 2 tablespoons of sugar and sprinkle over pita bread. Bake 15 to 20 minutes, until pita is crisp.

## Breakfast Sundaes

2 cups of plain nonfat yogurt
1 cup of frozen fruit
3 tablespoons of honey
1/2 cup of water
1 cup of Coconutty Blueberry Granola (see recipe in Chapter 11)

Bring frozen fruit, honey, and water to boil over medium heat in a pot. Cook for 15 minutes, until fruit is like jam. Put fruit into a bowl to cool.

To prepare sundaes: In a glass, place 1/4 cup of yogurt at the bottom. Place 1 tablespoon of fruit mixture. Place another 1/4 cup of yogurt on top, followed by 1 more tablespoon of fruit mixture. Sprinkle 1/4 cup of granola on top. Repeat with another 3 glasses.

## Crispy Spiced Chickpeas

1 can of garbanzo beans (chickpeas)
2 tablespoons of olive oil
Salt and pepper
1 teaspoon of cayenne pepper
1 teaspoon of cumin

Preheat oven to 400 degrees. Drain and place garbanzo beans into a colander and let dry. After they are dry, place garbanzo beans into a medium bowl. Drizzle olive oil and sprinkle spices over beans and mix well. Pour beans onto baking sheet and bake for 40 minutes, occasionally removing sheet to stir. Let cool and then serve.

## Cinnamon Vanilla Yogurt "Fondue" With Apple Banana Kabobs

1 1/2 cups of low-fat vanilla yogurt
1 tablespoon of cinnamon
2 apples (any variety)
2 bananas
8 wooden skewers

Place yogurt and cinnamon into a bowl and mix well. Wash apples, cut into quarters, and remove core. Slice each quarter across into 4 pieces/chunks and set aside. Peel bananas and slice into 1/2-inch pieces. Place apples and bananas alternating on the skewer. Serve with yogurt "fondue."

If serving to younger children, remove the fruit from the skewers before serving.

## References

1.  Yaffa, J. Forbidden nonfruit. (2009). *New York Times*. Available at http://www. nytimes.com/2009/01/04/magazine/04lives-t.html.
2.  Fisher, J.O., and L.L. Birch. (1999). Restricting access to palatable foods affects children's behavioral response, food selection, and intake. *Am J Clin Nutr. 69*(6): p. 1264-72.
3.  Birch, L.L. (1998). Psychological influences on the childhood diet. *J Nutr. 128*(2 Suppl): p. 407S-10S.

4.  Fisher, J.O., and L.L. Birch. (2000). Parents' restrictive feeding practices are associated with young girls' negative self-evaluation of eating. *J Am Diet Assoc. 100*(11): p. 1341-6.

5.  Birch, L.L., and J.O. Fisher. (2000). Mothers' child-feeding practices influence daughters' eating and weight. *Am J Clin Nutr. 71*(5): p. 1054-61.

6.  Klesges, R.C., R.J. Stein, L.H. Eck, T.R. Isbell, and L.M. Klesges. (1991). Parental influence on food selection in young children and its relationships to childhood obesity. *Am J Clin Nutr. 53*(4): p. 859-64.

7.  Costanzo, P., and E. Woody. (1985). Domain-specific parenting styles and their impact on the child's development of particular deviance: The example of obesity proneness. *Journal of Social and Clinical Psychology. 3*: p. 425-45.

8.  Markowitz, J.T., M.L. Butryn, and M.R. Lowe. (2008). Perceived deprivation, restrained eating and susceptibility to weight gain. *Appetite. 51*(3): p. 720-2.

9.  Fisher, J.O., and L.L. Birch. (1999). Restricting access to foods and children's eating. *Appetite. 32*(3): p. 405-19.

10. Kruger, J., D.A. Galuska, M.K. Serdula, and D.A. Jones. (2004). Attempting to lose weight: specific practices among U.S. adults. *Am J Prev Med. 26*(5): p. 402-6.

11. Killen, J.D., C.B. Taylor, C. Hayward et al. (1994). Pursuit of thinness and onset of eating disorder symptoms in a community sample of adolescent girls: A three-year prospective analysis. *Int J Eat Disord. 16*(3): p. 227-38.

12. Rosen, J.C., J. Gross, and L. Vara. (1987). Psychological adjustment of adolescents attempting to lose or gain weight. *J Consult Clin Psychol. 55*(5): p. 742-7.

13. Abramovitz, B.A., and L.L. Birch. (2000). Five-year-old girls' ideas about dieting are predicted by their mothers' dieting. *J Am Diet Assoc. 100*(10): p. 1157-63.

14. Carper, J.L., J. Orlet Fisher, and L.L. Birch. (2000). Young girls' emerging dietary restraint and disinhibition are related to parental control in child feeding. *Appetite. 35*(2):p. 121-9.

15. Mischel, W., and E.B. Ebbesen. (1970). Attention in delay of gratification. *Journal of Personality and Social Psychology. 16*: p. 329-37.

16. Daniels, S.R., D.K. Arnett, R.H. Eckel, S.S. Gidding, L.L. Hayman, S. Kumanyika, T.N. Robinson, B.J. Scott, S. St. Jeor, and C.L. Williams. (2005). Overweight in children and adolescents: Pathophysiology, consequences, prevention, and treatment. *Circulation. 111*(15): p. 1999-2012.

17. Saris, W.H., S.N. Blair, M.A. van Baak, S.B. Eaton, P.S. Davies, L. Di Pietro, M. Fogelholm, A. Rissanen, D. Schoeller, B. Swinburn, A. Tremblay, K.R. Westerterp, and H. Wyatt. (2003). How much physical activity is enough to prevent unhealthy weight gain? Outcome of the IASO 1st Stock Conference and consensus statement. *Obes Rev. 4*(2): p. 101-14.

18. *The 2010 Dietary Guidlines for Americans.* (2010). The United States Department of Agriculture and the United States Department of Health and Human Services. Available at http://www.cnpp.usda.gov/dietaryguidelines.htm.

19. Magarey, A.M., R.A. Perry, L.A. Baur, K.S. Steinbeck, M. Sawyer, A.P. Hills, G. Wilson, A. Lee, and L.A. Daniels. (2011). A parent-led family-focused treatment program for overweight children aged 5 to 9 years: The PEACH RCT. *Pediatrics. 127*(2): p. 214-22.

# 5
# Mistake #5— Dismissing "Packaging"

*"Sometimes, life gives us lessons*
*sent in ridiculous packaging."*
—Dar Williams, singer/songwriter

"Power peas," "X-ray vision carrots," "tomato bursts," and "dinosaur broccoli trees" may be the long-awaited answer to dealing with your chronically veggie-rejecting kids. Cornell researchers found that when vegetables were given a wacky name, consumption doubled![1] And the effect persisted even when the vegetables went back to having their old boring names.

Blogger Christopher Pepper of "Daddy Dialectic" put this claim to the test:

*"I thought this was a simple and intriguing idea, so I decided to try it with Cole, my 5-year-old, last night. I told him we were going to have some "Colossal Corn" and "Super Sweet Potatoes" along with soup for dinner, and his eyes decidedly widened. And when the food arrived on the table, he did indeed eat significantly more than usual. He hesitated about eating the carrots and onions [in his soup] … but I told him they were actually flavor packets that exploded to release delicious tastes when they entered someone's mouth. After hearing that, he enthusiastically slurped them up."[2]*

Packaging—the way a food is prepared, presented, and promoted—matters. This offers parents both an opportunity and a challenge. While parents can devise innovative packaging and "marketing" tricks to help support children in developing healthier eating habits, parents also must be armed against the multi-billion-dollar food industry targeted at shaping children's food preferences.

# The Effects of Food Marketing on Kids' Health

Do not underestimate the power of the food industry to pressure your children to beg, plead, and cajole for heavily advertised products that tend to be high in sugar, solid fats, and salt. The Robert Wood Johnson Foundation, by far the biggest funder of work on childhood obesity, spends about $100 million each year to tackle childhood obesity. As Kelly Brownell of Yale's Rudd Center for Food Policy and Obesity likes to point out, the food industry spends that much by January 4 each year to market unhealthy food to children.

Watch a Saturday morning cartoon with your kids one week. If it's anything like the typical show, you're bound to see about one ad every five minutes for foods of low nutritional value.[3] In all, the average child will see over 4,000 food-related ads per year[3]; 85 percent of them will be for foods high in fat, sugar, or sodium,[3] and a miniscule one percent will be for low-calorie, high-nutrient-density foods.[4] The ads may seem harmless enough, but those underlying messages are influencing your children's food preferences—whether they realize it or not. Kids exposed to these advertisements consistently choose advertised foods more, request them more (usually by name), and like them more than their peers that did not see the ads.[5] Because the vast majority of foods advertised are high in fat, sugar, or sodium,[3] television viewing is directly getting in the way of your efforts to get your kids to eat better. It's also getting in the way of your ability to raise your children in a peaceful environment. When your child begs you to purchase a product he saw advertised and you say "No," he's very likely to become upset or disappointed.[4] But it's not just TV anymore. Children are also bombarded with advertisements from multiple other venues, including schools, billboards, the Internet, movies, cell phones, and friends.

This massive marketing attack on children's food preferences comes at a price. As most people by now are well aware, childhood obesity has reached epidemic proportions in the United States, with about a third of children overweight or obese. You might think that easy access to high-calorie, low-nutrient-dense foods and a more sedentary lifestyle are the main culprits. But merely being exposed to TV food advertising is accountable for about one in seven cases of obesity.[5] That's even when factoring out all the mindless eating that tends to occur in front of the television. As nutritional gatekeepers, parents bear the primary responsibility to offer children a healthy diet, but it'd be a whole lot easier if you weren't up against expert mind manipulators investing billions of dollars to get your kids to eat more solid fats, sugar, and salt.

## Marketing and Packaging
## Strategies of the Gurus

Food marketing to kids is a multi-billion-dollar industry. Knowing this, the marketing gurus have invested extraordinary resources into research aimed at best understanding the child psyche and how to manipulate and entice kids into craving their products. These marketers are very skilled at influencing children's taste preferences. Figure 5-1 highlights some of the most commonly used strategies (and how you can use them to your advantage). A few of those prominent strategies and some other tactics are described here in more detail, along with tips to turn counterproductive marketing tricks into useful ways to help your kids eat better.

| Marketing Strategy | Healthy Application |
|---|---|
| *Family fun.* This type of ad shows a product as something that instantly helps families have fun together. If Mom serves this food, a regular weekday dinner turns into a party. | You can make healthy meals fun by making eating healthy a celebration. For example, for one dinner a month, let the kids help make appetizers and go a little out of your way to be festive—whether that includes decorations, special music, or a special guest (more on this in Chapter 12). |
| *Excitement.* The marketers want kids to believe this product is the key to amazing fun and adventure. One bite and you're surfing in the tropics or dancing onstage with your favorite band. | Create excitement with the names you give foods. You can do this by giving vegetables wacky names or even spicing up what you call your dinner menu. For example, researchers at the Cornell University Food and Brand Lab found that people at a restaurant were more willing to order traditional Cajun red beans with rice (vs. red beans with rice), succulent Italian seafood filet (vs. seafood filet), tender grilled chicken (vs. grilled chicken), homestyle chicken parmesan (vs. chicken parmesan), satin chocolate pudding (vs. chocolate pudding), and Grandma's zucchini cookies (vs. zucchini cookies). You can also create excitement by serving snacks with fun plates, napkins, cups, or straws or have a tasting party where children can vote for their favorite healthy snacks. |
| *Star power.* A huge celebrity eats this product, so it must be the best of its kind! | Cartoon characters and others of your child's favorite "stars" count. And kids love stickers. Place stickers with your kids' favorite characters, pastimes, or obsessions on healthy snacks, baggies, and containers to encourage consumption of healthy foods. |
| *Repetition.* Manufacturers hope that if you see a product or hear its name over and over again, you'll want it. Sometimes, the same ad is repeated several times during one hour. | Frequently offer the foods you want your kids to love. Prepare them in different ways, but continue to offer them. Remember, it takes 15 times for a child to accept a previously rejected food. |
| *Feel good.* This ad tells a story that makes you feel good. For example, a dad cheers up his daughter by taking her to lunch at their favorite fast-food chain. (This is the strategy used by the famous McDonald's Happy Meal, which also throws in an enticing toy for added appeal.) | "Package" favorite family activities with memories of healthy food offerings. For example, a family picnic reunion might always include cutting up a watermelon and having seed-spitting contests. Or try this idea offered by one mother in *Disney Magazine*: "On long car trips, our sons inevitably beg for fast-food kids' meals with plastic toys. I invented Mommy Meals as a healthier alternative. I bought reusable lunch sacks and ironed colorful patches on them. Now I just pack a homemade meal and inexpensive toy in each." |
| *Sounds good.* Manufacturers use music and other sound effects to grab your attention. | Make up fun songs to sing about your child's favorite healthy foods. For example, Sesame Street aired the catchy song and character "Captain Vegetable," who sings about his love of vegetables. |

Figure 5-1. Adopt the marketing strategies of the gurus

## Licensed Characters

Licensed characters are a secret weapon for food marketers who want to tap in to the multi-billion-dollar industry of advertising to the youngest consumers, who control about $30 billion dollars in food monies from their own discretionary spending.[6] Putting the faces of such licensed characters as Dora the Explorer, SpongeBob SquarePants, Hannah Montana, and various other popular children's icons on products is a surefire way to sell them. In one study, children were given the option of cereal with a plain box and the same cereal with the penguins Mumble and Gloria from Happy Feet on the box. The kids said they liked the cereal from the penguin-adorned box more, even though it was the exact same cereal.[7] Unfortunately, manufacturers typically decorate the packaging of highly processed unhealthy snack foods rather than the more nutritious foods.

Recognizing that licensed characters are a huge selling feature for a child, parents can try to avoid unhealthy purchases by refusing to purchase unhealthy products with "celebrity" character endorsements while simultaneously capitalizing on their popularity. For example, Sophia, a highly impressionable five-year-old, begs her mom to buy her the Dora the Explorer fruit snacks they happened to walk past in the grocery store as her mom was looking to buy diapers for Sophia's little sister. Sophia loves Dora and believes that anything Dora endorses is delicious and nutritious. Her mom holds strong—until she sees the edamame in the produce section adorned with a picture of none other than Dora! "Dora Beans!" Sophia squeals. Smiling, her mom places two packages in the cart.

Sophia's mom understands the power of packaging and has done her best to use the food marketer's tactics to her own advantage in trying to help her daughter to eat healthy. Of course, it's not often that food marketers stick licensed characters like Dora on the healthy food—usually the food targeting kids is disproportionately chocked full of sugar, salt, and artificial flavoring. But when Sophia's mom saw the opportunity to capitalize on Dora's fame, she went for it. She could apply this strategy at home by putting healthy foods in baggies and sticking a couple of Dora stickers on the baggies before offering them to Sophia.

## "Just for Kids"

In an editorial published in the *New England Journal of Medicine*, Marion Nestle, an outspoken nutrition advocate and professor of nutrition at New York University, describes the underlying agenda of food marketing: build brand loyalty by teaching children brand recognition, encouraging them to pester their parents to buy the advertised products, and convincing children they need special foods made "just for them." Manufacturers spend billions of dollars not only in advertising, but also in conducting research into the child and "mother as family gatekeeper" psyches and how to best manipulate them.[6] Their efforts work. An Institute of Medicine study on food marketing to kids found that at about two years of age, kids are able to recognize advertised products at supermarkets and ask for them by name.[8] And many children routinely report that they—not their parents—decide what they eat.[6] This strategy of promoting "special" foods that are "just for kids" extends well beyond the grocery store. Restaurants are notorious for their calorie- and fat-loaded children's menus (more on this in Chapter 7). Parents can counter this strategy in two ways: refuse to buy junk food—in stores and in restaurants—specifically targeted at children and present foods in ways that are appealing to children—"cute" small sizes, fun adornments, and multicolored. (Check out the recipes in this chapter for some ideas.)

## Faux Healthy Foods

Don't count on the food manufacturers to key you in to what products may be healthier than others. Nutrition claims on products are good business, and many manufacturers will slap on various different health claims in an effort to cloud your judgment. General Mills took out a one-page ad in the *New York Times* to boast about its huge effort to decrease sugar in its cereals. It proclaimed that Lucky Charms will now contain *only* 10 grams of sugar per serving (about three teaspoons) instead of the prior 11 grams. That's not much of a reduction and still is 1,000 percent more sugar than plain old Cheerios, which has just one gram of sugar. Manufacturers frequently try to mislead consumers by highlighting the content of single ingredients that are associated with health, such as vitamins A, C, and D; calcium; fiber; and omega 3s. But don't fall for it—just because a fruit snack has "100% of vitamin C" doesn't mean it's healthy. It could still be loaded with sugar and artificial flavoring. Many advocates are calling for uniform front-of-packaging labeling to help consumers compare products and choose the healthier items. But for now, it's on you to weed through the product claims and determine what truly is better for you and your family. And it's most likely not the foods that the food manufacturers are trying to convince you to buy.

To get an idea of what food manufacturers consider "better for you" foods, check out the list in Figure 5-2 that the industry put out to tout its pledge to devote 100 percent of child-directed advertising to these "healthier alternatives." The table also includes a list of foods that are actually better for you, but for the most part, still not really all that nutritious. After looking at this list of pseudo– "better for you" foods, your gut instinct might be to laugh (and wonder "better for you" than *what?*). Recognizing this potential deception, the Prevention Institute conducted a study to see whether front-of-package labels on these "better for you" foods marketed to kids actually promoted foods that were healthy. It turns out that 84 percent of the foods were considered unhealthy based on their saturated fat, sugar, sodium, and/or (lack of) fiber content. In addition, the researchers also found that 13 percent of beverages, 40 percent of cereals, and 50 percent of snack foods contained food dye additives to make foods more brightly colored and thus more appealing to kids.[9] This artificial coloring has been linked to hyperactivity, allergic reactions, and other harmful outcomes in kids. The coloring is often used to simulate fruits, but as an earlier Prevention Institute study showed, despite clear references to fruits on product packaging, nearly two-thirds of the most heavily advertised foods targeting kids contained little or no fruit at all.[10] The unfortunate reality is that it's very difficult to find processed foods that are nutritious, despite what the food manufacturers would like you to think.

# Counterstrategies

All parents, teachers, pediatricians, policymakers, and others looking out for children's health should fight against the pervasive and deceptive marketing strategies aimed to get kids to eat junk foods. In fact, the American Academy of Pediatrics put out a strong (though so far unsuccessful) statement in mid-2011 calling for pediatricians to work together with parents, schools, and other advocates to encourage Congress to put a ban on junk food advertising to young kids.[11] In the meantime, advocates can borrow proven marketing strategies to help kids prefer the healthy foods more and the less healthy foods less.

## Parents: The First Defense

As food marketers have become more sophisticated, product placement pops up everywhere, including the Internet, social media, movies, songs, toys, games, educational materials, text messages, celebrity endorsements, and even celebrity Twittering. It's unrealistic to expect to be able to fully protect a child from media

| A Sampling of "Better for You" Foods (According to Food Manufacturers) That Aren't Really Better for You | A Sampling of "Better for You" Foods That Really Are Better for You |
|---|---|
| Capri Sun® juice drinks:<br>6 ounces (1 pouch) = 60 calories, *16 grams of sugar*, 0 grams of saturated fat, and 15 milligrams of sodium | Capri Sun's Roarin' Waters drinks:<br>6 ounces (1 pouch) = 30 calories, 8 grams of sugar, 0 grams of saturated fat, and 15 milligrams of sodium |
| Pop-Tarts® brown sugar cinnamon toaster pastries:<br>1 pastry = 210 calories, *15 grams of sugar, 2 grams of saturated fat*, and 170 milligrams of sodium | Eggo® Homestyle waffles:<br>1 waffle = 100 calories, 2 grams of sugar, 1 gram of saturated fat, and 190 milligrams of sodium |
| Cheez-It® Scrabble Jr.™ shapes crackers:<br>28 crackers = 140 calories, 0 grams of sugar, *1.5 grams of saturated fat*, and 180 milligrams of sodium | Triscuit® Thin Crisps Quattro Formaggio crackers:<br>15 crackers = 140 calories, 1 gram of sugar, 1 gram of saturated fat, and 160 milligrams of sodium |
| Keebler® animal cookies:<br>Regular:<br>8 cookies = 130 calories, 7 grams of sugar, *1.5 grams of saturated fat*, and 135 milligrams of sodium<br>Frosted:<br>8 cookies = 160 calories, 13 grams of sugar, *5 grams of saturated fat*, and 80 milligrams of sodium | Teddy Grahams® honey crackers:<br>24 pieces = 130 calories, 8 grams of sugar, 1 gram of saturated fat, and 150 milligrams of sodium |
| Yoplait® Trix Triple Cherry/Wild Berry Blue yogurt:<br>4 ounces = 100 calories, *14 grams of sugar*, 0.5 grams of saturated fat, and 50 milligrams of sodium | Stonyfield Farms YoKids® yogurt:<br>4 ounces = 80 calories, 13 grams of sugar, 1 gram of saturated fat, and 70 milligrams of sodium |
| Item in *italic* indicates reason food doesn't meet nutrition standards. These standards are based on the Interagency Working Group on Food Marketed to Children standard to minimize harmful nutrients: ≤ 210 milligrams of sodium, ≤ 13 grams of sugar, 0 grams trans fat, ≤ 1 gram or 15% of calories from saturated fat. Most processed snack foods don't meet this group's criteria to make a meaningful contribution to a healthy diet. ||

Figure 5-2. "Better-for-you" food?

and advertising's vast influence. However, it's worthwhile to acknowledge how powerful advertising is in shaping children's food and beverage preferences, purchase requests, and beliefs. Recognizing the role of food marketing in dictating your child's food requests and preferences is the first step in defending against its influence. The next is aiming to purchase nutritionally dense foods for your kids. While no single agreed-upon standard for what constitutes a nutrient-dense food exists, a group of federal organizations, including the Federal Trade Commission (FTC), the United States Department of Agriculture (USDA), the Food and Drug Administration (FDA), and the Centers for Disease Control and Prevention (CDC) (known as the "Interagency Working Group on Food Marketed to Children"), has proposed the nutrition guidelines highlighted in Figure 5-3. Foods that don't meet these criteria are considered nutritionally-poor choices or low-nutrition foods. (More on the recommendations of this working group in the section "A Policy Approach to Fighting Against Undue Influence.") When shopping with your kids, keep these guidelines in mind. And remember not to automatically trust the front-of-package claims of health. Instead, check the detailed nutrition label and ingredient list to see if it really is "better for you." While they're hard to find, relatively healthy processed foods do exist; you just have to seek them out.

In addition to critically evaluating nutrition labels, some of the most powerful actions you can take to defend your children against harmful food advertisements include:

- Minimize your child's exposure to food advertisements as much as possible. Do this by limiting television time (ideally two hours or fewer per day for kids older than two and no screen time for kids younger than two) or at least DVR the programs that your child loves and fast-forward through

| Standard 1: Food Must be a Meaningful Contribution to a Healthful Diet | Standard 2: Food Must Minimize Amounts of Harmful Nutrients |
|---|---|
| Food must be at least 50% by weight of wholesome foods, including fruit, vegetable, milk, fish, lean meat, egg, nut, seeds, or beans.<br><br>Specifically, per serving (or 100 grams):<br>• > 0.5 cups of fruit or fruit juice<br>• > 0.6 cups of vegetable or vegetable juice<br>• > 0.75 ounces of 100% whole grain<br>• > 0.75 cups of milk or yogurt, 1 ounce of cheese, or 1.5 ounces of fat-free or processed cheese<br>• > 1.4 ounces of meat, fish, or poultry<br>• > 0.3 cups of cooked dry beans<br><br>Note: Individual foods need to have at least one of the above, main dishes at least two of the above, and meals at least three of the above. | Per serving (or per 100 grams in entrees and meals), food must not contain more than:<br>• 210 milligrams of sodium<br>• 13 grams of sugar<br>• 0 grams of trans fat<br>• 1 gram or 15% of calories from saturated fat |

*Source: Preliminary Proposed Nutrition Principles to Guide Industry Self-Regulatory Efforts.* (2011). Washington, DC: Interagency Working Group on Food Marketed to Children

Figure 5-3. Proposed nutritional standards for food marketed to children, according to the Interagency Working Group on Food Marketed to Children

the commercials or choose channels, such as Public Broadcasting Service (PBS), that don't have commercials. Strategically shop at the grocery store to decrease exposure to the battle-inducing heavily advertised candies and snacks (i.e., shop the perimeter, which is mostly produce and fresh food, and avoid candy and chip aisles).

- Hold firm when refusing to purchase the heavily advertised junk foods that your child so adamantly insists on buying. (You can make this easier by shopping at stores that don't carry heavily advertised and branded foods). This isn't to say your child should never be allowed to have a junk food snack. But you can make a point to buy the generic brand or refuse to purchase the most heavily marketed products.

Media literacy training—an organized effort to teach kids to question the validity of the media messages—is also a useful but fairly small piece of a multipronged strategy to protect children from the harms of advertisements. Teaching kids to be critical of advertisements isn't useful for younger kids because children younger than about eight do not have the cognitive ability to discern commercials from programming. (It's better to protect them from the advertisements altogether.) When a child is able to recognize that the advertiser has perspectives and interests that are different from that of the child; the advertiser aims to persuade; persuasive messages are inherently biased; and biased messages need to be taken with a grain of salt, then he may be ready to learn from media literacy training. But even then, everyone is constantly bombarded by advertisements from multiple sources. It would be impossible to exert the cognitive effort required to combat every one of these messages. Still, a comprehensive approach to countering the advertising messages includes teaching children to be critical of advertisements. One way to do this is to sit down with your child during a children's program and track the commercials together. Identify what strategies the advertisers use to try to persuade you. Are they compelling? What's the actual nutritional value of the product? Do healthier and less expensive alternatives that taste just as good exist?

## A Policy Approach to Fighting Against Undue Influence

Recognizing the powerful and negative influence food advertising has on children, several governments have taken action. Britain banned junk food advertisements during children's programs; Sweden and Quebec forbid all advertisements to children in general; and France requires that companies promoting unhealthy foods provide message disclaimers. The United States, on the other hand, has done very little.

While child health advocates have long rallied for government restriction of food marketing to kids, little headway has been made. The Federal Trade Commission proposed an outright ban on advertisements targeted to children in the 1970s, but those efforts were quickly abandoned due to political pressures. Instead, the main limitation on children's programming is that commercials can take up only 10 minutes and 30 seconds per hour of children's programming on weekdays and 12 minutes per hour on weekends. Stations that air children's programs must also air at least three hours of educational programming for children 16 and under each week. The industry has promised to self-regulate, but the guidelines are vague, voluntary, and do little to curb the effects of unfair advertising to children.

Renewed interest in regulating marketing to kids occurred in 2011, when Congress directed the FTC, the FDA, the CDC, and the USDA to establish a working group to develop a set of principles to guide industry to improve the nutritional value of foods marketed directly to children. Unfortunately, after a brutal push back by food marketers, plans for that report to be released have been mostly scrapped as of the time of this writing. The following were the goals of the working group, but it is unlikely these principles will take hold in the near future:

All foods heavily marketed to children should:
- Make a meaningful contribution to a healthy diet.
- Minimize the content of nutrients that can have a negative impact on health and weight.[12]

Refer to Figure 5-3 for more details.

### Applying the Tactics

While waiting for industries to step up, parents and communities will have to take matters into their own hands to protect kids from the food marketing and packaging wizards. One way to do this is to apply some of the experts' tactics to get kids to like the healthy foods.

Packaging matters. And the expert food marketers have something to offer parents interested in getting their kids to eat better. While healthy foods are a bit of a harder sell than the typical high-salt, high-sugar fare that food marketers push (after all, kids have an innate preference for sweet and salty), you can adopt expert marketers' tactics to make fruits, vegetables, and other healthy foods more appealing. (Review Figure 5-1 and check out some examples from real parents in the sidebar "Counterstrategies in Action: 'Marketing' Healthy Foods to Kids" to get started.)

# Developmental Considerations

Marketing tactics affect children differently depending on their age and developmental stage. Younger kids are extremely vulnerable, with few defenses to protect them from complete persuasion. As children get older, they have a better capacity to filter through the hype; however, even the most astute adults are persuaded by these expert mind manipulators. Parents are the first defense against harmful marketing to children. You can mount your defense against the unhealthy manipulations by targeting your child's developmental stage. You can also apply strategies most successfully if you keep in mind the following developmental considerations (Figure 5-4).

## Counterstrategies in Action:
## "Marketing" Healthy Foods to Kids

Check out some of these innovative strategies parents have used to "market" healthy foods to kids:

- Joshua, a rambunctious three-year-old, refused to eat the celery and raisins his mom gave him for his afternoon snack. Undeterred, Joshua's mom shuffled back into the kitchen, spread a dab of peanut butter over the celery, and stuck the raisins on top. She presented Joshua with his "ants on a log." He smiled and happily took a bite.

- Brad's two-year-old son Darren was a hesitant eater and obsessed with Thomas the Tank Engine. To encourage Darren to give clams a try, Brad told him that the clams were Cranky clams on top of Percy pasta with Bertie basil. Ryan gave it a try and realized that he actually loves clams!

- Debbie, mother of picky eater Ryan, figured out the perfect way to control portion sizes and use the power of marketing to her advantage. She served whole meals in a muffin tin. It's simple—you just adapt whatever meals you're making for the family to fit in the tin. For example, in a six-cup tin, you could fill three with veggies or salad or fruit, one with protein, one with whole grain carbs, and another with a calcium-rich product, such as cheese or yogurt. This is where the packaging comes in—Debbie suggests you could put a picture of a favorite character at the bottom of each cup and the kids will find the character when they finish the food or you could use colorful tin liners. You can even find cartoon character liners in the party section at any number of stores. How much you fill up each cup depends on your child's age and appetite.

- Jen makes sure the kids have positive thoughts and memories tied to eating healthy foods. For example, she says "Foods can be 'endorsed' by the kids' favorite people—if a certain food is a favorite of Grandpa's, we make sure to point that out when it's served. We also might bring up a good memory—saying, 'Remember when we saw the shrimp boat catching shrimp when we were on vacation? These shrimp are just like those ones!'"

- Homemade meals at the kitchen table may not have true marketing, but any type of special plates/kid silverware comes close to cool packaging and can make a healthy meal exciting. At Julie's house, they have some plates with fire trucks, some with Buzz Lightyear on them shaped like his rocket, Thomas the Tank Engine forks/spoons, some plates with the compartments (such as a frozen TV dinner), and some in all colors of the rainbow (to accommodate that week's favorite colors). When it's mealtime, the kids run to the drawer and try to get first pick.

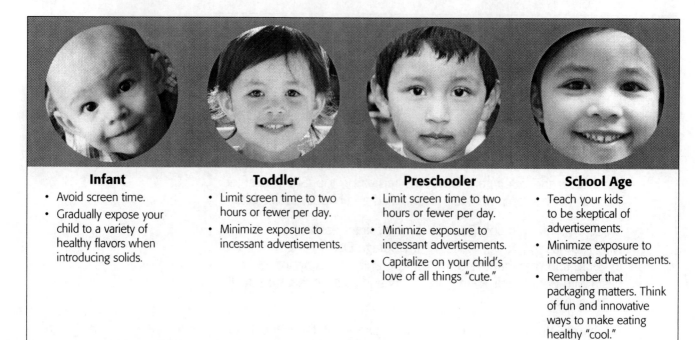

Figure 5-4. Developmental considerations

### Infant (0–1 years)

Developmentally, a child in the first year is minimally persuaded by advertisements. The most important actions at this stage are to avoid screen time (television, computer, movies) and to gradually expose the child to as many different healthy flavors and tastes as possible when introducing solids. This will set the stage for greater acceptance of vegetables and fruits when neophobia and tendency toward sugar obsessions begin around the age of two.

### Toddler (1–3 years)

Toddlers and even preschoolers are pretty lousy at telling the difference between TV advertisements and programming. SpongeBob blatantly trying to sell sugary cereal registers no differently than SpongeBob hanging out with his friends and playing around during his daily 30-minute TV slot. The fact that food marketing strategies have become so ingrained with product placements during actual programming further molds these impressionable minds. At this age, your best bet is to avoid exposure to these products as much as possible.

### Preschooler (3–5 years)

The typical four-year-old preschooler will for the first time start to realize that a difference exists between a television program and a commercial. But this understanding is limited. A child picks up that commercials may be funnier than programs or shorter than programs, but he doesn't get that the advertiser is employing persuasive strategies to try to sell him a product. As with toddlers, try to minimize exposure to incessant advertisements. You can also capitalize on your preschooler's love of all things "cute." Preschoolers love inherently packaged foods (such as edamame, which is fun to eat) and easy-to-eat single-serving snacks (such as yogurt tubes). You can also make significant progress if you give foods enticing names (such as "X-ray vision carrots") and package them well (such as baggies adorned with stickers).

## School Age (5–10 years)

To be able to defend against food advertisements, a child has to have the cognitive skills to differentiate an advertisement from regular programming and also be able to be somewhat critical of the motivators of the advertiser. Without these skills, which don't develop until about eight years of age, a child is left vulnerable and defenseless to powerful marketing strategies. But even at this age, most kids don't necessarily comprehend that not everything stated on TV is true. In other words, even though these kids can recognize that commercials intend to sell, many don't realize that they're biased messages that warrant some degree of skepticism. Media literacy training offers some opportunity to help counter these messages, but as nutritional gatekeepers, parents still play an important role in minimizing a child's exposure to the ads and trying to resist pressure to purchase heavily advertised, low-nutrition foods. And kids this age still dig your fun and innovative efforts to make healthy foods more appealing. (Check out the recipes in this chapter for a few ideas.)

# Chapter Summary

Packaging matters. Underestimate this power and you miss an opportunity to intervene in the unhealthy and unproductive mind manipulation of the manufacturers. But if you fully appreciate the power of packaging, you have one more tool at your disposal to inspire kids to eat healthy. The following points recap this chapter to help you get going:

- Don't underestimate the power of the food industry to pressure your children to beg, plead, and cajole for heavily advertised products that tend to be high in sugar, saturated fat, and salt. Counter the effects by refusing to succumb to marketing tricks.
- Harness the power of packaging by borrowing strategies from the marketing geniuses to promote healthy foods. (Review Figure 5-1 for several sample strategies.)
- Resist the temptation to buy your child heavily advertised foods with low-nutritional value—even if he begs and pleads. After you say "No," don't give in.
- Be skeptical of food advertisements. Ask yourself what the nutrition claims on packages really mean. Is the food actually a healthy choice or is it just a marketing gimmick? Let the nutrition guidelines in Figure 5-3 help you decide.
- Don't buy into the idea that some foods are "just for kids." Instead, make the same foods that the rest of the family eats appealing to the younger ones.
- Teach your older kids (eight and older) how to be skeptical of advertisements and marketing gimmicks.

- Limit screen time to fewer than two hours per day for kids older than two. Avoid TV and screen time for infants and toddlers zero to two.
- Make it fun to eat healthy by creating cute and simple concoctions, such as "ants on a log," "smiley face" veggie pizzas, and crazy-named vegetables.
- Ask your child's school to limit advertisements and incentives from food companies and restaurants that serve mostly low-nutrition foods.
- Advocate for legislation and policies that restrict advertising to children.

# Recipes: Appealingly "Packaged" Meals and Snacks

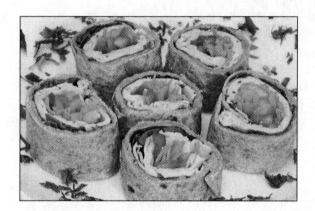

### Rainbow Pinwheels

2 whole wheat tortillas

1 cups of baby spinach, washed and dried

6 slices of deli-sliced turkey breast

1/2 cup of grated carrots

1 red bell pepper, julienned

1/2 cup shredded cheddar cheese

Place one tortilla in a pan over low heat. Sprinkle 1/4 cup of cheddar cheese over the tortilla. Remove tortilla from heat once cheese has melted and turn off stove. Place one layer of spinach over cheese and then place 3 slices of turkey breast. Next, place carrots and bell pepper in a single layer on one-half of the tortilla. Starting at one end with the carrots and peppers, roll the tortilla into a burrito. Slice into 1-inch rounds. Repeat this procedure with second tortilla.

### Goin' Nuts and Bananas! (Peanut Butter Banana Pancakes)

1 cup whole wheat flour

1 cup rolled oats

1 teaspoon of baking soda

1 teaspoon of baking powder

1/4 cup of brown sugar

3 ripe bananas, mashed

1/2 cup of buttermilk or plain yogurt

1/4 cup of peanut butter

2 eggs

2 tablespoons of butter, melted

1 tablespoon of cinnamon

1 teaspoon of salt

1 tablespoon of vanilla extract

*Toppings:*

Banana chips
Walnuts
Peanut butter

To prepare wet ingredients: Crack the eggs into a medium mixing bowl and beat lightly. Add the melted butter and peanut butter and then whisk until well incorporated. Mix in the brown sugar and stir. Add the buttermilk/yogurt and vanilla to the egg mixture and stir. Add the mashed bananas and stir until incorporated.

To prepare dry ingredients: Blend rolled oats in a blender until fine and then pour into a separate bowl. Add the whole wheat flour, baking soda, baking powder, salt, and cinnamon to the bowl and stir. Pour half of the dry ingredients into the wet ingredients and fold gently. Add the remaining dry ingredients and gently fold until just incorporated.

Prepare a shallow pan over low-medium heat. Spray with nonstick cooking spray. Pour approximately 1/4 cup of batter onto the pan. Cook for 3 to 4 minutes or until the top of the pancake has bubbles. Flip the pancake and cook for another 3 to 4 minutes.

Serve with crushed banana chips and peanut butter on top.

## Mean Green Pita Pockets

2 whole wheat pita breads
1 cup of cheddar cheese
1 cup of broccoli florets
1 chicken breast (see Simple Baked Chicken Breast in Chapter 10)
1 carrot, peeled and grated
Salt and pepper

Preheat oven to 375 degrees. Shred the chicken breast into small pieces—either using a fork or your hands if the chicken is cool to touch. Place shredded chicken into a bowl. Chop broccoli florets into small pieces and add to bowl. Stir the grated carrot into the bowl and mix well.

Split one pita bread into 2 pieces. Sprinkle 1/4 cup of cheddar cheese on one side of the pita bread. Place approximately 1/2 cup of chicken and vegetable mixture on top of the cheese. Sprinkle with another 1/4 cup of cheddar cheese and place remaining pita half on top and gently press to flatten the filling inside. Repeat with second pita bread. Reserve remaining filling in the refrigerator.

Place prepared pita bread on baking sheet and bake in oven for 15 minutes. Remove from oven, cut each pita sandwich in half, and serve.

### Eggs in a Nest (Zucchini Hash Browns With Maple Chicken Apple Sausage)

1 medium-sized potato

1 medium zucchini

1/4 cup all-purpose flour

1/4 cup of grated parmesan cheese

1/2 pound of ground chicken or turkey

1/2 apple (any variety)

1/4 cup frozen spinach (defrosted and squeezed)

2 tablespoons of maple syrup

Salt and pepper

Muffin tin

Nonstick cooking spray

Preheat oven to 400 degrees.

To prepare the "nests": Wash and dry the potatoes and zucchini. Using a cheese grater, grate the potatoes and zucchini into a clean kitchen towel. Sprinkle a teaspoon of salt on top of the vegetables and squeeze out the excess water from the zucchini and potatoes through the towel. Place the potatoes and zucchini into a mixing bowl. Place the flour and cheese into the bowl, along with a teaspoon of salt and pepper and mix well. Spray the muffin tin with nonstick cooking spray. Fill each muffin tin with the potato/zucchini mixture. Using the back of a spoon, press the vegetable mixture against the wall of each muffin tin, creating a well in the center of each nest. Bake for approximately 20 minutes while preparing sausages.

To prepare the "eggs": Grate the apple into a bowl. Add the ground chicken to the bowl. Add the spinach and maple syrup into the bowl. Mix ingredients well. Sprinkle with 1 teaspoon of salt and pepper and mix. Take approximately 2 tablespoons of meat mixture and roll into a ball. Heat a pan over medium heat. Place 2 tablespoons of olive oil into pan. Place sausages into pan approximately 2 inches apart, gently pressing down to slightly flatten each meatball. Cover the pan with a lid and cook for approximately 8 minutes. Flip the sausage over and cook covered for another 8 minutes.

Remove the muffin tin from the oven. Place one sausage on top of each vegetable "nest" and serve.

## References

1. Cuellar, S. (2009). Names turn preschoolers into vegetable lovers. *The Mindless Eater*. Available at http://foodpsychology.cornell.edu/pdf/newsletters/Newsletter_ Spring_09.pdf.

2. Pepper, C. (2007). Power Peas and Colossal Corn. Available at http://daddy-dialectic.blogspot.com/2007/10/power-peas-and-colassal-corn.html.

3. Powell, L.M., R.M. Schermbeck, G. Szczypka, F.J. Chaloupka, and C.L. Braunschweig. (2001). Trends in the nutritional content of television food advertisements seen by children in the United States: analyses by age, food categories, and companies. *Arch Pediatr Adolesc Med. 165*(12): p. 1078-86.

4. Kunkel, D., C. McKinley, and P. Wright. (2009). *The Impact of Industry Self-Regulation on the Nutritional Quality of Foods Advertised on Television to Children.* Oakland, CA: Children Now.

5. Veerman, J.L., E.F. Van Beeck, J.J. Barendregt, J.P. Mackenbach. (2009). By how much would limiting TV food advertising reduce childhood obesity? *Eur J Public Health. 19*(4): p. 365-369.

6. Nestle, M. (2006). Food marketing and childhood obesity--a matter of policy. *N Engl J Med. 354*(24): p. 2527-9.

7. Lapierre, M.A., S.E. Vaala, and D.L. Linebarger. (2011). Influence of licensed spokescharacters and health cues on children's ratings of cereal taste. *Arch Pediatr Adolesc Med. 165*(3): p. 229-34.

8. McGinnis, J., J.A. Gootman, and V.I. Kraak (eds.). (2006). *Food Marketing to Children: Threat or Opportunity?* Washington, D.C.: Food and Nutrition Board, Institute of Medicine.

9. Sim, J., L. Mikkelsen, P. Gibson, and E. Warming. (2011) *Claiming Health: Front-of-Package Labeling of Children's Food.* Oakland, CA: Prevention Institute.

10. Mikkelsen, L., C. Merlo, V. Lee, and C. Chao. (2007) *Where's the Fruit? Fruit Content of the Most Highly-Advertised Children's Food and Beverages*: Oakland, CA: Prevention Institute.

11. Strasburger, V.C. (2011) Children, adolescents, obesity, and the media. *Pediatrics. 128*(1): p. 201-8.

12. Interagency Working Group on Food Marketed to Children. (2011). *Preliminary Proposed Nutrition Principles to Guide Industry Self-Regulatory Efforts.* Washington, DC: Interagency Working Group on Food Marketed to Children. Available at http://www.ftc.gov/os/2011/04/110428foodmarketproposedguide.pdf.

# 6

# Mistake #6—
# Failing to "Live It"

*"Don't worry that children never listen to you;
worry that they are always watching you."*
—Robert Fulghum, author of *All I
Really Need to Know I Learned in
Kindergarten*

Joey and his mom are seated for dinner. Mom subtly encourages the four-year-old to taste the crunchy spinach salad she's prepared for him. Curious, Joey is about ready to give it a try. Dad takes his seat at the table, notices the salad, and says "Yuck. I hate spinach." Joey, always eager to impress and emulate Dad, says "Yuck" and sets down his fork. Welcome to the phenomena of modeling, a powerful strategy to raise healthy eaters—or not.

## For Better or Worse, Modeling Matters

As any parent who accidentally uttered a four-letter word and then heard that word boldly repeated by a loud-mouthed toddler at the most inopportune time and place knows, kids have an uncanny ability to learn by watching and listening—sometimes when adults have no idea that the child was even paying attention. One of the most potent ways that kids learn about their environment is by watching how other people that they look up to behave in different situations. And then, for better or worse, the kids repeat those actions. Understanding how modeling works gives parents an opportunity to capitalize on the power of modeling to get kids to eat better and be more active without coercion, begging and pleading, bribes, or threats of punishment.

## Bandura's Theory of Modeling

In a series of now classic experiments conducted in the late 1970s, psychologist Albert Bandura first described modeling (also known as *social learning theory* in the world of psychology). Bandura and his graduate students showed kindergartners a video of a graduate student beating up a bobo doll, an inflatable "clown" with a weighted bottom. The grad student punched, kicked, hit with a hammer, and otherwise aggressively abused the doll. The kindergartners overall seemed to think it was a pretty cool and entertaining clip. The researchers then let the kids out to play in a room that, conveniently, had a bobo doll and a few hammers. No one will be too surprised by what ensued: the kindergartners grabbed the hammers and beat up the doll. They punched, kicked, hit with a hammer, and otherwise aggressively abused the doll. In essence, they did exactly what they saw the graduate student in the video do. The children learned aggression by modeling. This study was a big deal at the time because up until then, psychologists believed that kids really only learned through a system of rewards and punishments (the essence of operant and classical conditioning described earlier in this book).

Bandura and others after him went on to conduct several follow-up experiments, which further demonstrated that modeling is a powerful way of learning. And it goes beyond learned aggression to all domains of a child's life, including learning to like fruits and vegetables and exercising. But kids don't just automatically copy everyone and everything they see. A few components are involved in the process:

- *Attention.* To be influenced by a model, kids have to be paying attention. If the model is particularly engaging, attractive, prestigious, or perceived to be similar to the child, the child is going to be paying more attention. This helps to explain some of the powerful effects of television on children's food preferences.
- *Retention.* The child has to remember the experience. It's very obvious a child has retained something he saw or heard when he acts out a behavior from a movie or TV show or recites lines from songs or repeats a phrase someone said.
- *Reproduction.* For an action to make an impression, the child needs to be physically capable of performing the action. For example, a two-year-old won't be much influenced by watching an older child skateboard if the two-year-old doesn't yet have the physical capability to do the activity.
- *Motivation.* As with anything, motivation is a necessary ingredient for modeling to work. Promises of rewards and punishments can influence a child's motivation to model, including what's known as *vicarious reinforcement,* when a child sees the actions of a model being rewarded (or punished).
- *Confidence (or self-efficacy).* The child has to believe he can actually successfully reproduce the behavior.

## Parents as Models

Parents are particularly influential models for their children. This is especially the case in the first few years of life—before peer models take over the number one spot. Parental modeling works because it inherently includes the five components necessary for modeling to occur: attention, retention, reproduction, motivation, and self-efficacy. Your kids are paying attention to what you do. The repeated opportunities to see how you eat and play make it easy for kids to remember the experiences. Around the age of one, kids are able to feed themselves; they're a little bit older when they start to pick up on your physical activity patterns. They're motivated to copy your actions because, at least early in life, children tend to idolize their parents. Self-efficacy is high because they have already learned the basics and feel confident in their ability to feed themselves and move their bodies.

It follows, then, that one of the most powerful and also most difficult actions you can take to help your children to eat healthy and engage in physical activity on a regular basis is to do those things yourself. In fact, time and again, research has shown that the most effective strategy to prevent and reduce childhood obesity is to focus exclusively on the parent.[1-4] One study found that specifically training parents in healthy lifestyle habits led to a 10 percent weight loss in moderately obese five- to nine-year-old children—and this loss was maintained for two years.[4] Another found that a parent-centered nutritional program that focused on parental goal setting, role modeling, and positive reinforcement was essential for sustainable weight improvements in obese kids.[5] In short, if you really want your kids to be healthy, you've got to be the primary driving force to make that happen. That includes practicing the healthy behaviors yourself.

## Barriers

This is easy to say but hard to do. Parenting young children is time consuming and stressful. Perhaps no more powerful of an example helps to show the struggles that parents face in "Do as I say and as I do" is a study published by researchers from the University of Minnesota comparing the health habits of young adults with young children and those without children. This study assessed the eating and physical activity behaviors of 1,500 socioeconomically and ethically diverse young adults. Results showed that mothers drank more sugary drinks; ate a whopping 400 more calories per day; ate more saturated fat; ate fewer dark green vegetables (the healthiest kind of vegetable); and exercised less than the nonmothers. With all that bad news, it's no surprise the mothers also weighed more than the nonmothers. Fathers had lower physical activity levels but no major nutrition changes and no difference in BMI than the nonfathers. From this study and others like it, it's pretty clear that parenthood can take quite a toll on the health habits of parents—particularly the mothers of young children.

Typically the primary caregiver at home (regardless of whether they work outside the home or not), mothers are counted on to feed, nurture, and care for their kids. These responsibilities may lend to decreased free time for physical activity, increased consumption of "kid friendly" junk foods, more interrupted sleep due to nighttime feedings and awakenings, and retention of the ever-nagging leftover pregnancy weight. Given all this, it's kind of surprising that any mothers regularly exercise, eat healthy, and maintain a healthy weight. But they do. While struggling to keep it all together themselves, many parents (especially mothers) feel an obligation to be sure their children eat healthy and exercise and consequently go to great efforts to encourage kids to eat their vegetables and get moving. This all adds up to a major discrepancy and the unspoken message of "Do as I say, not as I do." When kids pick up on this disconnect, the parent's power to influence lessens.

## Commit to Healthy Changes

For the sake of your children's health, now is the best time to commit to making healthy changes for yourself. Not only can you serve as an excellent role model for your children and thus make it that much easier to get your kids to adopt healthy behaviors, but it also gives you the chance to put any long-term struggle that you have had with healthy eating, exercise, or your weight to rest once and for all. Make the commitment today, and your life will change forever. It sounds dramatic, but it's true.

The following are a few tried and true strategies to consider as you get started. Many of the recommendations are rooted in findings from the National Weight Control Registry (NWCR) (http:/www.nwcr.ws), a database that tracks more than 5,000 people who have lost at least 30 pounds and maintained the loss for at least one year. Results from several observational research studies further highlight what works and what doesn't. The tips aren't just for people trying to lose weight. Parents already at a healthy weight could adopt some of these strategies to avoid the pound-per-year weight gain that plagues most adults. By the way, most of these strategies are described elsewhere in this book as ways to help your kids adopt healthier habits.

- *Ask yourself before eating "Am I hungry?"* If not, don't eat. Eat when you're hungry and stop when you're full. It's such a basic principle, but if we all followed it, very few people would be overweight or obese. It takes no extra time out of the day or any extra effort to adopt this strategy.
- *Control portions.* Twenty years ago, a bottle of soda was 6.5 ounces and 85 calories. Today, a standard bottle of soda is 20 ounces and 250 calories. To burn the extra calories, you'd have work strenuously in the garden for 35 minutes. A typical muffin was 1.5 ounces and 200 calories. Today, it's 5 ounces and 500 calories—the difference equates to 90 minutes of vacuuming. As standard portions get larger, so do Americans. The only remedy is to pay attention to serving sizes. In fact, research suggests portion control is the greatest predictor of successful weight loss.[6] Control portions by reading nutrition labels; measuring out servings; eating only one helping; using smaller serving dishes; and resisting the urge to "clean your plate." Some initial investment of your time is needed to follow this recommendation—learning to read nutrition labels and the time spent doing so while shopping, spending the time measuring servings (although once you get an idea of what a standard measurement looks like, you'll be better at "eyeballing"), and buying the smaller plates if you don't have some already. But after the initial effort, it really requires very little extra time or energy to control portions.
- *Exercise.* More than 94 percent of participants in the NWCR increased physical activity in order to lose weight.[7] In fact, many reported walking for at least one hour per day. And for those who kept the weight off, exercise was crucial. People who dropped their fitness program put on the pounds.[7]

The hugely important recommendation to be physically active may be the most difficult one to actually implement. In fact, study after study has shown that parents are much less physically active than their nonparent peers.[8] Exercise requires a time investment, and time for most parents of young kids is in short supply. The activities you engage in every day just to take care of and play with your children count, but finding the time to commit to an exercise program not only sets a great example for your children but also helps you feel better, achieve or maintain a healthy weight, and up your efficiency. The sidebar "Counterstrategies in Action: How a Few Busy Parents Stay Active" highlights how just a few really busy mothers find creative ways to stay active.

- *Eat breakfast.* Seventy-eight percent of NWCR participants eat breakfast daily; only 4 percent never do.[9] Research suggests that breakfast eaters weigh less and suffer from fewer chronic diseases than nonbreakfast

---

### Counterstrategies in Action:
### How a Few Busy Parents Stay Active

Finding the time and energy to fit in physical activity is no simple feat for most parents. The following very busy and highly active parents offer a glimpse into their workout routines, along with a few tips on how to stay active despite the time pressures and challenges of parenthood.

- "I do a combination of things to try to get some exercising in. Sometimes, I take Xavier with me on walks or let him play in the room while I do an exercise video. Other times, I have my husband watch him while I go running or I just wait until he is napping or in bed to work out. I still have a hard time myself finding the time and energy to exercise as much as I used to before I had a child. It's hard not to feel guilty taking time to exercise by yourself when I already feel like I don't get to spend enough time with Xavier. But it keeps me happier and less crazy, so I figure that benefits him as well. No one wants a nutty mother!"

    —Amber, mother of two-year-old
    Xavier

- "I heard on a show one day that a healthy person should be putting in 10,000 steps a day. I had no idea what my steps were. So, I went out and bought a pedometer and found I did only approximately 3,000 steps! So, when Samantha went to bed, I would finish my steps on the treadmill to reach 10,000 steps. Some days, I'd only have to walk for 30 minutes—some longer. Then, I graduated from walking to running. Then, my husband signed us up for the Shamrock Shuffle in 2010— first running event ever! And by May of 2010, I'd lost 20 pounds and two dress sizes."

    —Barb, mother of 12-year-old Zach
    and 10-year-old Samantha

eaters.[10] Plus, if you eat breakfast, your kids are more likely to eat breakfast. And research shows that kids who eat breakfast also have healthier overall diets, are less likely to be overweight or obese, and perform better academically.[11]

- *Monitor intake.* One of the strongest predictors of a successful and maintained lifestyle change is monitoring dietary intake.[12] While tedious, keeping a food log is a highly effective and proven strategy. You don't have to do this every day. Just pick out a typical day, go to an online food tracker (such as thedailyplate.com or the SuperTracker at choosemyplate.gov), and enter what you ate for a 24-hour period. If you have school-aged kids, it might be fun to do this together. This gives you a chance to spend some quality time with your child and also get a sense of how well you're eating.

- *Turn off the TV.* Time spent watching TV is time spent being completely sedentary—and thus expending minimal amounts of calories—and eating.

---

- "The best way for me to exercise is to take both kids out in the jogging stroller. Once or twice a week, I meet some other moms at the walking trail (which I think is a 5K). It is halfway between where we live, so that works out great, and having someone else to walk with is a huge motivator. Pushing 60-plus pounds of kids and stroller up and down hills for an hour is a pretty good workout for me! I bring snacks and books for the kids, and we always let them run around on the trail for a few minutes when we finish ... which they like. ... I have found that it's best not to get discouraged when I can't stick with any kind of regular exercise routine. ... I realize that whatever I can do is at least something."

  —Danielle, mother of four-year-old
  Owen and one-year-old Hannah

- "I think of exercising as an essential form of 'self-care.' Like they tell you in the airplane, put on your oxygen mask first before assisting others. I need to exercise and care for myself in order to be the best mom that I can be. I get up before Matthew wakes up, and I do a quick workout. I keep a blank calendar on the fridge, and I write in what I did each day for a workout. On the same page as the calendar is printed, I have my goal in bold letters—which says: Beth's goal: four days per week—so that I can see very clearly what I am shooting for. ... I also sign myself up for events, such as races or triathlons, so that I have something to work toward. I figure if I already spent the money, then I had better put in some training so I can finish it!"

  —Beth, mother of one-year-old
  Matthew

---

Most people mindlessly consume snacks while mesmerized in front of the television, not noticing the rapidly multiplying calorie intake. Successful NWCR "losers" watch fewer than 10 hours of television per week.[13] No doubt you need some time to decompress after a long day of work or taking care of kids, but what about taking a walk, going to the park, having a family game night, or reading a book after the kids have gone to bed?

- *Retrain your brain.* A study of successful NWCR "losers" found that people who lost and kept off the most weight were "lower left" brained: organized, controlled, methodical, and disciplined.[14] Not that those of us who thrive on spontaneity or embrace clutter are doomed—it's just a matter of retraining our brains. Start by writing a grocery shopping list and sticking to it. Improve timeliness by making a coffee or tea date with a friend and getting there early. Plan your workout schedule for the next week and make a promise to stick to it. These efforts will help solidify your lifestyle change and make eating healthy and exercising a lot easier. Plus, by planning ahead, you can open up some free time (by minimizing the amount of time wasted) and plan such activities as exercise, grocery shopping, and playing with your kids into your schedule.

- *Don't wait until tomorrow to start—and no "cheating."* It's easy to put off starting a serious lifestyle change to a later date. Likewise, it's also easy to "cheat" and eat an extra piece of cake here or go to a pizza buffet there. Instead, build the less healthy foods into an eating plan that overall is nutrient rich and emphasizes moderation. Some research shows that people who don't consistently give themselves a day or two off to cheat are 150 percent more likely to maintain their weight loss.[15] Adopt a healthy lifestyle that you can stick with so you don't feel compelling urges to unwittingly sabotage your lifestyle change success.

- *Know thy friend.* A study of 12,000 people followed over 30 years concluded that obesity spreads through social ties.[16] That is, obese people tend to have obese friends. Pairs of friends and siblings of the same sex seem to have the most profound effect. The study authors suspect the spread of obesity has a lot to do with an individual's general perception of the social norms regarding the acceptability of obesity. The logic works like this: if my best friend and my sister are obese and I love and admire them all the same, then maybe it's not so bad that I gain a few pounds. You can reverse this psychological phenomenon by inviting pals to work out at the gym or go for a bike ride to stay or get fit.

- *Be optimistic!* Research suggests that people who are optimistic—that is, they have perceived control, positive expectations, empowerment, a fighting spirit, and lack of helplessness—are more successful at changing behaviors.[12]

## Peers as Models

Just as parents influence the development and preferences of children, so do peers. As children grow up, they spend more and more time with peers—and less with their parents and other adults. Peers play an increasingly important role in shaping attitudes, preferences, and behaviors. In fact, starting around the age of two, children learn what behaviors are acceptable and desirable and which aren't just by watching the behaviors and actions of their peers.

Peers "reinforce"—pay attention to, praise or criticize, or share—each other's behaviors. This reinforcement—whether positive or negative—goes a long way in shaping a child's behavior. To illustrate this, researchers had adults instruct a child's peers to pay attention to a child's helpful and cooperative behaviors and ignore mean or aggressive behaviors. As a result, the child increased his helpful behaviors and decreased his mean behaviors.[17] The same can go for eating and activity behaviors. A child who hangs out with kids who like to play sports and be physically active is more likely to be active than a child who hangs out with kids who spend hours inside playing video games. He'll be even more likely to want to continue playing if he sees that kids who play sports get recognition and hold a higher social status among peers. Likewise, a child who spends time at a friend's house where only healthy snacks are available is more likely to try those snacks if his friend is eating and enjoying them. The opposite, of course, is also true. A child who likes vegetables but gets made fun of by his friends for eating them is less likely to want to continue to eat vegetables. Highly regarded older peers, such as siblings, mentors, and babysitters, tend to play a particularly important role in influencing a child's preferences.

# Counterstrategies

Modeling is a powerful way of influencing behavior. If used effectively, modeling can help you get your kids to eat healthier and be more physically active while altogether avoiding mealtime food fights, bribes, and coercion. But you've got to be careful because modeling can also backfire if the most influential people in your child's life express the opposite types of attitudes and behaviors than the ones you hope to reinforce. The following are a few ideas to maximize the chances that your child will be positively influenced by influential people.

## Maximize Modeling's Influence

As described earlier in the chapter, modeling is most likely to influence a child's behavior with five essential ingredients: attention, ability to remember the event, ability to reproduce the behavior, motivation, and confidence in his ability to imitate the behavior. You don't have to leave it to luck whether any or all of these ingredients are present. Set the stage. When "something big" is going to happen that you want your child to emulate (such as eating vegetables or participating in activity), make sure you're prepared to maximize the chances your child will take note:

- *Minimize distractions.* For example, if you're going to be eating a family meal together with a lot of vegetables and a child's favorite uncle (who also happens to be a veggie lover) as a guest, make sure during dinner the TV and cell phones are off, no one's rushing to go anywhere or finish up quickly, and that the child is seated in close proximity to his uncle.
- *Make the occasion worth remembering.* Pair the desired activity with something fun or some memorable jingle or experience. Fast food restaurants and food marketers do a great job at thinking up catchy

gimmicks that stick (and sometimes even incorporate role modeling), such as "Breakfast of Champions" from Wheaties® or the obese-to-thin-on-the-Subway® -diet ads starring Jared. You could do something as simple as thinking of wacky names for the vegetables that you're eating at dinner, such as the "X-ray vision carrots" and "power peas" described in Chapter 5.

- *Choose reproducible activities.* Really want to get your four-year-old into sports and outdoor activities? Try taking him along to a professional baseball game. Then, invest in a T-ball set and don't be shocked if he's thrilled to learn how to play. You might not get the same result from a sport that he developmentally isn't capable of playing yet, such as football or tennis.

- *Highlight major motivators.* Think about what most motivates your child. What does he say he wants to be when he grows up? Who are his best friends? Who does he look up to most? What skill or success is he trying to achieve? Use these motivators to help show your child why it's important to practice healthy behaviors. For example, if a best friend who has a real appreciation for seafood comes over and your otherwise picky child is willing to try some shrimp (which he's never had before), you could remark that you're impressed he's become such "an adventurous eater." This recognition might inspire your child to be a little more willing to venture outside his comfort zone.

- *Assess his self-efficacy.* Your child may not latch on to a model behavior because he doesn't think he's capable. For example, a four-year-old who by all means should love soccer (all his friends play, it's his dad's favorite sport, he loved going to a professional game, and he joined the local preschool team), but who refuses to play may be suffering from low self-efficacy. One easy way to assess self-efficacy is simply to ask him: How sure are you that you can kick the ball? How hard do you think it will be to run all the way across the field?

## Check Yourself

You're a very important role model for your child. Obviously, your behaviors, such as eating healthy and being physically active, make a big difference in your child's perception of what's normal and desirable. Practicing what you preach is important. But it goes beyond simply eating vegetables now and then and trying to be active most days. Your most ingrained attitudes permeate what you say and do, even without your realizing it. Everyone has some health-related holdup—whether it's a long-standing struggle with weight, constantly dieting and trying the latest "fad," unwittingly commenting "Does this make my butt look big?" in earshot of a self-conscious daughter, refusing to eat certain fruits and vegetables, having a serious sweet tooth (which makes the idea of keeping all junk food out of the house totally undoable), loving to watch TV, hating to exercise, and the list goes on. It would be unrealistic and, quite frankly, impossible to expect parents to be perfect and to have no personal issues, challenges, or struggles in trying to keep it all together to be great role models for kids. But it's critically important to at least be aware of your biggest struggles and then make small steps to overcome them. This is especially important when your actions may have long-standing impacts on your children, such as when dieting mothers raise dieting daughters. (This phenomenon is described in more detail in Chapter 4 in the section "Dieting Mothers Raise Dieting Daughters.")

You can start tackling your most challenging health struggles with goal setting. Try this exercise: write down three goals—a nutrition goal, a fitness goal, and a behavioral goal. Try to operationalize this goal as much as possible. One way to do this is by trying to make sure your goal is SMART:

- *S—specific.* What exactly do you hope to achieve?
- *M—measurable.* How will you know if you got there?
- *A—achievable.* Make sure it's something realistic that you're going to be able to achieve with some moderate amount of effort.
- *R—results-driven.* Choose a goal that's meaningful to you. You should feel like you've really accomplished something when you achieve your goal.
- *T—time-bound.* When exactly do you want to achieve this goal? Set a specific date.

A parent who's struggled with portion control and gets limited physical activity due to a very busy work schedule might set three-week goals, such as these:

- *Nutrition:* "I'm going to eat five servings of fruits and vegetables every day for the next three weeks. I'll make this easier by making sure to eat a fruit at breakfast, a vegetable and fruit at lunch, and two vegetables at dinner."
- *Physical activity:* "My goal is to accumulate 10,000 steps each day. I'm going to purchase a pedometer and wear it every day for the next three weeks. To help increase my activity, I'll take the stairs instead of the elevator, take walks whenever possible, and play with my kids. At the end of each day, I'll record my total number of steps."
- *Behavioral:* "For the next three weeks, I'm going to ask myself "Am I hungry?" before eating snacks during the day. If I answer "No," then instead of eating, I'm going to take three minutes to do some physical activity to burn energy and distract myself from the food."

Each of these goals is "process centered" instead of "outcome centered." Process-centered goals are the small steps that lead to achieving an outcome-centered goal. For example, if the aforementioned parent had a goal to lose 10 pounds (an outcome-centered goal), each of these smaller process-centered goals would help get him closer to the weight loss goal.

## Capitalize On the Power of Peers

Starting at the age of about three or four, your child will start to feel the effects of peer influence, with increasing importance each year up through adolescence. While the parent of a teenager has limited control over the teen's friends, in the younger years parents can strategically plan playdates and other events with peers to facilitate behaviors that the parent would like to encourage. For example, if a child's friend likes a healthy food, serving it during a playdate is the perfect way to increase the chances of acceptance for the child who would otherwise shun the snack. If a child spends time with friends from a soccer league who would rather play outside and run around than sit inside and play video games, then the child is more likely to spend his time being physically active. Ultimately, friends matter. The more you can do to encourage interaction with children who practice healthy habits, the more likely your child will do the same without your having to do or say anything. On the other hand, it is important for kids not to reject other kids who may not practice healthy habits or who may struggle with being overweight. Instead, you can help your kids to be the healthy models. Only serve healthy snacks when the kids come to your house and help the kids choose physically active, fun games to play that do not require a high level of skill or fitness for the child to feel successful.

## Set Up Systems

Kids are place-specific. They understand that different places may have different rules. One way you can set the stage for healthy eating without being overly restrictive or coercive is to set up systems or "rules" at home. For example, parents keep only the healthy habits that they want to encourage in the home (such as by using some of the strategies described throughout this book) and the others (such as licking frosting at a friends' birthday party) restricted to other people's homes. This also comes into play when trying to negotiate with grandparents. As one mother interviewed for this book said, "Although we'd love for the grandparents to follow all of our rules, we think it's equally important for our children to learn that different homes have different rules. ... If they are in our home, they follow our rules." More on this and handling grandparents in Chapter 11.

# Developmental Considerations

The extent and importance of parental and peer role modeling depends on a child's age and developmental stage. In the early years, the parent is the most important role model for a child. As a child grows up, the parent still plays an important role, but peers gain increasing importance and influence (Figure 6-1).

### Infant (0–1 years)

Even though an infant is simply trying to figure out how to do such things as eat and get around, by six months, he's already started to model behaviors of others. Smile and laugh at a six-month-old and you're likely to get a broad-faced smile and giggle in return. Despite an infant's evolving brilliance, his nutrition and activity patterns won't be influenced much by modeling, although the table foods your infant eats in the second half of the first year depends a lot on the types of foods you have around the house. But enter the second year of life—and everything changes.

### Toddler (1–3 years)

Toddlers rely heavily on their parents' role modeling and behaviors to figure out what is and what isn't acceptable. Even when parents don't think so or are unaware, children at this age are paying attention to what their parents are doing and increasingly try to reproduce those behaviors.

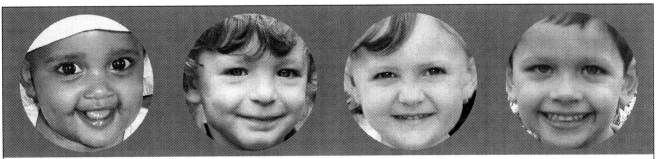

|  Infant  |  Toddler  |  Preschooler  |  School Age  |
|---|---|---|---|

- **Infant**
  - Enjoy spending time with your infant. Don't worry so much about setting a good example—yet.
  - Get ready to be a good role model as the toddler years fast approach.

- **Toddler**
  - Keep in mind that your toddler is watching and listening to you—even when you don't expect it.
  - Capitalize on peer influence by arranging playdates with friends who already do whatever it is you wish your child would do.

- **Preschooler**
  - Know your child's friends and their health behaviors.
  - Capitalize on peer modeling by encouraging your child to spend time with friends with good health habits.
  - Don't underestimate your influence as a parent.

- **School Age**
  - Consider all the role models in your child's life, including siblings, peers, teachers, parents, celebrities, and others.
  - Be a "life coach" for your child. That is, guide him as he makes decisions about activities to engage in and the friends he chooses.
  - Develop innovative ways to make eating healthy "cool."

Figure 6-1. Developmental considerations

A toddler may also have his first friends. At this age, friendship is more often a matter of convenience. Children who live near each other or whose parents are friends may spend time together. This actually provides parents a great opportunity to choose which kids a child will play with and the child is most likely to go along with it. Because kids at this age are beginning to model after peers, choosing to have a playdate with a child who's known to like a food or activity your child doesn't is a great way to try to increase acceptance in your child. Or, if a child's friend is less accepting of certain foods or activities, the next time he comes to your house, try a few of the strategies described in this book to help that child learn to try new foods and activities.

## Preschooler (3–5 years)

Developmentally, preschoolers move from the "parallel play" of toddlers—in which kids will play in the same vicinity with the same toys but pay little attention to each other—to "cooperative play"—where kids are very much paying attention to each other and are starting to develop imaginary play and scenarios that involve both kids. At this stage, peers become increasingly important in shaping the behaviors and beliefs of a child. Preschoolers also have the ability to begin choosing their friends (unlike toddlers, who tend to play with whoever is available). It is in the parents' interest to really get to know a preschooler's good friends and then take it to the next step to capitalize on the healthy behaviors of friends. For example, if a school friend really loves vegetables but your child doesn't, inviting the veggie lover over for a veggie-filled dinner might just get your kid to be a little more accepting of the veggies you offer at home.

On the other hand, spending a lot of time at a friend's house where junk foods are readily available could set your kid up for craving the food. In those cases, playdates at the park or at your house might be a better bet. Even though peers gain in importance at this age, don't underestimate your power as a parent. Kids at this age still adore their parents and want to be like them. They're watching what you're saying and doing.

### School Age (5–10 years)

As your child makes his way off to elementary school, he'll spend more time with his friends, older peers, teachers, and coaches. Each of these people will influence his health beliefs and behaviors. The role of the parent is still important, but as a child grows up, it becomes even more important for parents to think about the models in the various aspects of a child's life. While it's still imperative that the home be a place where a child sees healthy habits in action, a parent's role as "life coach" becomes more important. Your job is to help guide a child to make smart decisions with the activities he engages in and the friends he chooses. Keep this in mind as you and your child sit down to plan his activities.

# Chapter Summary

Children learn in many ways. One of them is by simply watching other people. You can skip the stress and mealtime battles of trying to get your kids to eat better and be more active by capitalizing on the power of modeling. As with any of the strategies described in this book, it's not going to "work" overnight, but over time, you'll see that your children will eat better and be more active if the influential people in their lives are committed to doing the same. Ultimately, to be successful, healthy lifestyle changes have to be a family affair, starting from the top (you) down. The following will help you move from understanding that modeling is important to actually doing it:

- Recognize that modeling is a powerful tool to help shape healthy behaviors in children.
- Don't underestimate your power as a parent in shaping your children's health behaviors. Parental goal setting, role modeling, and positive reinforcement are important components of a successful effort to optimize a child's nutrition and physical activity habits.
- Maximize the power of modeling by making sure the behavior you want modeled will stick. Remember that kids are most influenced by modeling when they're paying attention (so minimize distractions), remember what they see or hear (make mealtimes or activity times really fun), are physically and developmentally capable of reproducing the behavior (for the most part, as long as they're capable of feeding themselves and walking, you're good to go), are motivated (help them see the benefits of being healthy in the successes of potential role models), and think that they'll be successful (help them gain confidence in their abilities).
- To raise truly healthy and active kids, you've got to be healthy and active yourself. No shortage of barriers exists, but hopefully, by adopting a few of

the strategies that have worked for other parents and are described in this chapter, you'll be able to not only get your kids to eat better and be more active, but you'll also be able to optimize your own health.

- Set SMART (specific, measurable, achievable, results-driven, and time-bound) health goals and teach your school-aged children to do the same.
- Recognize your less-desirable habits and diligently strive to *not* model them for your children.
- Know your child's friends and their health behaviors. Capitalize on the power of peer influence by encouraging your child to spend more time with the friends who have the healthier habits (but don't necessarily tell your kid what you're up to.)
- Set up systems. Kids are place-specific. Because of this, you can make your home a health haven without restricting foods by allowing fewer healthy behaviors to occur as long as they're done *outside your home.*
- Tailor your strategies to your child's developmental stage.
- Partner with your child to make healthy lifestyle changes a family affair.

## Recipes: Delicious and Healthy Recipes That Adults Will Love

### Tuna Salad Lettuce Wraps

2 8-ounce cans of tuna, drained
1 15-ounce can of white cannellini beans, drained
2 celery ribs, diced
1/2 medium red onion, diced
1/4 cup sun-dried tomatoes, julienned
1/4 cup black olives, sliced in half
1/4 cup of Italian parsley, chopped
2 tablespoons of olive oil
Juice of 1/2 lemon
1 teaspoon of salt and pepper
1/2 head of red leaf lettuce, washed and dried

Mix all ingredients together in a bowl and stir. Serve on top of lettuce leaves.

### Balsamic Roasted Vegetables and Caramelized Onion Couscous Salad

*Balsamic Roasted Vegetables*

1/2 head of cauliflower, cut into small florets
2 cups of Brussels sprouts, halved
2 cups of butternut squash, cut into 1/2-inch cubes
4 tablespoons of olive oil
4 tablespoons of balsamic vinegar
1 teaspoon of salt and pepper

*Caramelized Onion Couscous Salad*

1 medium onion
1 cup of dried couscous
1 1/2 cups of water

To prepare the roasted vegetables: Preheat oven to 375 degrees. Place cauliflower, Brussels sprouts, and butternut squash into a bowl. Mix in the olive oil and balsamic vinegar until vegetables are coated. Pour vegetables onto baking sheet in a single layer. Bake for approximately 30 minutes, until vegetables are tender and browned.

To prepare the onion couscous salad: Cut onion in half and then slice lengthwise into thin slices. Heat a pot over medium heat. Place 2 tablespoons of olive oil into pot and then add onion slices. Cook onion for approximately 10 minutes, stirring occasionally, until soft and browned. Place water into pot, taking care while pouring the water, as it might spatter. Bring water to boil and then put couscous into pot. Immediately cover the pot with the lid and turn off the heat. Let sit for 7 minutes and then remove lid and fluff the couscous with a fork.

To serve, place 1 cup of couscous on a plate and then approximately 1 cup of vegetables mixture on top.

*Optional*: Sprinkle 1 tablespoon of goat cheese on top of the vegetables and serve.

## Cold Sesame Whole Wheat Noodle and Kale Salad

1/2 package of whole wheat spaghetti
1 red bell pepper, julienned
1 bunch of kale, destemmed and leaves cut into 1/2-inch ribbons
1/2 cup of chopped cilantro
1/4 cup soy sauce
Juice of 1 orange
2 tablespoons of sesame seeds
3 tablespoons of olive oil

Bring a large pot of water to boil. Add spaghetti to water and cook according to instructions on package. Approximately 5 minutes prior to the end of the cooking time for the pasta, add the kale to the water and cook for 5 minutes. Drain into colander and then put into a large mixing bowl. Add bell pepper julienned strips to the kale/pasta. Pour the soy sauce, orange juice, sesame seeds, and olive oil into bowl and mix until well coated. Add chopped cilantro and serve.

## Creamy Cauliflower Soup

1 head of cauliflower, cut into small florets
1 medium white onion, diced
1 medium potato, cut into 1/4-inch cubes
2 cloves of garlic, chopped
1 teaspoon of ground cumin
1 teaspoon of salt and pepper

Heat a large pot over medium heat. Place 2 tablespoons of olive oil into pot and then place onions into pot. Cook onions for 5 minutes and then add cauliflower, potato, and garlic. Sprinkle in cumin, salt, and pepper. Add water to pot to cover the vegetables by approximately 1/2 inch. Bring to boil and then turn to low and let simmer for 40 minutes.

Turn off stove, remove pot from heat, and let cool approximately 10 minutes. Blend soup in batches (taking care while removing the lid of the blender due to hot steam). Ladle into bowls and serve.

*Tip:* Don't have cauliflower? Substitute it with broccoli for a creamy broccoli soup.

## References

1. Golan, M., V. Kaufman, and D.R. Shahar. (2006). Childhood obesity treatment: Targeting parents exclusively v. parents and children. *Br J Nutr.* 95(5): p. 1008-15.
2. Golan, M., and S. Crow. (2004). Targeting parents exclusively in the treatment of childhood obesity: Long-term results. *Obes Res.* 12(2): p. 357-61.
3. Golan, M., A. Weizman, A. Apter, and M. Fainaru. (1998). Parents as the exclusive agents of change in the treatment of childhood obesity. *Am J Clin Nutr.* 67(6): p. 1130-5.
4. Magarey, A.M., R.A. Perry, L.A. Baur, K.S. Steinbeck, M. Sawyer, A.P. Hills, G. Wilson, A. Lee, and L.A. Daniels. (2011). A parent-led family-focused treatment program for overweight children aged 5 to 9 years: The PEACH RCT. *Pediatrics.* 127(2): p. 214-22.
5. Collins, C.E., A.D. Okely, P.J. Morgan R.A. Jones, T.L. Burrows, D.P. Cliff, K. Colyvas, J.M. Warren, J.R. Steele, and L.A. Baur. (2011). Parent diet modification, child activity, or both in obese children: An RCT. *Pediatrics.* 127(4): p. 619-27.
6. Logue, E.E., D.G. Jarjoura, K.S. Sutton, W.D. Smucker, K.R. Baughman, and C.F. Capers. (2004). Longitudinal relationship between elapsed time in the action stages of change and weight loss. *Obes Res.* 12(9): p. 1499-508.
7. The National Weight Control Registry. (n.d.). NWCR facts. Available from http://www.nwcr.ws/Research/default.htm. Retrieved September 14, 2011.
8. Bellows-Riecken, K.H., and R.E. Rhodes. (2008). A birth of inactivity? A review of physical activity and parenthood. *Prev Med.* 46(2): p. 99-110.
9. Wyatt, H.R., G.K. Grunwald, C.L. Mosca, M.L. Klem, R.R. Wing, and J.O. Hill. (2002). Long-term weight loss and breakfast in subjects in the National Weight Control Registry. *Obes Res.* 10(2): p. 78-82.

10. Timlin, M.T., and M.A. Pereira. (2007). Breakfast frequency and quality in the etiology of adult obesity and chronic diseases. *Nutr Rev. 65*(6 Pt 1): p. 268-81.

11. Rampersaud, G.C., M.A. Pereira, B.L. Girard, J. Adams, and J.D. Metzl. (2005). Breakfast habits, nutritional status, body weight, and academic performance in children and adolescents. *J Am Diet Assoc. 105*(5): p. 743-760; quiz: p. 761-2.

12. Tinker, L.F., M.C. Rosal, A.F. Young, M.G. Perri, R.E. Patterson, L. van Horn, A.R. Assaf, D.J. Bowen, J. Ockene, J. Hays, and L. Wu. (2007). Predictors of dietary change and maintenance in the Women's Health Initiative Dietary Modification Trial. *J Am Diet Assoc. 107*(7): p. 1155-66.

13. Raynor, D.A., S. Phelan, J.O. Hill, and R.R. Wing. (2006). Television viewing and long-term weight maintenance: Results from the National Weight Control Registry. *Obesity (Silver Spring). 14*(10): p. 1816-24.

14. Mithers, C. (2005). The mind of the successful dieter. *O, The Oprah Magazine.* Available at http://www.oprah.com/health/Inside-the-Minds-of-Successful-Dieters-How-to-Think-Thin.

15. Gorin, A.A., S. Phelan, R.R. Wing, and J.O. Hill. (2004). Promoting long-term weight control: Does dieting consistency matter? *Int J Obes Relat Metab Disord. 28*(2): p. 278-81.

16. Christakis, N.A., and J.H. Fowler. (2007). The spread of obesity in a large social network over 32 years. *N Engl J Med. 357*(4): p. 370-9.

17. Furman, W., and L. Gavin. (1989). *Peers Influence on Adjustments and Development.* New York: Wiley.

# THE EVERYDAY MISTAKES

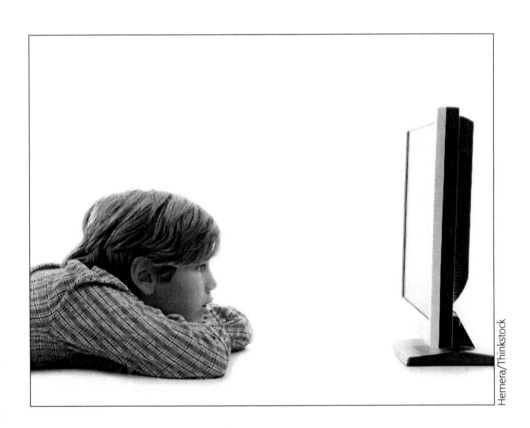

Hemera/Thinkstock

## Part Three

# 7

# Mistake #7— Catering to Picky Eaters

June Cleaver:  *"Dear, do you think all parents have this much trouble?"*

Ward Cleaver:  *"No, just parents with children."*

*—Leave It to Beaver*, late 1950s and early 1960s family sitcom

Marion, 10, eats mostly carbs. She recently declared herself a vegetarian and has since refused all meat products. Her sister, Annie, 8, loves meat—and a lot of it. She hates pizza, won't touch pasta, and frequently insists on a very specific breakfast of one egg sunny-side up, three slices of bacon, and a cup of fruit. When eating out, she's quick to order steamed mussels (to the surprise of anyone who doesn't know her), while her sister carefully scans the children's menu, which is usually full of her favorite white carbs, such as French fries, pasta with marinara sauce, cheese pizza, or macaroni and cheese. Although they're sisters who share their genetic makeup and home environment, these two kids have very different eating preferences. If their mom always tried to accommodate each of their requests, she might as well give up her day job and become a short-order cook. But if she ignores the requests, she may be setting the stage for unpleasant mealtime battles. With some very focused and consistent parenting strategies, both kids can learn to choose and enjoy a healthy and balanced eating plan, even when their parents aren't looking over their shoulders.

## Picky Eating

Picky eaters—the kids with a limited repertoire of "acceptable" foods (and these are usually high-saturated-fat, high-salt, low-nutrient-density foods) and a blatant refusal to even try any other type of food to the point that it interferes with normal family functioning—can wreak havoc on a peaceful family meal.

The problem is exceedingly common; about one-third of toddlers are "picky," while about two-thirds of parents with toddlers describe one or more eating problems, such as not enjoying mealtimes, strong food preferences, refusal to eat, requests for specific foods but then refusal to actually eat those foods, and ending a meal after only a few bites.[1] While these troubles are most pronounced in toddlerhood (with about 50 percent of kids described by their parents as picky between 19 and 24 months), they often can extend into preschool and elementary school years (about 20 percent of kids are described by their parents as picky at 8 years of age).[1]

Parents have historically taken one of two approaches when dealing with these picky eaters—either coerce them into trying other foods (which ends up being counterproductive, as previously described in this book) or cater to a child's food demands (i.e., rely on a child's "preferred foods" in an attempt to ensure the child doesn't otherwise starve). It turns out that parents can start to overcome picky eating by refusing to buy into "just for kids" foods. These are the foods that manufacturers have carefully formulated to appeal to a child's innate taste for sweet and salty—frequently with a disregard for a child's nutritional needs.

## The Mistake of Resorting to "Just for Kids" Foods

Food marketers, restaurants, and other outlets in the business of selling food to easily influenced and demanding children want you to believe such a thing as "just for kids" food exists. Not only does this perception resonate with kids who like the idea of something being made just for them, but it also makes it easy on parents, especially those who have picky kids—"Finally, something that he'll eat!" The problem is that these foods that are "just for kids" are usually of a low nutritional value. The food tends to be fried, highly processed, full of additives, and void of fruits and especially vegetables. But these are the foods that kids like. If parents give into their children's requests and resort to "just for kids" foods, they pretty much guarantee that the child will eat a nutrient-poor meal. It will also further solidify their unwillingness to try anything new. The most effective way to break this cycle is twofold: refuse to prepare separate meals and don't trust children's menus.

## Banishing Separate Meals

An unscientific ParentCenter.com poll asked: do you make separate meals for your child? With nearly 8,000 replies, half said "Yes." The true number is probably higher. No one likes mealtime food battles, and managing picky eaters is no simple feat. It's one thing to advise someone to adopt the mealtime rule of "Take it or leave it," but it's another thing to actually deal with the outcomes. It's possible that a child may decide to "leave it" and begrudgingly refuse to eat or may "take it" and complain with every bite. But as Nancy Gibbs of *Time* magazine wrote in an excellent piece describing the benefits of the family meal, "The food-court mentality—Johnny eats a burrito, Dad has a burger, and Mom picks pasta—comes at a cost."[2] And that cost seems to be a lot more than a few extra empty calories.

## Value of a Family Meal

Researchers from the University of Illinois explored just what role the family meal has on the health status of children and adolescents. They compiled the results of 17 studies, which together assessed the relationship between family meals and eating patterns, obesity, and disordered eating on over 180,000 children and adolescents. They found that kids who ate at least three meals per week with at least one adult family member had healthier overall eating habits, including fewer sweets, fried foods, and soda and decreased rates of obesity and eating disorders.[3] Other studies also support that eating meals with family is associated with greater consumption of fruits, vegetables, and other nutritious foods—especially when the child eats food similar to his parents.[4] Family meals also offer parents an excellent opportunity to model healthy eating habits and a healthy relationship with food. In fact, one study found that parents who ate more fruits and vegetables had kids who ate more fruits and vegetables—and the association between parent and child intake strengthened with an increasing number of family meals.[5] On the other hand, if a parent gives in to the begging for a "special" meal, the family misses out on the opportunity to broaden a child's tastes and promote the willingness to try new foods.

Kids who regularly eat meals with their families are not only healthier, but they also do better in school, develop more advanced language skills, and are less likely to drink alcohol or experiment with other drugs as teenagers.[6]

## Finding Time to Eat Together

While many obstacles can get in the way of eating a meal together as a family, parents can make efforts to minimize them. The following is a five-step plan to help organize the family's hectic schedules to make family meals a frequent occurrence at your house:

- *Commit to making eating together a priority.* That sounds obvious and simple enough, but if you don't commit to at least three meals per week together (or whatever number is doable at your house), then barriers to eating together will become overwhelming and you may fall into the old habits.

- *Set a time for dinner.* Choose a time that's most likely to have everyone present, even if that means you push off dinner until 7:30 or eat earlier at 5:00. Kids can adjust snack times and amounts to make sure that they're hungry (but not ravenous) for dinner. If at all possible, parents should plan their work schedules so that, whenever possible, at least one parent is home for a sit-down dinner on most nights. Think twice before signing a child up for yet another activity that will extend into dinnertime.

- *Plan meals ahead.* The chances of coming home after a long day of work and exerting the mental focus and energy to think up what to make for dinner and then find all the right ingredients are low for most people. Spend an hour once per week to come up with a menu of meals for the coming week. Consider putting together a family calendar where not only do you write down everyone's activities, but you also write down the planned menu for each day. This way everyone knows what to expect and you can maximize the chances that you'll be able to quickly put together a healthy meal for the family on most days.

- *Shop efficiently.* On your weekly shopping trip, buy all the ingredients you'll need for the week so you can save time by not having to make repeated trips to the store. Increase the likelihood that your picky eater will actually eat what you prepare by bringing him along to the store and giving him choices of which healthy foods he'd most like to eat. (For example, if you're planning a steamed vegetable as a side for a dinner, give him the choice between carrots or squash or the choice between broccoli or cauliflower.)

- *Multitask preparation time.* The time required to make a meal after a long day can be a major barrier to cooking a family meal when it's much easier to get takeout or go for fast food. Make it easy on yourself by choosing easy-to-prepare meals. (See the recipes in this chapter for some dinner ideas that are simple and sure to be well received by the kids.) And involve your kids in meal preparation. You can speed up meal prep time, teach them how to prepare healthy foods, and spend some quality family time together and catching up on what's going on in their lives.

# Dealing With Children's Menus

The good news is that many families figure out ways to eat meals together. The less exciting reality is that a large proportion of these meals are eaten outside the home, where families have a lot less control or knowledge of what exactly is in the food. Most Americans spend nearly half of their food budget and a third of total calories eating out. On any given day, about 30 percent of children eat fast food at least once.[7] While it's still possible to experience many of the benefits of a family meal even when the food is eaten at a restaurant or fast-food place, parents must be more conscientious to ensure that the child has a balanced meal. Considering that fast food is typically higher in calories, saturated fat, sugar, quantity, and oftentimes palatability than prepared-at-home meals, how can parents eat out with their kids without blowing their efforts to feed their children healthy foods? The first step is to not trust children's menus because they typically consist of hamburgers, chicken nuggets, macaroni and cheese, and French fries—foods that cater to a child's love of grease, free toys, and catchy packaging.

## The Biggest Culprits

The Center for Science in the Public Interest (CSPI) assessed the nutritional quality of children's menus at the 25 largest chain restaurants in the United States. The researchers evaluated the nutritional quality of all possible combinations of each entree, side item, and beverage from each restaurant's children's menu. While unhealthy high-saturated-fat, high-sodium entrees and sides, such as fried chicken and French fries, dominated the menus, some healthier options frequently were available, including grilled chicken, seafood, fruits, and vegetables. Alarmingly, soft drinks were most often paired with children's menus. Soft drinks not only contain large amounts of sugar (and calories), but they also often contain caffeine and other additives. Many restaurants offered milk, but half offered only the high-fat whole and 2% versions. Ninety-three percent of studied meals were high in calories, 45 percent exceeded recommendations for saturated and trans fat, and 86 percent were high in sodium.[8] Figure 7-1 offers a summary of the study results. In most cases, it's difficult but not impossible to choose a healthy meal off the children's menu at many restaurants. Figure 7-2 highlights a few of the healthier children's meals the researchers uncovered.

Two popular movements may make navigating restaurant menus somewhat easier for parents. First off, restaurants are increasingly required to provide nutrition information in an easy-to-see location. Parents can use this information to ensure healthy food choices for children. When this information is available, parents tend to guide their kids toward choosing healthier meals.

| Rank (by revenue of chain) | Restaurant | Meal/ Combo Name | Total Number of Meal Combos | Number of Meals That Exceed Calorie Limit (>430 calories) | Percent of Meals That Exceed Calorie Limit (>430 calories) |
|---|---|---|---|---|---|
| 2 | KFC* | Kids Laptop Meal | 440 | 440 | 100% |
| 13 | Sonic | Wacky Pack | 48 | 48 | 200% |
| 18 | Jack in the Box | Kid's Meal | 24 | 24 | 100% |
| 24 | Chick-fil-A | Kid's Meal | 3 | 3 | 100% |
| 8 | Taco Bell | Kid's Meal | 3 | 3 | 100% |
| 12 | Chili's | Pepper Pals | 700 | 658 | 94% |
| 7 | Wendy's | Kids' Meal | 30 | 28 | 93% |
| 1 | McDonald's | Happy Meal and Mighty Kids Meal | 40 | 37 | 93% |
| 3 | Burger King** | Kids Meal and Big Kids Meal | 49 | 45 | 92% |
| 22 | Dairy Queen | Deeqs Kids' Meal | 18 | 16 | 89% |
| 15 | Arby's | Kids Meal | 32 | 22 | 69% |
| 22 | Denny's *** | The D-Zone at Denny's | 52 | 31 | 60% |
| 5 | Subway | Fresh Fit for Kids | 18 | 6 | 33% |
| Total/Average | | | 1,474 | 1,378 | 93% |

*For KFC, the items offered for the children's menu vary between outlets.

**Burger King's children's meal (macaroni and cheese, apple, fries, and 1% milk) was introduced after this study's data collection was complete and was not included. This meal would qualify as a healthier option.

***Includes breakfast and lunch/dinner combos, and beverages aren't included as a part of children's meals.

*Source*: Wootan, M, A. Batada, and E. Marchlewicz. (2008). *Kids' Meals: Obesity on the Menu*. Washington, DC: Center for Science in the Public Interest.

Figure 7-1. Nutritional quality of children's meals at the largest chains

| Restaurant | Meals That Met Nutrition Standards # (%) | Description of Meals That Met Standards |
|---|---|---|
| Subway | 8 (44%) | • Ham mini-sub with juice box and apple slices or raisins<br>• Roast beef mini-sub and juice box with any side (apple slices, raisins, yogurt)<br>• Turkey mini-sub and juice box with any side (apple slices, raisins, yogurt) |
| Chili's | 3 (<1%) | • Grilled chicken sandwich with apple juice and corn kernels or mandarin oranges or pineapple |
| Denny's* | 2 (4%) | • Pancakes with meat and with maple syrup<br>• Macaroni and cheese with grapes |
| Arby's | 2 (6%) | • Popcorn chicken or junior roast beef sandwich with fruit cup and fruit juice |

*At Denny's, beverages are sold separately, thus nutrition totals for meals don't include beverages.

*Source*: Wootan, M., A. Batada, and E. Marchlewicz. (2008). *Kids' Meals: Obesity on the Menu*. Washington, DC: Center for Science in the Public Interest.

Figure 7-2. Healthier children's meals at top restaurants

For example, one study comparing theoretical restaurant ordering with a menu that contained calorie information versus one that didn't, parents with the labeled menu chose 102 fewer calories for their children than parents who weren't privy to calorie information.[9]

Secondly, more restaurants are beginning to turn to the healthier choices as the default menu option. For example, McDonald's now offers apple dippers and low-fat milk as a default side and drink for a Happy Meal® (though, unfortunately, the standard meal still includes a side order of French fries as well). This change makes it a little bit easier for parents and kids to identify and choose healthier options.

### Best Chances

The best chances to get your kids to eat healthy while eating out occur when you set the stage for a successful experience. First off, when deciding where to take the kids, consider choosing from a premade list of kid-friendly restaurants that offer healthy options. This way, you can minimize mealtime stress (because you don't have to feel like you're putting anyone out if the kids don't behave) but also know you'll be able to help the kids find something reasonably healthy to eat. If you want to frequent a fancy restaurant, no problem. Try to choose a time when the kids are the most cooperative, and you may even consider offering them a light and healthy snack before you head out. That way, they won't be too hungry and impatient while waiting for the food; you can minimize the splurge on bread or other appetizers; and you can be sure they'll at least be exposed to something healthy.

While it's great if you can go to a restaurant that offers a healthy children's menu, in many cases, the restaurant will either not offer a children's menu or the items will be the typically nutrient-poor and calorie-dense "standard fare." In these cases, don't be scared to order off the adult menu. In fact, you and your kids may be better off if you choose a meal together and share it. By ordering from the adult menu, you have the chance to maximize a child's exposure to different foods and teach a basic life skill about how to choose a healthy meal.

# The School Lunch

While eating at school is a little bit different from eating out, it's worth discussing the status of foods served at school. Historically a saturated- and trans-fat-laden, nutrient-poor makeup of surplus food products, the school lunch was a source of excessive calories and was at least as bad as fast food restaurants in its limited healthy offerings. But these days, a revolution is under way in the nutritional composition of the school lunch. With the publication of the Institute of Medicine Report on school lunch[10] and subsequent passage of the Healthy, Hunger-Free Kids Act in 2011, the new school lunch is more of a balanced, healthy meal. The USDA has set calorie limits and offers more fruits, vegetables, and whole grains and less salt. In fact, it turns out that in many cases, school lunches are healthier than the typical packed lunch a child brings from home. So much so that one Chicago school has even banned homemade lunches while one Tucson school only allows packed lunches if their contents are free of white flour, refined sugar, or other processed foods. While this may be overreach by some school districts, the point is well taken. We all need to do better to ensure that our kids are eating a healthy, balanced diet. While that starts at home, it extends into the school day, where a child spends nearly one-third of his time. The sidebar "The Healthy Lunchbox" offers a few tips on how to prepare a healthy, balanced lunch for your child. It's also worth taking a look at your child's school menu and deciding for yourself if your child is better off purchasing a school lunch.

# Counterstrategies

So, how do you turn all this information into action to get your picky eater to be a little bit more adventurous? The following are a few ideas.

## Get to the Root of It

People will typically reject foods for one of three reasons: they dislike the flavor and/or appearance of the food; they have a fear of negative consequences from eating the food (such as stomach upset); or they're disgusted by the food (due to potential contamination or the thought of where it came from).[1] If a child consistently rejects particular healthy foods, try to understand "why."

Two reasons that "just for kids" foods appeal to children are that they typically taste good (because they usually are loaded with salt, sugar, and/or fat) and because they're usually packaged in some creative kid-friendly way. You can make a "boring" healthy food delicious and highly appealing to a child if you make it taste good (see Chapter 8 for more strategies on how to do this) and make it fun to eat (review Chapter 5 for tips). The recipes in this chapter are designed to help you give it a try.

## The Healthy Lunchbox

You might have considered on more than one occasion what to put in your child's lunchbox or really whether to make a lunch at all and instead opt for hot lunch. While a hot lunch is certainly easier, sending your child to school with a lunch at least a couple of times per week gives you an excellent opportunity to help shape his eating habits. (By the way, that goes for you too. Bring your own lunch to work instead of eating out and you're likely to have a much more balanced, lower-calorie, less-expensive meal.) Of course, it's a delicate balance. The decision between what you would like your child to eat versus what you think he or she will actually consume influences your choices. Should you put in the carrots you know Johnny will reject just so he's exposed to the vegetables? How about his favorite chocolate chip cookies simply because you know how happy it will make him? Without you there looking over your kids' shoulders and supervising intake, the school lunch really is their opportunity to exert some control over food choices. (They can choose to trash, barter, or eat your carefully planned meal.) And now might just be your chance to further solidify your efforts to raise healthy eaters—free of food battles and junk food binges.

### Some Basic Tips

- *Aim for balance.* Try to include something from each of the major food groups—a whole grain; a protein-containing food, such as meat, beans, or legumes; a fruit; a vegetable; and a dairy product or another calcium-containing food—in your child's lunchbox every day. Even if he chooses not to eat it all, your child will start to pick up on what a balanced meal includes. Consider allowing one portion-controlled sugary or "junk food" item to be included on occasion depending on your feeding philosophies and your child's preferences.

Perhaps a child refuses a specific food or type of food due to a food allergy or intolerance. If this is the case, eating the food will cause a child physical discomfort, such as abdominal pain or diarrhea. If you notice patterns of refusal (for example, a child refuses only milk products or certain textures of foods) or if a child complains of physical pains after eating a food, it's worth mentioning to a pediatrician to better assess if your child suffers from an underlying condition.

Around seven or eight, a child may begin to refuse certain foods due to concern where the food came from. For example, Marion decided to become a vegetarian once she realized that meat came from cows, like the ones that she sees grazing in the fields on her way to school. After that, the idea of eating a burger disgusted her. In these cases, a parent may prefer to cater to a child's avoidance of certain foods. However, without understanding *why* Marion all of the sudden decided to refuse meat, her mom might chalk it up to her pickiness and then either force her to eat certain meat products or begrudgingly prepare her something separate at mealtimes. When accommodating preferences such as these, a parent should still aim to provide a balanced and wholesome diet for the whole family.

- *Increase exposure to healthy foods.* A prepared lunch gives you a perfect opportunity to continue to expose your child to a variety of healthy foods. As stated in a review article advocating that children be repeatedly exposed to a variety of healthy foods, "[C]hildren like what they know and they eat what they like."[11] One of the best ways that parents can help their children to develop healthy eating habits is to repeatedly expose them to a wide variety of foods. While children may not accept the novel food on the first try, with repeated attempts and familiarity with the food, they'll become more likely to develop a preference for it. Use lunchtime as an opportunity to expose your children to a small amount of a previously rejected food. Even if they choose not to eat, mere exposure may help to increase the chances they'll appreciate it in the future. It usually takes 15 to 20 tries for a child to accept a previously rejected food.

- *Teach portion control.* A study of preschool-aged children found that when portion size was doubled, the children ate 25 to 29 percent more than the age-appropriate portions of the foods, even though they consumed only two-thirds of smaller portions of the meal.[12] Preparing a lunch gives you a perfect opportunity to pay attention to portion control. Use baggies; attempt to measure out what a standard portion of the food actually is; and try to pick up some inherently portion-controlled items for the lunchbox, such as applesauce and string cheese.

- *Involve your child.* The best way to ensure your kids will actually eat the food you put in their lunchbox is to give them some control of what goes in there. Even the pickiest eaters enjoy some healthy foods. Be sure to include at least one healthy item your child loves. And next time you head out to the grocery store, ask for your kids' input into what *healthy food* they'd like to have in their lunchboxes. The mere exercise

*(cont.)*

## Undo Picky Eating

Just because a child is a picky eater now doesn't mean it always has to be that way. You can begin to undo picky eating with a few of the following strategies:

- *Keep mealtimes relaxing and enjoyable.* Have fun together as a family and don't dwell on the food. If the child refuses the meal, don't make a big deal out of it.
- *Choose at least one food you know your child will like.* This way, not only do you assure that your child will eat something during the meal, but it also shows your child you do care about his preferences when planning meals.
- *Engage your child in meal preparation.* For example, while grocery shopping, ask your child to pick out one fruit or vegetable that he would like to try at dinner that night. Or invite your children into the kitchen to help prepare the meal.
- *Use food bridges.* Once a food is accepted, find similarly colored or flavored "food bridges" to expand the variety of foods a child will eat. For example, if a child likes pumpkin pie, try mashed sweet potatoes and then mashed carrots.

---

### The Healthy Lunchbox *(cont.)*

of helping them sort through their favorites (many of which are likely sugar- and salt-ridden) will help them learn what types of foods are healthy for their bodies and which ones are less healthy. But don't make the sugary and salty favorites completely off limits, as this will encourage going for the stuff when you're not looking. Just remember portion control and moderation. When you ask your child how his day went, also consider asking about lunch. What did he eat and what did he throw out? You might be surprised by what your kids tell you.

- *Make eating healthy fun.* Kids, especially preschool- and elementary-aged children, love foods that are packaged in a fun way. Perhaps your child will be more likely to eat the baby carrots if you package them in a funnily decorated baggy. Or maybe your child will totally reject celery and raisins if offered separately, but when presented as "ants on a log" (celery with peanut butter and raisins), he might eat the food up. Just be careful to avoid marketing tricks in which junk foods are packaged with your child's favorite characters (such as SpongeBob fruit snacks). This just helps your child love the sugary stuff even more. These foods are acceptable but might be better offered in their own boring, clear plastic baggy.

  If you have older kids, work on transitioning the job of preparing lunch from you to them. Share with them the lunchbox requirement of balance and let them decide what goes in. Before transitioning the responsibility, you could give them a quick lesson on the things you consider when making a lunch, such as going for high-fiber whole grain rather than the highly processed white version, leaner meats, fruits and vegetables of different colors, etc. Initially, you might inspect to make sure lunch doesn't just include several Twinkies and a soda, but eventually, you might want to slowly transition to trusting their choices and periodically giving a surprise inspection. Remember, for the most part, kids will only have available to them items they can find in the house. This offers you a good opportunity to double-check whether you're maximizing access to healthy foods versus

- *Spice it up.* Do your best to make the foods taste good. It sounds simple enough, but ask around and you'll quickly find people permanently turned off to fresh fish after childhood meals of unappetizing frozen fish sticks or others unwilling to try fresh steamed vegetables after too many dinners forced to eat the limp and overcooked kind.
- *Offer it often.* Children learn to like what's familiar to them. Just because a child rejects a food once, don't label it "rejected." Instead, continue to reintroduce it and expect that it will take about 15 times before the child will accept it.

Despite all this, if kids still continue to refuse healthy foods, it's not worth a fight. Hold firm on refusing to make "just for kids" foods and then patiently

the more highly processed and less healthy versions. (Don't forget to also teach your kids to throw in a couple of ice packs to keep perishable foods cold. One study of preschoolers' lunches found that a lot of kids go to school with a lunch at risk for high spoilage. By the time the kids actually ate their food, more than 90 percent of lunches contained items that were above the safe zone, leaving those kids highly susceptible to food-borne illness.[13])

**Some Sample Lunches**

Out of lunch ideas? The following are some easy-to-make lunches that follow the preceding suggestions (including an *optional* relatively healthy sweet snack which you may choose to include or leave out depending on your preferences) and could help your children expand their food preferences:

- Peanut butter and banana sandwich with natural peanut butter, sliced banana, and whole grain bread cut into fun-sized heart shapes to show your child a little extra love. Include a few baby carrots and a(n) (optional) package of fruit snacks. Throw in 50 cents to buy milk.
- Turkey sandwich with hummus and tomato on whole grain bread. Add some string cheese, some crackers, an apple, and a(n) (optional) couple of fig bars. Include a child-sized water bottle with a squirt of lemon.
- Try last night's leftovers. Don't forget to include a plastic fork/spoon/knife (if needed) and an ice pack to keep it cold. Add a few cherry tomatoes, a hard-boiled egg, and some applesauce. Consider a low-sugar pudding cup.
- How about a little adventure with a couple California rolls and edamame along with red grapes, an (optional) cup of low-sugar Jell-O®, and some milk money?

These are just a few ideas to help you get started. But don't feel limited—consider these tips as well as other food priorities that are important to you. Be creative! You and your child might just uncover a few fun new creations that get you even closer to your goal of raising healthy eaters.

continue to practice some of the strategies to undo picky eating while also providing a multivitamin with iron at bedtime. Think of it as a type of fruit and vegetable insurance while you're working on teaching your children to prefer a healthy, balanced diet.

**Choose Foods Wisely**

Eating out is a major activity of modern life. While food eaten away from home tends to be less healthy than food prepared at home, eating out doesn't have to interfere with your efforts to teach children to eat a healthy, balanced diet. The following are a few tips to help you and your family eat healthy when eating out:

- Ask for water or order fat-free or low-fat milk, unsweetened tea, or other drinks without added sugars.
- Ask for whole wheat bread for sandwiches.
- In a restaurant, start your meal with a salad packed with veggies to help control hunger and feel satisfied sooner. Ask for salad dressing to be served on the side.
- Choose main dishes that include vegetables, such as a stir-fry, kebobs, or pasta with a tomato sauce.
- Order steamed, grilled, or broiled dishes instead of fried or sautéed dishes.
- Avoid creamy sauces and gravies.
- Choose a small or medium portion.
- Avoid the all-you-can-eat buffet.
- Order an appetizer or side dish instead of an entree.
- Share a main dish with a friend (or child).
- If you can chill the extra food right away, take leftovers home in a "doggy bag."
- When your food is served, set aside or pack half of it to go immediately.
- Resign from the Clean Plate Club—when you've eaten enough, leave the rest.
- Choose fruits for dessert most often.
- On long commutes or shopping trips, pack some fresh fruits, sliced vegetables, low-fat string cheese sticks, or a handful of unsalted nuts to help you avoid stopping for high-calorie, low-nutrition snacks.

See the sidebar "Counterstrategies in Action: Creating Peaceful and Healthy Mealtimes" for tips and ideas from parents who have refused to cater to picky eaters.

# Developmental Considerations

Picky eating and the effects of foods marketed to kids vary based on a child's developmental stage. What's normal at two years of age can be detrimental at eight. A basic understanding of child development goes a long way toward tailoring your approach to help broaden your child's food preferences (Figure 7-3).

### Infant (0–1 years)

Breastfed infants are less likely to be picky once solids are introduced compared with formula-fed babies. While about 20 percent of babies are "picky" at four to six months of age, the majority of infants are eager to try a variety of new foods.[1] Consider it a golden opportunity to expose your baby to as many flavors as possible before neophobia sets in during toddlerhood.

Introduce new flavors to an infant slowly and one at a time. Help your child's cognitive and language development by saying aloud the names of foods. Meals at this age should last at least 10 to 15 minutes.

## Counterstrategies in Action:
## Creating Peaceful and Healthy Mealtimes

Picky eating is a way of life for many young children. But that doesn't mean it has to make your life miserable. Check out some tips from parents who have successfully dealt with picky eaters without mealtime battles and heartache.

- *Get to the root of it.* Sometimes, picky eaters are picky for a reason. Take four-year-old Anthony, who refused to eat eggs. Trying to get him to take even a bite led to intense food battles. Incidentally, Anthony also had a severe case of eczema, for which he was evaluated by a pediatric allergist. The allergist did a skin test, which revealed that Anthony is allergic to eggs. This may explain, at least in part, Anthony's intense egg refusal.

- *Undo picky eating.* Sarah, mother of three children (ages three, four, and seven), shares her approach to dealing with picky eaters: "I always ask each kid to pick out one ingredient each, and I will customize an entire meal around that ingredient. They go shopping with me, and they help me prepare, make, and serve the meal. I am a personal chef [lucky kids!], so I have my kids put on my apron and chef hat. They really love that!"

- *Choose foods wisely.* Eating out has become commonplace for American kids. That reality doesn't have to be a nutritional disaster. In fact, you can even use it as an opportunity to broaden your kids' nutritional repertoire. Take it from Janice, mother of three young kids (ages two to six): "We eat out relatively often with our kids. We avoid kids' menus at most restaurants since the options tend to be unhealthy and of poor quality. Our children will share an adult entree or we will order two entrees and an appetizer and our family of five will share everything. This gives the kids an opportunity to try more new foods and increases the chances of them finding something they really like!"

## Toddler (1–3 years)

Toddlers are infamous for their strong-willed resistance to trying new foods. With about half of 18-month-olds showing picky traits, the number continues to climb until about three years old, when the rate of pickiness slowly tapers. During this trying time, parents will do best if they're patient with their toddlers, recognize neophobia is normal at this age, and continue to attempt to expose a child to a wide variety of foods while also being prepared for the reality that the child may not accept those foods. Resist the temptation to prepare the same requested food day in and day out and instead try to pair favorite foods with other types of foods. (For example, a child who insists on peanut butter and jelly might be willing to try a peanut butter and banana sandwich. A child hooked on macaroni and cheese might not mind if you add a small amount of canned tuna. Then, how about some finely chopped cooked broccoli?)

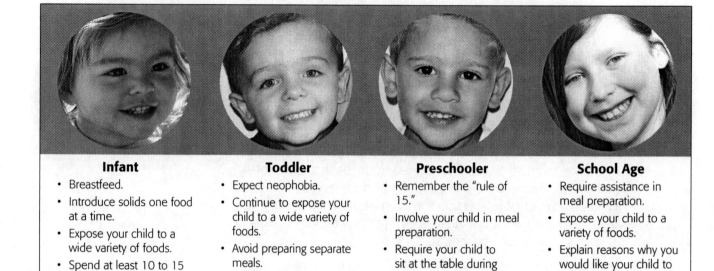

| Infant | Toddler | Preschooler | School Age |
|---|---|---|---|
| • Breastfeed.<br>• Introduce solids one food at a time.<br>• Expose your child to a wide variety of foods.<br>• Spend at least 10 to 15 minutes on meals.<br>• Name the foods your child is eating to help him develop language skills. | • Expect neophobia.<br>• Continue to expose your child to a wide variety of foods.<br>• Avoid preparing separate meals.<br>• Keep mealtimes relaxing and enjoyable.<br>• Keep the TV off during meals. | • Remember the "rule of 15."<br>• Involve your child in meal preparation.<br>• Require your child to sit at the table during mealtimes for at least 15 to 20 minutes, but don't force him to eat. | • Require assistance in meal preparation.<br>• Expose your child to a variety of foods.<br>• Explain reasons why you would like your child to try a particular food.<br>• Use mealtimes to share stories and experiences. |

Figure 7-3. Developmental considerations

Even though this is a highly stressful stage of development for many families, it's important to keep mealtimes as relaxing and enjoyable as possible. Require that children sit at the table for at least 15 to 20 minutes, even if your toddler refuses to even take a bite of any foods. Turn the television off and begin to teach your child mealtime manners. Also, help your child's speech development by continuing to use family mealtimes as an opportunity to expose your child to conversation and language.

### Preschooler (3–5 years)

Around the time of preschool, most kids outgrow their pickiness and become willing again to try some new foods. The key is to remember the "rule of 15"—it takes about 15 to 20 exposures for a child to learn to like a previously rejected food. After about four years of age, a child becomes increasingly less interested in trying new foods and may be less likely to learn to like previously rejected foods.

Many of your strategies for toddlers can carry over to the preschool years. Start by making mealtimes fun and low stress. Encourage your preschooler to help in some way with meal preparation—whether by helping pick which foods to prepare, choosing serving size, or putting napkins on the table. Again, make sure to turn the television off and require that the child stay seated during the mealtime. Use the time to talk about what happened in the neighborhood or at preschool. Keep the focus off of what or how much the child is eating, although it's appropriate to remind a distracted child to eat (for example, "Dylan, would you like to try those carrots?" but not "Dylan, eat your carrots!").

### School Age (5–10 years)

By the time a child is ready to start school, his eating habits are fairly well established. In fact, after about age eight, it's increasingly difficult to undo picky eating habits.[1] That's not to say to give up on your older kids. Rather, it will require a little bit of extra patience and some effective strategies to help kids at this age become more willing to try new foods. A couple of ideas include capitalizing on the power of peer influence and providing information on the reasons why you would like a child to try a particular food.

The school-aged child can play an increasingly active role in family mealtimes. Encourage (or require) your child to assist in meal preparation at least once per week—whether by helping make the food, setting or clearing the table, or washing the dishes. Use your mealtime together to talk about each other's day and plan for fun activities during the weekend. Be sure to provide a wholesome and balanced family meal, but then leave it at that. Resist the urge to focus the attention around food or what someone did or didn't eat.

# Chapter Summary

A goal of this chapter was to help you develop foolproof ways to encourage healthy eating (no matter where your child ends up eating) while also being able to avoid mealtime battles when a picky eater refuses to eat.

The following recaps the major points of this chapter:
- Recognize that most foods that cater to children are unhealthy. Refuse to buy "just for kids" foods or at least stop and do a quick nutrition evaluation of the product first.
- Don't prepare separate meals for picky eaters. Instead, make sure to include at least one healthy item your child likes at each meal and gently encourage (but don't force) him to try new tastes.
- Commit to eating a family meal together at least three times per week or, ideally, more frequently.
- Make mealtimes relaxing and enjoyable. Think of the time as an opportunity to connect as a family and facilitate optimal child development. Don't waste your energy on mealtime food fights.
- When eating out, be careful when ordering off of the children's menu. When possible, share a healthy adult entree with a child instead.
- Stay well informed of what your children are eating at school. If you help them prepare a packed lunch, make sure it's a wholesome and balanced meal—even if they do end up tossing the good food when you're not looking.
- Make an effort to understand why your child continues to reject healthy foods. Is it because it doesn't look or taste good? Does he have an underlying food sensitivity? Does your older child have some aversion to certain food for moral or other reasons?

- Try to undo picky eating with covert strategies, such as bridging, repeated exposure, and pairing items a child likes with new items, rather than using coercion or bribing to induce eating healthy foods.
- Accept that picky eating and neophobia can be a normal part of a child's development. Take it in stride, but don't give up on continuing to offer previously rejected healthy foods.
- Keep kids involved in choosing and preparing meals. They're much more likely to eat something they helped make.

# Recipes: Healthy Foods Even the Pickiest Eaters Will Love

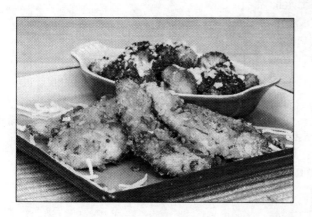

### Baked Honey Mustard Chicken Fingers

2 cups of crispy brown rice cereal

3 skinless and boneless chicken breasts

Salt and pepper

2 teaspoons of dried parsley or oregano

1/4 cup Dijon mustard

3 tablespoons of honey

Olive oil

Preheat oven to 400 degrees. Cut chicken breasts lengthwise into 1/4-inch strips. Sprinkle the chicken strips with salt, pepper, and the dried parsley or oregano. Mix mustard and honey together in a bowl and then pour into a large resealable plastic bag. Place the chicken strips in the bag and seal. Lightly coat the chicken strips with the mustard/honey mixture on both sides.

Place cereal into a large resealable plastic bag. Gently crush the cereal into smaller bits (but not into a flour-like consistency). Transfer 4 to 5 chicken strips from the honey mustard mixture into the bag with the cereal. Coat the chicken with cereal and then place on a baking sheet that has been sprayed with nonstick cooking spray. Place the chicken pieces approximately 2 inches apart. Drizzle 2 tablespoons of olive oil over chicken and place in the oven.

Bake for approximately 20 to 25 minutes (depending on the thickness of your chicken pieces).

*Tip*: Serve with Roasted Garlicky and Cheesy Broccoli (see Chapter 10 for recipe).

### Crispy Green Bean "Fries"

1 pound green beans (preferably haricot verts), washed, dried with ends trimmed

2 tablespoons of olive oil

Salt and pepper

Preheat oven to 425 degrees. Place green beans on a baking sheet in a single layer. Put olive oil over beans. Sprinkle salt and pepper. Bake for 20 minutes, until crispy.

## Whole Wheat Spinach Macaroni and Cheese

1/2 pound of whole wheat elbow macaroni
8 ounces of frozen spinach, defrosted
4 cups of skim milk
2 tablespoons of butter
1/4 cup all purpose flour
1 1/2 cups low-fat cheddar cheese
1 teaspoon of mustard

Cook elbow macaroni according to package instructions. Drain pasta after cooking and set aside. Melt butter in a pot over medium heat. After butter has melted, add the flour to the butter and continuously whisk to form a roux. Cook for 2 to 3 minutes and then slowly add the milk to the roux, continuously stirring while pouring the milk to make the béchamel sauce. Let cook for 5 to 7 minutes or until the béchamel sauce has thickened, stirring occasionally. Next, add the mustard and cheese. Cook for another 5 minutes and then remove from heat.

Squeeze excess water out of defrosted spinach and add to cooked pasta. Mix spinach into pasta. Pour cheese sauce over pasta and mix until well incorporated and then serve.

## Cheesy Apple and Chard Quesadillas

4 whole wheat tortillas
1 cup low-fat cheddar cheese
1 large apple (any variety)
1 bunch of Swiss chard
Olive oil

Wash and dry the Swiss chard. Remove the leaves from the stems and discard the stems. Cut the Swiss chard into ribbons, approximately 1/4-inch strips. Place 2 tablespoons of olive oil in a pan over medium heat. Add the chard ribbons to the pan and cook for 4 to 5 minutes, until chard has wilted. Remove chard from pan and wipe the pan clean. Drain the excess liquid from cooked chard.

Wash and cut the apple in half. Remove the core and cut each piece in half again, lengthwise. Then, cut across each apple piece into very thin slices.

To assemble the quesadillas, place 1/4 cup of cheddar cheese on top of one tortilla. Place 1/2 cup of cooked chard in an even layer on top of the cheese. Next, place a single layer of apples on top of the chard. Sprinkle 1/4 cup of cheddar cheese on top of the apples and cover with another tortilla. Repeat with remaining tortillas.

Reheat pan over medium heat with 1 tablespoon of olive oil in the pan. Place one quesadilla in pan and cook for 4 to 5 minutes. Flip the quesadilla over to the other side and cook for another 2 to 3 minutes.

Serve with plain yogurt or guacamole.

*Yogurt Guacamole*

3 ripe avocados
1/2 cup of nonfat plain yogurt
1 garlic clove, finely chopped
1/4 cup of chopped onion, finely chopped
1/4 cup of chopped fresh cilantro
Juice from 1 lime
1 teaspoon of salt

Mash avocados well in a bowl with a fork. Add yogurt and stir. Add garlic, onion, cilantro, and stir. Mix in lime juice and salt.

## Pineapple Teriyaki Chicken

8 chicken drumsticks or thighs
1 15-ounce can of diced pineapples
1 1/2 cups of soy sauce
1/4 cup honey
2 cloves of garlic, chopped (or 1 tablespoon of garlic powder)
1 tablespoon of fresh ginger root, grated
Olive oil

In a large bowl, mix 1 cup of soy sauce, ginger, and garlic. Remove pineapples from the can and pour pineapple juice into the bowl with soy sauce. Add chicken to bowl. Wrap bowl with plastic wrap and let sit in refrigerator 1 to 2 hours or overnight. Reserve pineapple pieces in a separate container and place in refrigerator.

To cook chicken: Preheat oven to 400 degrees. Remove chicken from bowl and place on baking sheet that has been lined with foil. Drizzle chicken with 2 tablespoons of olive oil. Bake for 35 to 40 minutes.

To make sauce: Bring 1/2 cup of soy sauce and honey to boil over medium heat for 15 minutes. Add reserved pineapple pieces to sauce.

Once chicken is cooked, remove from oven. Pour teriyaki-pineapple sauce over cooked chicken. Serve with cooked brown rice and steamed broccoli.

## References

1.  Lumeng, J. (2011). Picky eating. In M. Augustyn, B. Zuckerman, and E. Caronna (eds.), *The Zuckerman Parker Handbook of Developmental and Behavioral Pediatrics for Primary Care* (3rd. ed.). Philadelphia: Lippincott Williams & Wilkins.

2.  Gibbs, N. (2006). The magic of the family meal. *Time*. Available at http://www.time.com/time/magazine/article/0,9171,1200760,00.html.

3.  Hammons, A.J., and B.H. Fiese. (2011). Is frequency of shared family meals related to the nutritional health of children and adolescents? *Pediatrics. 127*(6): p. 1565-74.

4.  Sweetman, C., L. McGowan, H. Croker, and L. Cooke. (2011). Characteristics of family mealtimes affecting children's vegetable consumption and liking. *J Am Diet Assoc. 111*(2): p. 269-73.

5.  Hannon, P.A., D.J. Bowen, C.M. Moinpour, and D.F. McLerran. (2003). Correlations in perceived food use between the family food preparer and their spouses and children. *Appetite. 40*(1): p. 77-83.

6.  Fiese, B.H., and M. Schwartz. (2008). *Reclaiming the Family Table: Mealtimes and Child Health and Wellbeing*. Ann Arbor, MI: Society for Research in Child Development.

7.  Bowman, S.A., S.L. Gortmaker, C.B. Ebbeling, M.A. Pereira, and D.S. Ludwig. (2004). Effects of fast-food consumption on energy intake and diet quality among children in a national household survey. *Pediatrics. 113*(1 Pt 1): p. 112-8.

8.  Wootan, M., A. Batada, and E. Marchlewicz. (2008). *Kids' Meals: Obesity on the Menu*. Washington, DC: Center for Science in the Public Interest.

9.  Tandon, P.S., J. Wright, C. Zhou, C.B. Rogers, and D.A. Christakis. (2010). Nutrition menu labeling may lead to lower-calorie restaurant meal choices for children. *Pediatrics. 125*(2): p. 244-8.

10. Food and Nutrition Board. (2009). *School Meals: Building Blocks for Healthy Children*. Washington, DC: Institute of Medicine.

11. Cooke, L. (2007). The importance of exposure for healthy eating in childhood: A review. *J Hum Nutr Diet. 20*(4):p. 294-301.

12. Orlet Fisher, J., B.J. Rolls, and L.L. Birch. (2003). Children's bite size and intake of an entree are greater with large portions than with age-appropriate or self-selected portions. *Am J Clin Nutr. 77*(5): p. 1164-70.

13. Almansour, F.D., S.J. Sweitzer, A.A. Magness, E.E. Calloway, M.R. McAllaster, C.R. Roberts-Gray, D.M. Hoelscher, and M.E. Briley. (2011). Temperature of foods sent by parents of preschool-aged children. *Pediatrics. 128*(3): p. 519-23.

# 8

# Mistake #8— Sacrificing Taste

*"The most remarkable thing about my mother is that for thirty years she served nothing but leftovers. The original meal has never been found."*
—Calvin Trillin, journalist

Although now an adult, Scott fondly remembers well-intentioned but unappealing childhood dinners, including one that was an iceberg lettuce salad, microwaved breaded fish sticks, limp vegetables, and an orange soda. It has taken him years to ever want to order fish from a restaurant menu or consider preparing it at home. Nine-year-old Sarah says she likes the food they eat at home, but she's getting kind of tired of grilled chicken, steamed vegetables, and brown rice at every meal.

Most adults can think back to some memory of a well-intentioned healthy dinner gone terribly wrong or of health-conscious but somewhat cooking-impaired parents trying their best to get something tasty and healthy on the table with varying degrees of success. With all the multiple schedules to balance, jobs to work, and homework to do, you can't really blame anyone for thinking of mealtimes as a chore and declaring success when an edible assortment of food makes it to the dinner table, even if the meal isn't the healthiest or tastiest. No one has much time to cook gourmet meals despite what seems to be a national obsession with cooking shows and gadgets.

This haphazard approach to meal preparation may be part of the reason for an extreme disconnect between what Americans know is a healthy meal and what they actually eat. The number one predictor of whether a kid chooses to eat a food is taste. And most people think that healthy food doesn't taste as good as the fat- and sugar-laden alternatives. But it doesn't have to be that way. The good news is that any standard healthy meal can simply and tastefully be made over into an even healthier gourmet delight with little added expense or effort. For example, Scott's questionable fish dinner could easily be transformed into a simple spinach salad with tomatoes and carrots, grilled tilapia, steamed mixed vegetables, and a glass of cold milk. Or you could make more grand changes and end up with grilled salmon tacos with mango black bean salsa and quinoa spinach salad. Simple cooking modifications can change everything.

# How Humans Experience Food

Food preferences evolve from in utero throughout childhood and adult life. Babies exposed to a wide variety of healthy foods (first in utero, next through maternal breast milk, and then in the first several months of exposure to solid foods) acquire a taste for a wide variety of foods. In addition to the taste of a food, social and cultural factors play a large role in determining a person's food preferences (Figure 8-1). As you learn how to prepare foods that taste great, you can create the context and mood to help your family members develop a liking for the healthy foods. Plus, if from a young age you expose your children to a wide variety of food types from around the world, you'll raise kids with not only a more sophisticated palate but also a higher tolerance for trying new foods.

## Taste

The first step to transforming your potentially bland meals into delicious masterpieces is to develop a fundamental understanding of what and how we taste.

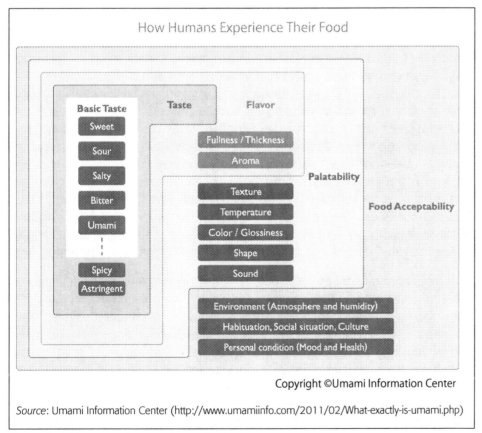

Source: Umami Information Center (http://www.umamiinfo.com/2011/02/What-exactly-is-umami.php)

Figure 8-1. How people experience food

The sense of taste comes from what are known as papillae on the tongue. These are little bumps on the outside border of your tongue. These papillae house taste buds which allow us to experience five different types of taste: sweet, sour, bitter, salty, and *umami* (see the section "Flavor Enhancers" for more on umami). The taste buds at the tip of the tongue are more sensitive to sour, while those at the back of the tongue are more sensitive to bitter. When a sweet, sour, bitter, or salty substance touches the tongue, a message is rapidly sent to the brain to help identify the taste.

Taste is the best predictor of whether a child will eat a food. Enhance taste with a touch of spice.

## Seasonings: Salt and Pepper

Seasonings are the ingredients added to a food that enhance the food's flavor without being specifically tasted themselves. The judicious use of seasonings can significantly enhance a meal. Salt and pepper are basic seasonings that improve the flavor of a food. Salt is an ancient commodity that's greatly overused by present-day Americans. While it does add flavor to foods, it also comes loaded with sodium, which can increase blood pressure and cause hypertension. It's best to use salt sparingly and in very small increments. Both black and white ground pepper add flavor to foods without any increased risk of negative health effects.

## Flavor Enhancers

Flavor enhancers don't bring flavor to a dish. Instead, they enhance other flavors. Two commonly used flavor enhancers are monosodium glutamate (MSG) (derived from the amino acid glutamic acid) and compounds known as 5'-ribonucleotides. MSGs used to be a major ingredient in Chinese restaurant food and are common ingredients in many processed foods; however, foods marketed specifically to children don't contain MSGs due to theoretical negative health risks. Although MSG does occur naturally in many foods (these are glutamic acid–rich foods, such as cheese, tomatoes, cured meat, and wine), the most readily available compound is synthetically produced from the fermentation of molasses. MSG has been heavily criticized for causing what's known as the "MSG symptom complex" in some individuals. The MSG symptom complex—which may or may not truly be a reaction to MSG—includes tingling and burning in the head and neck and a feeling of pressure in the upper body.

The 5'-ribonucleotides occur naturally in some foods, such as beef, chicken, fish, and mushrooms. These compounds may also be synthetically produced from yeast and added to many processed foods to enhance flavors. When combined with MSG, they create a "fifth taste," known as *umami*. Umami is derived from a Japanese word meaning "delicious" or "savory." Umami occurs naturally in many vegetables, such as mushrooms and tomatoes. It's also found in foods that are aged, including soy sauce, aged cheeses, and fermented products. For a taste of umami, check out the Grilled Portabella Mushroom Burgers With Sundried Tomato Yogurt Aioli and Roasted Parmesan Sweet Potatoes recipes in this chapter.

*Spices and Herbs*

Spices and herbs can work miracles in transforming a bland meal to a truly gourmet experience. Spices are components of aromatic plants, such as bark, roots, buds, flowers, fruits, and seeds, that are grown in the tropics and add a sweet, spicy, or hot flavor to foods. Herbs are leaves and stems of plants that grow in temperate climates. Such seeds as caraway and sesame, which come from tropical and temperate regions, and dehydrated vegetables (such as celery and garlic salt) also add flavor to foods. Test your herbs and spices know-how with the quiz in Figure 8-2.

*Sweeteners*

Sugar is an innately preferred taste. Many food manufacturers capitalize on this by adding sweeteners, such as raw sugar, granulated sugar, powdered sugar, and honey, to foods. Noncaloric sweeteners—calorie-free because the body can't metabolize them—are also processed compounds used to add sweet taste to food and beverages. Aspartame, also known as Equal® in packaged sweetener and NutraSweet® in foods and beverages, acesulfame K (called Sunett® in cooking products and Sweet One® as tabletop sweetener), saccharin, sucralose (Splenda®), and neotame are all approved for use in the United States. While early studies in laboratory rats found that certain sweeteners may cause bladder cancer, subsequent studies of humans haven't found an association. Americans can now get their calorie-free sugar fix from an all-natural alternative to artificial sweeteners. Once limited to the health food market as an unapproved herb, the plant-derived sweetener known as stevia is now widely available and rapidly replacing artificial sweeteners in consumer products. Stevia is 30 times sweeter than sugar and has no effect on blood sugar and little aftertaste, making it a popular all-natural, noncaloric sweetener. A sizeable amount of research supports that sweeteners are generally safe for adults, but parents should tread carefully when providing children with sweetened snacks and drinks as there is a lack of research on the safety of sweeteners for children.

## Flavor and Smell

At the same time the brain is processing a food's taste, it is getting another message from the smell center in the nose. The sense of smell is pretty powerful—it can differentiate hundreds of distinct odors. That makes it 10,000 times more sensitive than the sense of taste. Simply smelling a delicious food or a familiar scent can rapidly bring back memories of another time when you smelled that food (for example, a whiff of fresh-baked cookies might immediately bring you back to when you were a child visiting Grandma's house and how every time you arrived at her house it was just in time to pull the cookies from the oven). This is the perfect example of the intersection between eating and being hungry—and how sometimes people may eat for reasons other than hunger, such as to bring back fond childhood memories. Of course, you can also use this to your advantage. If you make your children's meals smell *and* taste good when they're children, they'll prefer those tempting smells and delicious flavors when they're older. Pair this with a pleasant experience at family mealtimes and you're inching closer to your overall goal to raise healthy eaters who prefer healthy foods even when you aren't looking.

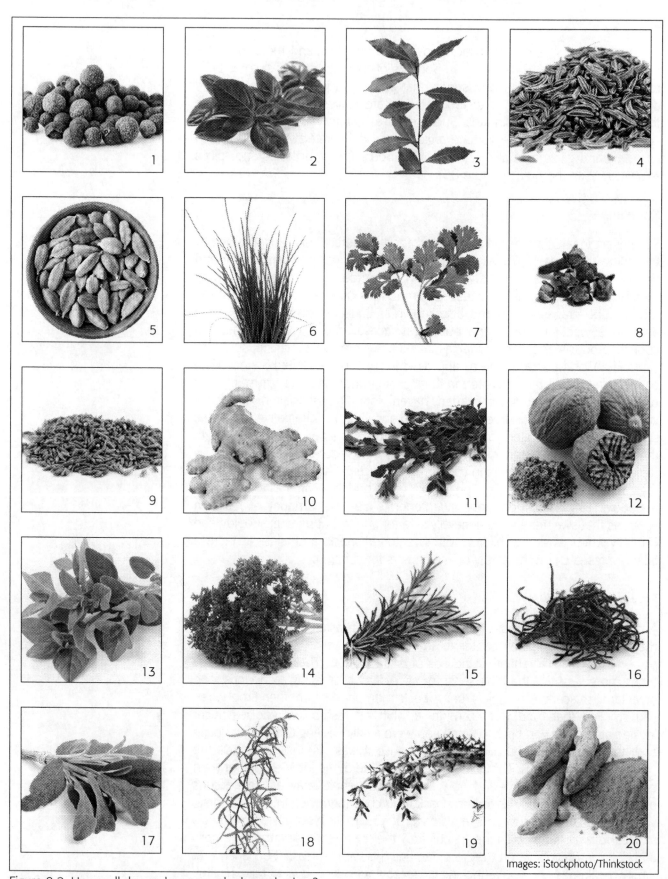

Figure 8-2. How well do you know your herbs and spices?

Images: iStockphoto/Thinkstock

1. *Allspice*: Berry of the evergreen "pimento tree"; commonly used in Jamaican cooking. Tastes like a mix of cinnamon, nutmeg, and cloves, thus the name "allspice." Uses: Chicken, beef, fish (key ingredient in "jerk" dishes), fruit desserts, cakes, cookies, apple cider.

2. *Basil*: Aromatic leaf of the bay laurel. Pungently aromatic, sweet, spicy flavor. Uses: Essential ingredient in Italian and Thai dishes, main ingredient in pesto.

3. *Bay leaf*: Leaf of evergreen laurel. Aromatic, bitter, spicy, pungent flavor. Uses: Soups, stews, braises, and pâtés, used often in Mediterranean cuisine.

4. *Caraway seed*: Fruit of biennial herb of parsley family. Warm, biting, acrid but pleasant, slightly minty. Uses: Rye breads, baked goods, often used in European cuisine.

5. *Cardamom*: Seeds from fruit of perennial herb of ginger family; grown mostly in India; very expensive. Sweet and pungent flavor, highly aromatic. Uses: Indian curry dishes, lunch meats.

6. *Chives*: Smallest species of the onion family. Onion flavor. Uses: Soups, salad dressings, dips.

7. *Cilantro (coriander)*: Annual flowering herb, can be cultivated for leaves, seeds, flower, and roots. May have "soapy" versus "herby" taste, based on genetics of taster. Uses: Often used in Latin American, Indian, and Chinese dishes, in salsa and guacamole, stir-fry, grilled chicken or fish. Best when used fresh.

8. *Cloves*: Dried flower buds from evergreen of myrtle family. Warm, spicy, astringent, fruity, slightly bitter flavor. Uses: Whole cloves on ham or pork roast; ground cloves to season pear or apple desserts, beets, beans, tomatoes, squash, and sweet potatoes.

9. *Cumin seed*: Seeds of flowering plant of parsley family. Earthy and warming flavor. Uses: Curry powder, chilis, used throughout the world (second most common seasoning after black ground pepper).

10. *Ginger:* Underground stem of perennial tropical plant. Biting flavor, fragrant. Uses: Asian dishes, marinade for chicken and fish, gingerbread, cookies, processed meats.

11. *Marjoram*: Leaves and flowers of perennial of mint family. Sweet pine and citrus flavor. Uses: Meats, fish, poultry, vegetables, soups.

12. *Nutmeg*: Seed of fruit of evergreen tree. Sweet, warm, pungent, aromatic, bitter flavor. Uses: Eggnog, French toast, cooked fruits, sweet potatoes, spinach.

13. *Oregano*: Leaves of perennial of the mint family. Related to marjoram, but very different flavor. Strong, pungent, aromatic, bitter flavor. Uses: Italian dishes, chili, beef stew, pork, and vegetables.

14. *Parsley*: Leaves of a biennial herbaceous plant; curly and flat leaf varieties. Grassy, bitter flavor. Uses: Widely used throughout the world, including in meat, soup, vegetables; often used as garnish.

15. *Rosemary*: Woody perennial herb of evergreen shrub of mint family. Sweet, spicy, peppery flavor. Uses: Flavoring in stuffing and roast lamb, pork, chicken, and turkey.

16. *Saffron*: Spice derived from flower of iris family; very expensive. Earthy, sweet flavor. Uses: Baked goods, rice dishes.

17. *Sage*: Medicinal plant of mint family. Slightly peppery flavor. Uses: Often used to flavor fatty meals.

18. *Tarragon*: Flowering tops and leaves of a perennial herb, often called "dragon herb." Minty "anise-like" (resembles licorice) flavor. Uses: Chicken, fish, egg dishes, one of four "fine herbs" of French cooking.

19. *Thyme*: Leaves and flowering tops of a shrub-like perennial of the mint family. Biting, sharp, spicy, herbaceous flavor; blends well with other herbs. Uses: Meats, soups, and stews.

20. *Turmeric*: Stem of plant of tropical perennial herb. Mild, peppery, mustardy, pungent taste. Uses: Curry powders, mustards, condiments.

*Sources*:
- Bennion, M. and B. Scheule. (1999). *Introductory Foods*, 11th ed. Upper Saddle River, NJ: Prentice Hall.
- University of Tennessee Extension Expanded Food and Nutrition Education Program (2002). *Eat Smart: Get Your Family to the Table—Cooking Basics*. Available at https://utextension.tennessee.edu/publications/Documents/SP732.pdf.

## Palatability

A palatable food is appealing enough to try and is then perceived to taste good. It's critical that the foods you prepare for your family are highly palatable if you want everyone to continue to be willing to try new foods. Texture, temperature, color, shape, and sound all affect a food's palatability.

### Texture

Texture encompasses the qualities you can feel with your fingers, tongue, palate, or teeth. Universally liked textures include crispy, crunchy, tender, juicy, and firm. Generally disliked textures are tough, soggy, crumbly, lumpy, watery, and slimy. Keep this in mind when preparing your meals. For example, when steaming vegetables, err on the side of not cooking enough (leaving a little bit of crunch) rather than cooking too much (leading to soggy).

### Temperature

Temperature affects how tastes are experienced. The same amount of sugar tastes sweeter at higher temperatures, while the opposite is true for salt—the same amount of salt tastes saltier at lower temperatures. Serve foods at their ideal temperature to optimize their flavor and acceptance. Also, if you combine cold and hot temperatures in the same dish (like mango salsa on baked mahimahi) or mix hot and spicy foods, your food will be more flavorful.

### Color

A food's appearance can determine whether a kid is interested in giving it a try or if he'll reject it outright. You could make a relatively bland-appearing but balanced meal (brown rice, grilled chicken, applesauce, roasted potatoes, and skim milk) that no one wants to try or a highly attractive meal that contains an array of different colors (wild rice, tomato and basil chicken, red grapes, roasted sweet potatoes, and skim milk). When putting together a meal, try to include as many different colors as you can. This will help increase the appearance of the meal as well as ensure you have ample fruits and vegetables (because these are the most colorful foods) containing a balanced mix of nutrients.

### Shape

The shape of food is especially important when trying to encourage kids to eat certain foods. Mickey Mouse whole wheat pancakes are going to be a much bigger hit with the kids than the standard circular kind. A heart-shaped turkey sandwich holds much more appeal than the cut-down-the-middle sandwich.

### Sound

You may not think much about how your food "sounds," but food marketers do. The "snap, crackle, pop" of Rice Krispies, the crinkle of a potato chips bag, and the distinctive sound of opening a soda trigger an emotional reaction to the food—and ultimately may affect your perception of the food's palatability. You can capitalize on the appeal of "foods that make noise" with your young kids by having a carrot crunching contest or awarding a prize to whoever guesses how many "pops" the boiling cranberries will make.

## Acceptability

A food's acceptability depends on many factors that extend beyond the actual properties of the food, such as the surrounding environment, habituation, social and cultural factors, and mood and health.

### Environment

In a movement to return back to choosing local and in-season foods, the environment where a family lives determines which foods are available fresh at various times throughout the year. Of course, most foods can be purchased anytime at the local grocery store, in which case environment plays a lesser role, although the freshest and best-tasting foods are often the ones grown and purchased locally.

### Habituation, Social Factors, and Culture

Kids learn to eat and appreciate the same foods their parents eat and appreciate. Family meals offer the ideal opportunity to expose children to the same healthy tastes the rest of the family enjoys. Cultural preferences and norms also shape a child's early eating practices and which flavors are most readily accepted and rejected.

### Mood and Health

An understanding of what foods and food combinations promote ideal health greatly influences food purchases in health-conscious families. At the same time, emotional and psychological factors play an important role in a child's food experiences. An infant learns security and attachment when his tears of hunger are met with food. Familiar foods bring back memories and increase security. Food is a symbol of hospitality, an opportunity to bond with a friend or family member, and a perfect gift for a special occasion.

# Counterstrategies

So, how do you apply all this information to make your healthy meals taste delicious?

## Apply Basic Cooking Essentials

Start with these three basic cooking essentials:
- *Prepare.* Do this by completely cleaning out your pantry and refrigerator and starting fresh. This ensures you have fresh ingredients, you have food on hand that will actually be eaten, and you're well aware of the arsenal of ingredients you have at your fingertips (and those you may need to go to the store to pick up).

• *Follow a recipe.* As you're getting started, rely on high-quality cookbooks and recipes. (Check out the various recipes throughout this book for ideas to get started.) Choose basic recipes that don't contain too many ingredients and are easy to follow. Make sure you read the entire recipe before starting. Once you feel comfortable in the kitchen, get creative with the recipes. Try substituting ingredients and experimenting with spices and herbs. For example, instead of ground beef for taco night, try baking mahimahi with cumin and lemon for a lighter, healthier, and more adventurous version. Or try using thinly sliced eggplant and zucchini as substitutes for pasta in your favorite lasagna recipe.

• *Remember that timing is everything.* The temperature, texture, and overall taste of a food depend in large part on timing. Make sure you serve hot foods hot and cold foods cold. Steam vegetables to the point where they still hold a bit of crunch and aren't soggy.

Additional basic cooking essentials and tips are included in the appendix.

*Make It a Meal They'll Love*

The first goal when cooking is to make a delicious meal the family will love. You can maximize a food's acceptance by considering factors that may make it more appealing in general. The following are a few tips:

• *Choose flavorful ingredients that also smell delicious.* Such ingredients as onions, garlic, and many herbs and spices create a mouth-watering aroma that's sure to encourage the kids to give the food a try.

• *Remember to include at least one food your picky eater likes at each meal.* This way, you don't have to worry about him refusing to eat everything; he'll be happy and you can avert unpleasant mealtime battles. With this, however, don't hesitate to add a new fresh ingredient to an old favorite to try to help your child to be a little more open minded in food preferences. For example, add broccoli and canned tuna to macaroni and cheese or tomatoes and spinach to freshen up grilled cheese.

• *Make it look good.* If your meal looks attractive and appealing, it's much more likely that family members will eagerly give it a try.

• *Spice it up.* Create a cultural masterpiece by mixing a few special spices. For example, the following vegetable, herb, and spice combinations can give a basic meal a cultural flare:
  ✓ Indian: garlic + onion + curry powder + cinnamon
  ✓ Asian: garlic + scallions + sesame + ginger + soy sauce
  ✓ Italian: garlic + basil + parsley + oregano
  ✓ Middle Eastern: garlic + onion + mint + cumin + saffron + lemon
  ✓ Mexican: cumin + onion + oregano + cilantro

See this chapter's recipes for some ideas to get started.

## Optimize Health

The second goal is ensuring that the food optimizes health and, if preparing a full meal, that the meal is healthy and balanced. Do this by including each of the major food groups at every meal. You can use MyPlate to guide your choices. That is, aim for a plate of 25 percent high-quality protein, 25 percent whole grain, 50 percent fruits and vegetables, and one serving of low-fat dairy.

Use cooking methods that create delicious-tasting food without an excess of calories. For example, simmering, boiling, stewing, steaming, braising, and poaching all use water as the primary cooking medium. Roasting, baking, broiling, and grilling use heated air as the main cooking medium. Both of these types of cooking methods add no extra calories. On the other hand, sautéing, panfrying, and deep-fat frying all use calorie-dense fat as the main cooking medium and add hundreds of excess calories.

Choose the healthiest cuts of meat. The leanest cuts of meat are the round and loin. The most tender cuts of beef include the short loin and sirloin (as well as the very fatty ribs). The round is a medium tender cut. Poultry and fish are generally healthier than red meat and beef. Fish is very high in protein and essential nutrients, such as omega-3 polyunsaturated fats. While the typical American gets nowhere near this, eating fish two times per week goes a long way toward optimizing health.

Seek out the most colorful and freshest fruits and vegetables. If possible, choose produce that's locally grown and in season. Not only do you support the local farmer, but you ensure that your family gets the freshest produce available (which will help increase consumption of these oft-rejected foods). See the sidebar "Should I Buy Organic?" and Figure 8-3 for suggestions on how to choose the tastiest fruits and vegetables.

## Make It Easy on You

As a parent of young kids, you have little time to spare, and you certainly don't have the time to spend hours making meals for the family. One of the most important considerations as you make a commitment to prepare healthier, more delicious meals is to make sure that it doesn't add a significant amount of time in the kitchen. The following are a few suggestions to make it easier on you:

- *Plan meals ahead of time.* Create the weekly menu right before you go to the grocery store. While you're at the store, make sure you pick up all the necessary ingredients for the week. This will save you time pondering what to make on your way home from work at 5:30 when you're already exhausted and the last thing you want to do is spend a lot of time making a meal.

- *Do the prep work when you're not already tired.* If you do your grocery shopping on the weekend, consider washing and cutting the vegetables you'll need for some of the week's recipes ahead of time. This way, you make it easier for the family to snack on the produce and you save yourself time when you're already exhausted. You may even consider making portions of the week's meals over the weekend and then freezing them for easy reheating when they're needed.

- *Stick with the simple recipes.* If you're in a crunch for time, stick with easy but healthy and delicious recipes. Check out a few of the recipes included at the end of this chapter for some ideas.

## Should I Buy Organic?

Organic food choices fill supermarket shelves—and it's not just at the Whole Foods and other natural food stores where you would expect to find them. Even Walmart now offers organic selections. Many people happily cough up the almost double it sometimes costs to go organic, whereas others balk at such a high price for a food that may taste no different from its conventional counterpart. So, who's right? Well, it turns out that it depends.

To get the USDA organic seal, foods need to have been grown, handled, and processed by certified organic facilities. These facilities must be wholly organic. Meat, poultry, eggs, and dairy products need to be produced from animals that have never been given antibiotics or hormones and who have been fed organic crop. Organic crops must be grown free of conventional pesticides, free of fertilizers made with synthetic ingredients or sewage sludge, and without bioengineering or use of ionizing radiation. The USDA is careful to note than an organic seal doesn't mean that a food is healthier or safer than its conventionally grown equivalent.

In fact, a review looking at studies of organic foods and health benefits over the past 50 years determined that not enough good data exist to say one way or the other if organic foods are healthier.[2] Of the studies that have been done, the only one that found a health difference showed that the risk of eczema was decreased in infants who ate strictly organic dairy products. Overall, not enough good information exists for anyone to say for sure.

As for safety, a study of preschool children in Seattle found that kids who ate conventional diets had significantly higher levels of urine pesticides than the kids who ate organic.[3] But higher urine pesticides haven't been connected to real health outcomes, although intuitively, it seems like a good idea to minimize the consumption of toxic chemicals.

Ultimately, it may not be the health and safety for the consumer that will tip you one way or the other with organic foods, but it's worth considering the broader health and environmental outcomes. For example, farm workers overall are afforded minimal rights and often work in horrendous conditions. Those working on conventional farms are often exposed to massive levels of pesticides, which can contribute to serious health outcomes, including birth defects and cancers. Furthermore, an extraordinary amount of environmental resources and energy go into shipping a crop from halfway around the world to your local grocery store, although these days, it's not unusual to see organic food that was grown abroad. This becomes more common as an increasing number of massive companies jump on the organic bandwagon.

At the end of the day, everyone has to make his own decision as to whether to buy organic based on the limited information we have on whether organic foods are worth it. It may be that the spirit of organic foods (which you can often tap into at a local farmers' market or by nurturing your own garden)—such as a good use of natural resources, minimal use of toxic compounds, sustainable farming, supporting local business—is more important than whether the food is actually grown organic.

The Environmental Working Group (EWG) conducted a study to see which fruits and vegetables had the highest and lowest levels of pesticides, and found the following results.

*The "dirty dozen" (in other words, try to buy these organic)*
- Celery
- Peaches
- Strawberries
- Apples
- Blueberries
- Nectarines
- Sweet bell peppers
- Spinach
- Kale/collard greens
- Cherries
- Potatoes
- Grapes (imported)

*The "clean 15" (lowest in pesticides; probably don't need to buy organic)*
- Onions
- Avocado
- Sweet corn (frozen)
- Pineapples
- Mango
- Sweet peas (frozen)
- Asparagus
- Kiwi fruit
- Cabbage
- Eggplant
- Cantaloupe (domestic)
- Watermelon
- Grapefruit
- Sweet potatoes
- Honeydew melon

*Reference*: Environmental Working Group (http://www.ewg.org/pesticidesorganics)

| How to Choose Fresh Fruits and Vegetables | | | | | | | | | | | | | |
| --- | --- | --- | --- | --- | --- | --- | --- | --- | --- | --- | --- | --- | --- |
| Note: Shaded boxes indicate the months the fruit or vegetable is in season. | | | | | | | | | | | | | |
| Fruit/Vegetable | January | February | March | April | May | June | July | August | September | October | November | December | Characteristics to Look For |
| Apple | ■ | ■ | ■ | | | | | | ■ | ■ | ■ | ■ | Firm with no soft spots |
| Apricot | | | | | | ■ | | | | | | | Golden yellow, plump, and firm; not yellow or green, very hard or soft, or wilted |
| Artichoke | | | ■ | ■ | | | | | | | | | Plump and compact; green, fresh-looking scales |
| Asparagus | | ■ | ■ | ■ | ■ | ■ | | | | | | | Straight, tender, deep green stalks with tightly closed buds |
| Avocado | ■ | ■ | ■ | ■ | ■ | ■ | ■ | ■ | ■ | ■ | | | Firm but yields to gentle pressure |
| Banana | ■ | ■ | ■ | ■ | ■ | ■ | ■ | ■ | ■ | ■ | ■ | ■ | Firm with no bruises |
| Bell pepper | ■ | ■ | ■ | ■ | ■ | ■ | ■ | ■ | ■ | ■ | ■ | ■ | Firm skin and no wrinkles |
| Blueberry | | | | | ■ | ■ | ■ | ■ | | | | | Firm, plump, brightly colored |
| Broccoli | ■ | ■ | ■ | ■ | | | | | ■ | ■ | ■ | ■ | Dark green bunches |
| Brussels sprout | | | | | | | | | ■ | ■ | ■ | ■ | Tight outer leaves; bright green color and firm body |
| Cantaloupe | | | | | ■ | ■ | ■ | ■ | ■ | | | | Slightly golden with light fragrant smell |
| Carrot | ■ | ■ | ■ | ■ | ■ | ■ | ■ | ■ | ■ | ■ | ■ | ■ | Deep orange; not cracked or wilted |
| Cauliflower | | | | | | | | | ■ | ■ | ■ | | Bright green leaves enclosing firm and closely packed white curd |
| Celery | ■ | ■ | ■ | ■ | ■ | ■ | ■ | ■ | ■ | ■ | ■ | ■ | Fresh, crisp branches with light green to green color |
| Cherry | | | | | ■ | ■ | ■ | | | | | | Fresh-appearing, firm |
| Coconuts | ■ | ■ | ■ | | | | | | ■ | ■ | ■ | ■ | Good weight for size with inside milk still fluid |
| Cranberry | | | | | | | | | ■ | ■ | ■ | ■ | Firm, plump, brightly colored |
| Corn | | | | | ■ | ■ | ■ | ■ | ■ | | | | Green, tight, and fresh-looking husk; ears with tightly packed row of plump kernels |
| Cucumber | | | | | ■ | ■ | ■ | ■ | | | | | Firm with rich green color and no soft spots |
| Eggplant | | | | | | | | ■ | ■ | ■ | | | Firm, heavy, smooth, uniformly dark purple |
| Grapefruit | ■ | ■ | ■ | ■ | ■ | | | | | | | | Firm, well rounded, heavy for size; avoid puffy/rough-skinned |

Figure 8-3. Choosing fruits and vegetables

## How to Choose Fresh Fruits and Vegetables
*Note*: Shaded boxes indicate the months the fruit or vegetable is in season.

| Fruit/Vegetable | January | February | March | April | May | June | July | August | September | October | November | December | Characteristics to Look For |
|---|---|---|---|---|---|---|---|---|---|---|---|---|---|
| Grape | | | | | ■ | ■ | ■ | ■ | ■ | | | | Firm, plump, well-colored clusters |
| Honeydew | | ■ | ■ | ■ | ■ | ■ | ■ | ■ | ■ | | | | Creamy yellow rounds and pleasant aroma |
| Kiwi | | | | | | ■ | ■ | ■ | ■ | ■ | | | Soft |
| Lettuce | ■ | ■ | ■ | ■ | | | | | | ■ | ■ | ■ | Fresh, crisp leaves without wilting |
| Mushroom | ■ | ■ | ■ | ■ | ■ | | | | | | | | Firm, moisture- and blemish-free |
| Onion | ■ | ■ | ■ | ■ | ■ | ■ | ■ | ■ | ■ | ■ | ■ | ■ | Dry and solid with no soft spots or sprouts |
| Orange | ■ | ■ | ■ | ■ | | | | | | ■ | ■ | ■ | Firm, heavy for size, and brightly colored skin |
| Peach | | | | | | ■ | ■ | ■ | ■ | | | | Soft to touch with fragrant smell |
| Pear | ■ | ■ | | | | | | ■ | ■ | ■ | ■ | ■ | Should yield gently to pressure at stem end |
| Pea | | | | ■ | ■ | ■ | ■ | | | | | | Bright green, full |
| Pepper | ■ | ■ | ■ | ■ | ■ | ■ | ■ | ■ | ■ | ■ | | | Firm with thick flesh and glossy skin |
| Persimmon | ■ | | | | | | | | | ■ | ■ | ■ | Firm, plump, orange-red |
| Pineapple | | ■ | ■ | ■ | ■ | ■ | ■ | | | | | | Slightly soft; ripe when leaves easily removed with small tug |
| Plum | | | | | | ■ | ■ | ■ | ■ | | | | Plump, yields to slight pressure |
| Pomegranate | | | | | | | | | ■ | ■ | ■ | | Thin-skinned, bright purple-red |
| Spinach | | | ■ | ■ | ■ | | | | ■ | ■ | ■ | | Large, bright leaves; avoid coarse stems |
| Strawberry | | | | ■ | ■ | ■ | ■ | | | | | | Dry, firm, bright red in color |
| Summer squash | | | | | | ■ | ■ | ■ | ■ | | | | Firm with bright and glossy skin |
| Sweet potato | | | | | | | | ■ | ■ | ■ | ■ | ■ | Firm, dark, smooth |
| Tomato | | | | | ■ | ■ | ■ | ■ | ■ | | | | Plump with smooth skin and no blemishes |

*Sources*:
- www.fruitsandveggiesmatter.gov
- Greer, B. (2009). A Guide to Buying Fresh Fruits & Vegetables. Knoxville, TN: University of Tennessee Extension. Available at https://utextension.tennessee.edu/publications/Documents/SP527.pdf.

Figure 8-3. Choosing fruits and vegetables (cont.)

• *Solicit help.* Give the other family members tasks in helping prepare food, whether that's setting the table, washing and cutting the produce, mixing the salad, or cleaning the dishes. Having help not only saves you time, but it also gets the other family members involved in cooking and thus they'll be more likely to want to eat the foods you offer.

**Sneak It In**

While it's great if you can get your kids to love fruits and vegetables, you might sometimes have to sneak it in just to get your kids to give it a try so they ultimately acquire a taste for vegetables and fruits. Studies suggest this method actually works. For example, in one study, pureed zucchini, cauliflower, broccoli, tomatoes, and/or squash were added to several standard meals, such as zucchini bread, pasta with tomato sauce, and chicken noodle casserole. When the pureed vegetables were added to the dishes, the kids ate 50 percent more vegetables that day than their typical intake.[1] Experiment with foods and see

---

### Counterstrategies in Action: Making It Taste Good

**Apply Basic Cooking Essentials**

Nicole may not have the time, energy, or know-how to come up with great recipes on her own, but she realizes that she doesn't need to: "I'm not all that creative in coming up with new, healthy, and tasty meals, but with all of the excellent cookbooks available these days, I don't need to be! … My husband and daughter keep complimenting me on our healthy and delicious dinners, as if I came up with it myself. It's not hard for us to eat healthy—all I have to be able to do is find a really good cookbook and then be able to follow the recipe."

**Make Meals They'll Love**

Courtney, mother to four-year-old Lila and two-year-old Lorenzo, knows that a major key in getting her kids to be happy at mealtimes but also be willing to venture outside their comfort zones is to pair new tastes with the old "tried and true": "I make certain that new dishes or ones that were greeted without enthusiasm the first time are paired with other options that I know they like. Usually, when it's a whole plate or new or different foods, it's more difficult to get a good reaction. If I mix a favorite vegetable dish with a new protein, they will usually tolerate it pretty well."

**Optimize Health**

Amber may be strapped for time and energy after she gets home from a long day of work, but she's discovered several tried-and-true dinner menus that not only optimize health (they're pretty much in perfect alignment

---

what kind of superhealthy concoction you can put together that your kids will love. It's not so far fetched. One mother shared how she saw a recipe that called for adding three cups of spinach to a fruit smoothie. She gave it a try, called it a "shamrock smoothie," and offered it to her kids, who eagerly gobbled it down.

Check out the sidebar "Counterstrategies in Action: Making It Taste Good" for some more ideas from creative parents on how to make dinners taste better.

# Developmental Considerations

Ultimately, taste dictates food preferences at most any age. However, you can employ some age-specific strategies to help maximize the chances you'll find just the right taste to encourage a child to eat and enjoy a healthy diet (Figure 8-4).

with the MyPlate recommendations) but are also well-received favorites of her husband and two-year-old. They include baked fish (tilapia, cod) with steamed green beans, brown rice or baked sweet potatoes, and garden salad; pasta with ground turkey and mixed vegetables in a tomato sauce; roasted chicken, steamed broccoli, sliced tomatoes, and fresh whole wheat bread with olive oil and parmesan cheese. Each dinner comes with a glass of skim milk, and most are followed by a whole fruit dessert.

**Make It Easy**

At Jessica's house, it's easy to get the kids to eat healthy foods. She just makes sure it tastes good and the kids are having fun. It doesn't hurt that the kids have also picked up along the way that eating good-for-you foods helps make for strong bodies. When Jessica asked four-year-old Kevin why he tries to eat healthy things he said: "Because my brain tells me to. I am trying to be big and strong, and the dentist doesn't want cavities in my mouth, and I like making fruit smoothies." His mom adds: "Letting Kevin make the smoothies makes him pumped to be drinking it, even though it is made of yogurt and fruit!"

**Sneak It In**

The boy doesn't feel like eating his vegetables today? No problem. Shannon has the perfect backup plan for when her toddler decides to be picky. She just blends some veggies into his favorite foods. She's had remarkable success with a red pasta sauce that includes a mix of pureed veggies, mashed potatoes that have steamed red pepper and zucchini mixed in, and toast with a mashed cannellini beans and avocado spread.

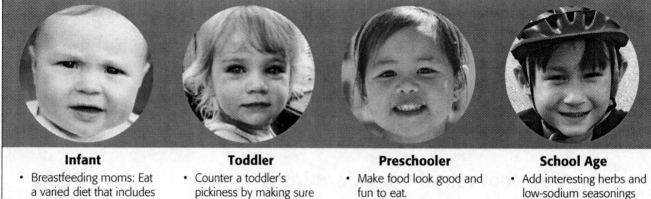

| Infant | Toddler | Preschooler | School Age |
|---|---|---|---|
| • Breastfeeding moms: Eat a varied diet that includes many different flavors.<br>• Capitalize on an infant's willingness to eat anything by exposing him to a wide variety of flavors. | • Counter a toddler's pickiness by making sure the healthy food tastes good.<br>• Bridge familiar tastes to newer tastes by slightly modifying favorites. | • Make food look good and fun to eat.<br>• Continue to introduce a variety of new and interesting foods. | • Add interesting herbs and low-sodium seasonings to give old favorites a new taste.<br>• Make sure the healthy food tastes great to encourage independently healthy eaters down the road. |

Figure 8-4. Developmental considerations

### Infant (0–1 years)

The sense of taste in infancy is very poorly developed and nondiscriminating. That is, you can get a zero- to one-year-old to try just about anything. Breastfeeding mothers can take advantage of this by eating a varied diet, which includes many different flavors. This early exposure to many tastes helps to avoid picky eating later on. Once solids are introduced around six months, gradually introduce an increasing variety and quality of flavors. This way, when your child develops neophobia (the fear of trying new foods) around two years, not all that many flavors will be "new."

### Toddler (1–3 years)

The toddler years are the toughest when it comes to getting the average kid to be willing to try—much less like—healthy foods. Everyone knows of a toddler who gets into a macaroni and cheese or peanut butter and jelly rut. Remember, toddlers like tastes that are familiar to them. Bridge familiar tastes to newer tastes and textures by slightly modifying a mealtime favorite.

### Preschooler (3–5 years)

The presentation and visual appeal of meals and snacks take center stage in the preschool years. Presenting food in cool shapes, multiple colors, and adornments entices a preschooler to give it a try. If you also make sure it tastes good, you're likely to have long-term success in raising a child who prefers the healthy foods.

## School Age (5–10 years)

By now, your child's taste preferences are fairly well established. This is great news if you have a veggie lover who prefers simple foods with few added tastes and textures. However, if you have a child with a preference for greasy or highly processed foods, then you've got a little more work to do. To transition this child to preferring a wholesome fruit and veggie–rich diet, you'll have to make sure the food you're making tastes great. Instead of adding a lot of salt, sugar, or fat to achieve this objective, consider experimenting with seasonings and herbs to give an old taste a new flare.

# Chapter Summary

A goal of this chapter was to help you easily prepare nutrient-dense meals that taste delicious. The following is a 10-point recap of the highlights from this chapter:

- Remember that taste is the number one predictor of whether a child will eat a food.
- Multiple characteristics determine whether a person likes a food, including taste, texture, temperature, shape, color, smell, and social, cultural, and personal factors.
- The sense of smell is 10,000 times more sensitive than taste and is a major determinant of how positively a food is received. If you make your meals smell good, you greatly increase the chances that the kids will eat them.
- Many seasonings, flavor enhancers, herbs, and spices add a great deal of flavor to your meals without sacrificing nutritional value (except for the addition of a lot of salt) or increasing caloric content.
- When shopping, aim to choose the highest-quality ingredients to maximize flavor and taste and thus how well the family members will like them. You don't need to spend a ton of money to do this. Rather, be aware of what products are in season (and thus less expensive and more flavorful) and know how to pick the freshest offerings.
- Plan ahead for meals and shopping trips. This will help decrease the prep time and frustration surrounding cooking and increase the chances that you'll have the ingredients you need to quickly throw together a meal after a long day at work or taking care of the kids.
- Start with simple recipes. Once you get used to cooking and comfortable with the recipes, experiment with substitutions and additions.
- Solicit help. Involving the kids in meal preparation, serving, and clean up not only makes your job easier, but by including them in meal preparation, they'll be more likely to actually eat what they help make.
- Sneak it in. Help your kids acquire a taste for a consistently refused food by pureeing it and adding it in to a mealtime favorite. You might be surprised that they don't even notice.
- Have fun with it. Cooking need not be a dreaded ritual. Try to have fun experimenting with different ingredients and recipes. You might be surprised how diverse your family's taste preferences become.

# Recipes: Who Knew Healthy Tastes This Good?

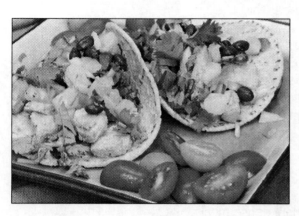

### Grilled Salmon Tacos With Mango Black Bean Salsa

2 6-ounce salmon filets
8 corn tortillas
1 lime, cut into wedges
Olive oil

*Mexican Spice Marinade*

1 teaspoon ground cumin
1 teaspoon of dried onion
1 teaspoon of ground oregano
1/2 cup of fresh cilantro

To prepare the fish: Mix all the spices in a large bowl and add 2 tablespoons of olive oil. Cut the fish into 1/2-inch cubes and place into marinade. Let sit in refrigerator for 1 hour. When ready to cook, place 2 tablespoons of olive oil in a pan over medium heat. Remove the fish from the refrigerator and into the pan. Cook for 10 to 12 minutes, stirring occasionally, until fish has cooked through.

Serve with warm corn tortillas and mango black bean salsa.

*Mango Black Bean Salsa*

2 small mangos or 1 1/2 cups of defrosted frozen mangos
1 15-ounce can of black beans, drained
1/4 medium onion (any color), finely diced
1 red bell pepper, finely diced
1/2 cup of fresh cilantro, chopped
Juice of 1 lime

If using fresh mangos, peel the skin and slice fruit off on either side of the seed. Cut mangos into small pieces, approximately the same size as the peppers and onions. Mix all ingredients together in a bowl and serve with tacos.

### Grilled Portabella Mushroom Burger With Sun-Dried Tomato Yogurt Aioli

4 portabella mushrooms, washed and dried
4 whole wheat buns
2 cups of baby spinach, washed and dried
Olive oil

*Asian Spice Marinade*

1 teaspoon of ground dried garlic (or 1 tablespoon of fresh garlic)
2 bunch of scallions, chopped
1 tablespoon of sesame seeds
1/2 inch of fresh ginger (or 1 teaspoon of dried ginger)
1/2 cup of soy sauce

*Sun-Dried Tomato Yogurt Aioli*

1 garlic clove
10 sun-dried tomatoes (in oil)
1/4 cup of plain yogurt
2 tablespoons of mayonnaise

On a large baking tray, mix the marinade ingredients. Place cleaned portabella mushrooms on the baking tray and let marinate for 30 minutes.

While mushrooms are marinating, prepare aioli. Place garlic clove and sun-dried tomatoes in a food processor and blend until smooth. Remove from blender and place into a small bowl. Mix yogurt and mayonnaise with sun-dried tomato mixture until well blended.

Prepare grill or large pan. If using large pan, place 1 tablespoon of olive oil into the pan. Once pan or grill is heated, remove mushrooms from marinade and let cook for 5 minutes. Flip mushrooms onto opposite side and let cook for another 3 to 4 minutes.

To prepare burgers, place 1 to 2 tablespoons of aioli on one side of the hamburger bun. Next, place cleaned and dried baby spinach and then mushroom on top of spinach. Top with remaining hamburger bun and serve.

## Mahimahi Pitas With Cucumber and Tomato Salad

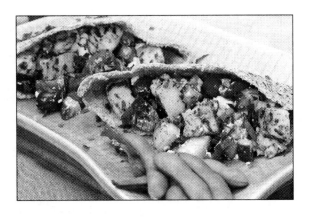

1/4 cup of plain nonfat yogurt
2 6-ounce mahimahi filets
4 whole wheat pita breads

*Middle Eastern Spice Marinade*

1 teaspoon of ground dried garlic (or 1 tablespoon
  of fresh garlic)
1 teaspoon of dried onion
1/4 cup of fresh mint
1 teaspoon of ground cumin
Pinch of saffron

Mix the spice marinade together with yogurt and 2 tablespoons of olive oil and place into a mixing bowl. Cut mahimahi filets into 1/2-inch cubes and place in marinade. Refrigerate for 1 hour. When ready to cook, remove the fish from the refrigerator. Place 2 tablespoons of olive oil in a pan over medium heat. Place the fish in the pan and cook for 10 to 12 minutes or until fish is cooked through.

Serve with warm pita bread and top with feta, cucumber, and tomato salad.

*Feta, Cucumber, and Tomato Salad*

1 English cucumber, seeded and chopped into 1/8-inch cubes
3 Roma or vine ripened tomatoes, seeded and chopped into 1/8 inch cubes
1/4 cup of crumbled feta cheese
1/2 red onion, chopped
1/2 cup black olives, seeded and halved
Olive oil

Mix all ingredients in mixing bowl. Drizzle with 2 tablespoons of olive oil. Serve with Mahimahi Pitas.

## Eggplant Zucchini "Pasta" Lasagna

1 large eggplant
3 medium zucchinis
1 jar of marinara sauce
2 cups of low fat ricotta cheese
1 egg
1 1/4 cup of low fat mozzarella cheese

*Italian Spice Marinade*

1 teaspoon of ground dried garlic (or 1 tablespoon of fresh garlic)
1 teaspoon of dried basil (or 1/4 cup of fresh basil, chopped)
1 teaspoon of dried parsley (or 1/4 cup of fresh parsley, chopped)
1 teaspoon of dried oregano

Preheat oven to 400 degrees.

To prepare the vegetables: Wash and dry the vegetables. Using a mandolin, slice the eggplant and zucchinis lengthwise into thin strips (mimicking the pasta used for lasagna). If you don't have a mandolin, carefully slice the eggplant and zucchinis lengthwise into very thin strips. Sprinkle the vegetable slices with 1 teaspoon of salt and pepper and set aside.

To prepare the herbed ricotta: Mix the spices for the marinade in a bowl. Mix in the ricotta and egg and stir well.

To assemble the lasagna: Place 1/4 cup of marinara sauce on the bottom of a 9x13 baking dish. Place a layer of zucchini/eggplant on the bottom. Next, sprinkle a layer of mozzarella cheese, followed by a layer of the ricotta, and then a layer of marinara sauce. Place another layer of zucchini/eggplant and repeat the layers. Once complete, cover the baking dish with foil.

Bake for approximately 45 minutes. Remove the foil and sprinkle with 1/4 cup of mozzarella cheese. Return to oven and bake for another 10 minutes, until cheese has melted.

## References

1. Spill, M.K., L.L. Birch, L.S. Roe, and B.J. Rolls. (2011). Hiding vegetables to reduce energy density: An effective strategy to increase children's vegetable intake and reduce energy intake. *Am J Clin Nutr. 94*(3): p. 735-41.
2. Dangour, A.D., K. Lock, A. Hayter, A. Aikenhead, E. Allen, and R. Uauy. (2010). Nutrition-related health effects of organic foods: A systematic review. *Am J Clin Nutr. 92*(1): p. 203-10.
3. Curl, C.L., R.A. Fenske, and K. Elgethun. (2003). Organophosphorus pesticide exposure of urban and suburban preschool children with organic and conventional diets. *Environ Health Perspect. 111*(3): p. 377-82.

## Resource

www.fruitsandveggiesmatter.gov—A website hosted by the Centers for Disease Control and Prevention that provides excellent information and resources for how to increase the number of fruits and vegetables in your daily eating plan.

# 9

# Mistake #9— Enabling the Couch Potato

*"It's just hard not to listen to TV: It's spent so much more time raising us than you have."*
—Bart Simpson

Newspaper reports buzz about the crisis of a generation of electronic media–obsessed kids. A 2010 Kaiser Family Foundation survey found that the average child spends a whopping 53 hours a week—that's 7 hours and 38 minutes per day—with such electronic media as TV, video games, computers, cell phones, iPads®, and iPods®.[1] Presumably, a child who's in front of the television for hours on end isn't getting the recommended minimum 60 minutes of physical activity per day. In fact, if you're like 80 percent of parents, your kid gets nowhere near this amount of physical activity.[2] But that doesn't mean that kids of this generation are destined for a lifetime of physical laziness—not even those who already spend a large majority of their free time in sedentary activity and who refuse to get moving. With a little bit of parental foresight and nudging, you can get your kid off the couch and out there truly loving being active. And, in reality, for the health and well-being of your children, you have no other option. Physical activity is essential for more than just preventing and treating obesity. Your kids also need it for optimum academic performance, socialization, and mental health.

So, how do you get a physically inactive child to exercise? Isn't it kind of like trying to get an unwilling kid to like broccoli? If you push too hard, he'll just push back and refuse. After all, you can't move a kid's muscles for him. You'll have to take a similar approach as you do with healthy eating—empower your child to actually like the activities. Consider these examples:

- Chris is a six-year-old first-grader enthralled by video games. He used to spend several hours every Saturday intent on winning the Super Bowl from the comfortable confines of his living room. Alarmed by his disdain for the great outdoors and any type of physical activity if it occurred at the expense of playing his video games, his parents began their pursuit to get Chris moving by investing in Kinect™, a video game system requiring user interaction and physical exertion. The average "active video gamer" gets light-to-moderate activity while playing and increases energy expenditure by about 222 percent. The results are even better for games that require more lower-body versus upper-body exertion.[3]

- Anna, a normal-weight but physically inactive fourth-grader, suffers from shyness. At her parents' urging, she's tried several sports but has dropped out of each of them. Recently, she joined Girls on the Run, a program that uses running as a vehicle to teach girls life skills. She brags to her friends that she finished her first 5K. The boost in her physical activity not only improves her overall health, but research suggests that higher levels of physical activity also increase feelings of self-efficacy and confidence.[4]

- Jimmy is an obese fifth-grader who's always picked last for the games at school and who's never been interested in sports, although he's told his parents on many occasions he wishes he were thinner. When his parents saw flyers for a weight training program for youth at their health club, they asked Jimmy if he wanted to give it a try. Over the course of a month in the program, Jimmy's increased strength (and realization that he's a lot stronger than many of his peers) was matched by a dramatic increase in confidence. Now he says he can't wait to try out for the sixth-grade football team.

# Motivators

Kids receive many benefits from being physically active, including the obvious ones, such as maintenance of a healthy weight and improved health and fitness, and some less well-known ones, such as improved academic performance, "executive function" (more on this later), and mental health. But regardless of each of these benefits, if your kid doesn't want to move his body, you can't force it. Just as with empowering your kids to *choose* healthy foods, the goal is to also empower your kids to *want* to be active. The key to making this happen is to first identify and address the barriers (see the sidebar "Barriers to Physical Activity and How to Overcome Them") and then work with your child's strengths and motivators to come up with an activity plan that he'll enjoy. Remember—your motivators as a parent may be different from your child's.

## Exercise for Fun!

Typically, kids just want to have fun! This fun usually comes from free play and sports.

### Play

Fifty-thousand people gathered for New York City's inaugural Ultimate Block Party in October 2010. The brainchild of the Play for Tomorrow coalition of educators, health professionals, and parents whose main focus is to champion the importance of play in children's lives, the event showcased the art and science of play.

## Barriers to Physical Activity and How to Overcome Them

The following are the top five perceived barriers to physical activity in overweight and obese children (and strategies to overcome them).[17] Many of the barriers may also apply to normal-weight children. (Rated on a scale of 1 = never to 5 = often.)

*Barrier:* Have too much homework (2.7) and not enough time for physical activity (2.5)

*Potential solution:* Suggest exercises, such as calisthenics, that can be done quickly in short bouts during homework breaks. Also, encourage weekend activity and walking or biking to and from school—if feasible.

*Barrier:* Self-conscious about looks (2.6) and body (2.55) when doing physical activity

*Potential solution:* Choose activities that focus on how to make their bodies work better and become more fit rather than activities that focus on how to make their bodies look better.

*Barrier:* Don't have anyone with whom to exercise (2.46)

*Potential solution:* Choose and plan for activities you can do together as a family that are appropriate for your child's age.

*Barrier:* Feel too overweight to do physical activity (2.37)

*Potential solution:* Help your child begin an exercise program that starts low and goes slow. Encourage fun, lower-intensity, everyday activities, such as walking the dog, playing hopscotch, gardening, and dancing.

*Barrier:* Chosen last for teams (2.35)

*Potential solution:* Avoid pushing your child into activities with excessive focus on skill level. Instead, consider bringing your child with you to the gym and doing a resistance training circuit together. This can help improve self-efficacy, as oftentimes, overweight children are very strong.

The social movement pushing for more child's play comes at a critical time. With an alarming number of schools eliminating recess and failing to reinstate regular physical activity in the school day, today's children are largely inactive and lacking a regular opportunity to just play. The Alliance for Childhood published a scathing report of the current state of kindergarten, where academic pressures have virtually eliminated playtime from the average five-year-old's school day.[5] Meanwhile, behavior problems and anxiety disorders have skyrocketed.[6]

We all can reminisce back to our childhood years and recall what seemed like endless hours of playing—playing pickup games with friends, riding bikes across town, rollerblading several miles, and participating in any number of made-up activities with the rest of the neighborhood kids. Our parents were probably even more active as they grew up with even less competing demands for a child's limited attention. But our kids have it much harder. The streets aren't as safe. The games aren't as fun when compared with today's toys, which are products of extraordinary technology advances. Parents are working more, coming home exhausted after a long day of work and wanting nothing more than a few minutes of respite; TV is a surefire way to keep the kids quiet and content.

Schools have replaced physical education classes with more "academic" subjects, such as English and math, even in the youngest grades. Recess is absent from many school agendas. (Although 96 percent of elementary students had at least one recess in 1989, only 70 percent of kindergarteners today get a recess period.[6]) Not to mention suburban sprawl and the difficulty to walk anywhere from many residential neighborhoods, including to school. These factors together help explain why kids are so sedentary. The numbers are startling: children today have lost 12 hours per week of free time, with 25 percent less play and 50 percent fewer outdoor activities compared with children in the late 1970s.[6] Our children have been deprived of play.

Play encompasses more than physical activity. The Ultimate Block Party broke it down into six domains: physical, creative, music and dance, make-believe, technology, and language. All components of play are essential for a child's optimal development. While physical play is only one domain, many of the other domains, such as music and dance and creative play, overlap and provide opportunities for a child to get moving. During free play, children learn problem-solving skills, practice leadership, expend energy, and develop important social and cognitive skills. Play is most powerful when it's child directed, child driven, and somewhat spontaneous. Overly scheduled children doing largely adult-directed activities have few opportunities for true play.

The United Nations High Commission for Human Rights believes child-driven play to be so important that it considers play a right of every child. In contrast to passive, sedentary entertainment, such as watching television or playing a video game, play demands creativity and innovation. Children who play together can create and explore their world while developing skills in sharing, decision making, conflict resolution, teamwork, and language. Play also offers engaged parents a glimpse into a child's world.

Studies of innovative curricula that incorporate and emphasize play have been shown to be superior in helping children develop *executive function* skills. Executive function is a marker of cognitive control comprised of inhibitory control (resisting habits, temptations, or distractions), working memory (retaining and using information), and cognitive flexibility (adjusting to change).[7] Executive function skills are essential for success in school and in life. A brief play period during the school day provides children with the opportunity to engage in physical activity, release energy, and get a mental break. Several studies have shown that this mental break actually increases retention of new information and produces more attentive and less fidgety students.[8] Studies have also found that having at least one recess period of at least 15 minutes was associated with better class behavior scores.[8]

The epidemic of lack of creative play and inactivity is alarming. While it would require massive environmental and policy changes to truly make a dent in solving the crisis, the solution for each individual child starts at home and in the nearby community.

---

### Eating for Sport

**My 10-year-old plays soccer competitively. What should she eat for optimal health and performance?**

A lot of attention has focused on the problem of childhood obesity and inactivity, but little mention has been made about the growing number of highly active kids engaged in competitive sports. These youth athletes push themselves physically and mentally to achieve impressive levels of athletic performance. While serious competition tends to develop during preadolescence, some 10-year-olds do take their sports very seriously and physically challenge their bodies. In these cases, it's critical to provide the right nutrition and fuel—for the sport and to support a rapidly growing body. A high training load creates unique nutritional demands. Kids aren't just "little adults," and the rules of adult sports nutrition don't necessarily apply.

First and foremost, a highly active youth athlete requires an adequate number of calories to fuel not only the strenuous exercise regimen but also optimal growth and development. Athletes involved in endurance sports, aesthetic sports (such as gymnastics and cheerleading), and weight-class sports are at the highest risk of not consuming adequate calories. Athletes can go to choosemyplate.gov to get a general idea of how many calories they need per day based on their age, weight, height, and activity level. The website also provides users with an individualized eating plan, which can help athletes consume an optimally healthy diet, including all the essential nutrients they need, such as iron and calcium, which are deficient in many preteens and teens. This individualized plan will work for most kids, although athletes should be sure to let hunger be their guide and choose nutrient-dense meals and snacks to fuel their activity.

While adults are advised to consume a carbohydrate-rich food within 30 minutes of finishing exercise for optimal recovery and then to have an overall increased protein intake to help rebuild muscles, nutrient recommendations for kids are a little less clear. The Recommended Dietary Allowance of carbohydrates for most kids is 130 grams per day. Ideally, athletes will get this from a diet rich in whole grains, such as cereals, rice, and pasta; fruits and vegetables; and limited in simple sugars. This recommended amount is based on the body's needs to provide glucose for brain development and doesn't include the needs for active children to replenish glucose stores. But kids metabolize sugars differently from adults, and it's not entirely clear if and how much more carbohydrate youth athletes need for optimal performance. Likewise, it's not clear if kids involved in long-distance endurance events

## Sports

Regardless of natural ability or level of athletic competition, nearly every child has some experience with sports during childhood. Many participate for the pure joy and fun of the sport and friendly competition. Others play sports competitively in hopes of making the high school team, playing in college, or one day becoming a professional athlete. (See the sidebar "Eating for Sport.")

---

benefit from carbohydrate-loading the same way adults do. Generally, most youth athletes will do well eating a healthy, nutrient-dense diet that contains at least 50 percent of calories from carbohydrate. As far as protein intake goes, most athletes will meet their protein needs with the standard recommendation of 0.8 to 1.2 grams of protein/kg/day (0.4 to 0.5 grams of protein/lb/day). Some athletes may have higher needs, but most will spontaneously increase their caloric and protein intake. Any protein consumed in excess of what the body needs will likely be used as energy or stored as fat.

In addition to healthy eating habits, staying hydrated is extremely important for young athletes. It's well known that kids have a more difficult time regulating body temperature, especially in extreme environments, such as on a hot and humid summer day. In general, kids should aim to drink as much in fluids as they lose in body weight during an exercise session. That is, they would ideally weigh themselves pre- and post-exercise and make up the difference with fluid intake. Even a 1 percent decrease in body weight from sweating decreases endurance in kids. Or more simply, kids should be reminded and encouraged to stay adequately hydrated while exercising and let thirst be their guide. While millions of adolescents in the United States consume sports drinks, the limited amount of research that's been done suggests that although athletes feel like the drinks are helping them, little effect on performance occurs, except in cases of athletes exercising for prolonged periods in hot temperatures.

So, how should you put all this into action? Check out a sample meal plan for your athlete at choosemyplate.gov. Then, divide the recommended types of food into a daily plan based on the athlete's exercise schedule. Pregame meals should be eaten about 1.5 to 3 hours before the event. Go for easily digestible, high-carbohydrate meals with moderate protein options, such as some pasta with ground turkey. Your child athlete might do well with a glass of low-fat chocolate milk or a granola bar with an orange shortly after a moderately strenuous practice or game. Or if an all-day tournament is under way, snacks like these that contain about 200 to 300 calories spaced throughout the day will help sustain energy. Fluids should be emphasized throughout the game or practice, and sports drinks might be a good idea for events in warm temperatures lasting longer than about an hour. A postgame dinner of pizza loaded with veggies on a whole grain crust would give an athlete a decent number of calories and nutrients to get her ready for the next day.

Ultimately, when it comes to youth sports nutrition, the goal is for your youth athlete to consume enough calories and fluids to fuel the exercise and enough nutrients to meet the body's demands for growth and strength.

In any case, participation in sports offers children tremendous health, social, and developmental benefits. Children who play sports not only have a regular opportunity to engage in physical activity, but they also develop life skills including leadership, teamwork, self-discipline, cooperation, and how to overall be a "good sport" whether the game is won or lost.[9]

Parents should take extra care to help facilitate a child's overall positive experience with sports while recognizing it's not possible to shield a child from all uncomfortable experiences. Repeated failures, criticism, excessive pressure, and negative peer interactions can leave a child permanently turned off to sports. Sometimes, parents themselves need to step back from the game and refocus on what's important. Consider this example of an interaction with a Little League baseball player and his coach. Six-year-old Josh was devastated after he struck out. Trying to console him, his coach shared that Pete Rose, the player with the most hits in baseball history, struck out more than 1,000 times. The kid responded with "Yeah, but Pete doesn't have to ride home with my dad."[9]

It's important to keep in mind a child's level of physical, social, and emotional development when enrolling a child in a sport and when setting behavior expectations. The typical progression is described in more detail in the "Developmental Considerations" section of the chapter. If you're considering encouraging your child to join a sport's team but aren't quite sure which sport(s) would be best, check out the sidebar "How to Find Your Child's Own Perfect Sport" for information on how to help your child find his own perfect sport.

## Exercise Health, Fitness, and Weight Loss

Kids who are physically active have higher levels of fitness and stronger muscles than their inactive peers. They also have decreased body fat, stronger bones, and are less anxious and depressed. Active kids also are less likely to have chronic diseases later in life, such as heart disease, high blood pressure, diabetes, and osteoporosis.[10] The ongoing epidemic of childhood obesity doesn't affect active kids quite as much as those who are inactive. And if an obese kid starts regularly moving his body, he's more likely to lose the extra weight (or maintain the weight as he grows taller), and has a better chance of entering adolescence and adulthood at a normal weight. Clearly, all parents want these advantages for their children. So, how do you go about making activity happen?

First, when you're thinking about strategies to help your children become more physically active, it's important to remember kids aren't little adults. While an adult may participate in prolonged endurance activities even if these "activities" are sometimes tortuous (such as a 5 a.m. appointment with the treadmill), kids aren't going to do activities that aren't fun. And they certainly aren't going to voluntarily participate in exercises that are incompatible with their short attention span and natural tendency to exercise in periods of short bursts, such as when they run, hop, skip, and jump during spontaneous play. Health and fitness gains are made in the context of brief periods of moderate-to-vigorous physical activity interspersed with brief periods of rest.

In 2008, the Federal Government released its first Physical Activity Guidelines for Americans. The idea was to reiterate the importance of physical activity and

## How to Find Your Child's Own Perfect Sport

With dozens of sports to choose from, you and your child may not be sure which one to try first. While the only way to know for sure if a child likes a sport or not is to get out there and try it, you should take a few steps to help you narrow down the playing field. Ask yourself:

- *What are my child's greatest athletic strengths?* Is it a remarkable ability to run far distances? If so, maybe soccer is a good place to start. Is it increased strength and bulk compared with peers? In this case, football could be a nice fit. Is it a fearless drive for constant stimulation and an adrenaline rush? You could try mountain biking or snowboarding (depending on where you live). Is it really good hand-eye coordination? If so, how about baseball or softball? The key is to guide your child to a sport that's most likely to boost confidence and provide for a positive experience. Also, don't forget to make sure that your child wears the proper sports and protective equipment such as a helmet for biking, skiing, baseball, or football to minimize the risk of serious injury.

- *Does my child gravitate toward team activities or individual activities?* Team sports help children develop social skills and leadership abilities, while individual sports help a child to build self-confidence and self-reliance. A child doesn't have to pick one or the other. Many kids thrive in team and individual sport environments.

- *Am I pressuring my child to play a particular sport because it's my favorite?* It's a natural tendency to encourage your children to play the same sport you grew up with and still love to watch and play. But remember, not everybody has the same interests—even if the child is 50 percent your genetic makeup. As your kids get older, give them the opportunity to pick which sport(s) they'd most like to try out.

- *What's my child's level of coordination and skill?* If a child is strongly resisting participation in a particular sport, it may be because his skill set is different from the skill set required to do well in the sport. Brush it off and give him the opportunity to explore other types of sports and physical activities.

- *Is my child having fun?* The goal of sports participation is to have fun! Try to resist the temptation to raise the next the Tiger Woods or Michael Jordan. When a kid becomes too specialized too soon, the game stops being fun and deprives the child of other equally enriching experiences.

put together a report based on the latest and most credible research to advise Americans how much and what kind of activity they need for optimal health. Although the guidelines pertaining to kids focus on ages six and older, many of the recommendations also apply to younger children. The recommendations advise that kids should get about one hour per day of physical activity. These activities can come in the form of aerobics (running, hopping, skipping, jumping rope, dancing, swimming, and bicycling); muscle strengthening (playing on playground equipment, climbing trees, playing tug-of-war, and more traditional strength training); and bone strengthening (running, jumping, basketball, tennis, hopscotch). (Refer to Figure 9-1 for additional activity examples.) Overall, the quantity of activity is more important than the particular types of activities, although the guidelines do recommend at least three days per week of vigorous aerobic activity and three days per week of muscle and bone strengthening.[10] Check out the sidebar "Meeting the Guidelines" for a sample plan for a seven-year-old who meets these guidelines.

*Exercise for Strength*

Weight lifting could be one piece of a well-rounded physical activity program for some children. Until recently it was thought that resistance training was unsafe and ineffective for children. Early research suggested that young boys didn't develop strength gains, and in 1983, the American Academy of Pediatrics (AAP) released a position statement saying that resistance training for children

| Type of Physical Activity | Activity Examples |
|---|---|
| Moderate-intensity aerobic | • Active recreation, such as hiking, skateboarding, rollerblading<br>• Bicycle riding<br>• Brisk walking |
| Vigorous-intensity aerobic | • Active games involving running and chasing, such as tag<br>• Bicycle riding<br>• Jumping rope<br>• Martial arts, such as karate<br>• Running<br>• Such sports as soccer, ice or field hockey, basketball, swimming, tennis<br>• Cross-country skiing |
| Muscle strengthening | • Tug-of-war and similar games<br>• Modified push-ups (with knees on the floor)<br>• Resistance exercises using body weight or resistance bands<br>• Rope or tree climbing<br>• Sit-ups (curl-ups or crunches)<br>• Swinging on playground equipment/bars |
| Bone strengthening | • Hopscotch and similar games<br>• Hopping, skipping, jumping<br>• Jumping rope<br>• Running<br>• Such sports as gymnastics, basketball, volleyball, tennis |

*Source: Physical Activity Guidelines.* (2008). Washington, DC: Department of Health and Human Services.

Figure 9-1. Examples of moderate- and vigorous-intensity aerobic physical activities and muscle- and bone-strengthening activities for children

## Meeting the Guidelines

### Harold: A Seven-Year-Old Child

Harold participates in many types of physical activities in many places. For example, during physical education class, he jumps rope and does gymnastics and sit-ups. During recess, he plays on the playground—often doing activities that require running and climbing. He also likes to play soccer with his friends and family. When Harold gets home from school, he likes to engage in active play (playing tag) and ride his bicycle.

Harold gets 60 minutes of physical activity each day that's at least moderate intensity. He participates in the following activities each day:

- *Monday:* Walks to and from school (20 minutes), plays actively with family (20 minutes), jumps rope (10 minutes), does gymnastics (10 minutes).
- *Tuesday:* Walks to and from school (20 minutes), plays on playground (25 minutes), climbs on playground equipment (15 minutes).
- *Wednesday:* Walks to and from school (20 minutes), plays actively with friends (25 minutes), jumps rope (10 minutes), runs (5 minutes), does sit-ups (2 minutes).
- *Thursday:* Walks to and from school (20 minutes), plays actively with family (30 minutes), plays soccer (30 minutes).
- *Friday:* Walks to and from school (20 minutes), plays actively with friends (25 minutes), bicycles (15 minutes).
- *Saturday:* Plays on playground (30 minutes), climbs on playground equipment (15 minutes), bicycles (15 minutes).
- *Sunday:* Plays on playground (10 minutes), plays soccer (40 minutes), plays tag with family (10 minutes).

Harold meets the Physical Activity Guidelines for Americans by doing vigorous-intensity aerobic activities, bone-strengthening activities, and muscle-strengthening activities on at least three days of the week:

- *Vigorous-intensity aerobic activities six times during the week:* Jumping rope (Monday and Wednesday), running (Wednesday), soccer (Thursday and Sunday), playing tag (Sunday)
- *Bone-strengthening activities six times during the week:* Jumping rope (Monday and Wednesday), running (Wednesday), soccer (Thursday and Sunday), playing tag (Sunday)
- *Muscle-strengthening activities four times during the week:* Gymnastics (Monday), climbing on playground equipment (Tuesday and Saturday), sit-ups (Wednesday)

*Reference*: Physical Activity Guidelines for Americans, 2008.

was essentially useless.[11] Other myths circulated, suggesting, for example, that resistance training would stunt a child's growth and worsen cardiovascular health and the flexibility and range of motion necessary to excel in sports.[12]

Today, we know that children and teens who participate in resistance training experience a variety of physical benefits, such as increased strength, decreased risk of injury, improved long-term health, and increased sports performance.[12] In addition, resistance training can increase children's self-esteem and confidence.[13] The American Academy of Pediatrics (AAP), the American College of Sports Medicine (ACSM), the National Strength and Conditioning Association (NSCA), and the American Orthopedic Society for Sports Medicine (AOSSM) have all released position statements emphasizing the benefits of resistance training for children and adolescents.

Can your child accept and follow directions? A position stand from the ACSM points out that seven- and eight-year-olds have benefited from resistance training programs and suggests no reason exists why younger kids who can follow directions couldn't benefit from an age-appropriate program that includes such exercises as push-ups and sit-ups. In fact, as a general rule, ACSM says a child who's ready for organized sports or activities, such as Little League baseball, soccer, or gymnastics, is also ready for some type of supervised strength training.[14] More on this in "Developmental Considerations."

Children who are highly motivated to participate in resistance training may benefit from a couple of sessions with a certified and competent personal trainer to learn good technique, reduce risk of injury, and get access to a safe and effective program. If you decide to hire a trainer, first check out the sidebar "Parent Tips for Hiring a Personal Trainer." Overall, the benefits are further enhanced and the risks of resistance training are lessened when youth are under the supervision and instruction of a competent adult. But before signing your kid up for the next possible class at the local Y or your gym, find out your child's overall goals. Often, they're not the same as your goals as a parent. Parents tend to enroll their kids in personal training because they want the child to either excel in a sport or lose weight. That is, parents tend to be results oriented. Kids, on the other hand, usually just want to have fun.

*Exercise for Weight Loss*

A summary analysis of the studies conducted on the role of exercise in the treatment of childhood obesity found substantial benefit, including about a six-and-a-half pound weight loss (3 kg) over 14 weeks at 155 to 180 minutes of moderate-intensity exercise per week—about 20 to 25 minutes per day.[15] While it's desirable to build up to an hour of activity per day, children can start slowly with lesser amounts of exercise and still achieve significant benefits. And remember, the goal isn't necessarily weight loss but rather decreased body mass index (BMI) (children "growing into" their weight) and, ideally, a lifelong interest in physical activity. Refer to Chapter 10 for a more detailed discussion of BMI in kids and what it means.

---

### Parent Tips for Hiring a Personal Trainer

When you're hiring a personal trainer for your child, the trainer should be able to answer yes to all these questions:

- Does the trainer have a certification from a nationally recognized organization and/or a bachelor's degree in a fitness-related field?
- Does the trainer have several years' experience working with children/teens?
- Is the trainer certified in CPR/first aid?
- Does the trainer have a network of professionals, such as physicians, dietitians, physical therapists and other health professionals?
- Does the trainer require a health screening or physician's release before working with your child?
- Can the trainer provide references to other parents you can call?
- Will the trainer keep track of your child's workouts and chart his progress?
- Are the costs and cancellation policies clearly stated?
- Does the trainer have liability insurance?
- Is the trainer aware of guidelines for children's fitness programs from the American Academy of Pediatrics and the American Orthopedic Society for Sports Medicine?
- Does the trainer/facility have an emergency plan in place that ensures that events are handled safely and effectively?

*Source*: Kathie Davis, executive director, IDEA Health & Fitness Association

---

Kids can easily meet the physical activity recommendations and achieve a healthy weight by integrating physical activity into everyday life; it doesn't need to come from organized sports or a physical education class (although those activities count toward the 60 minutes per day). A stop at the playground, an evening walk around the block, and taking the stairs instead of the elevator are easy ways to add a few steps to a child's day. The sidebar "Five Everyday Ways for Families to Increase Physical Activity" offers a few simple, everyday ways for the whole family to increase physical activity.

As you consider how to best go about increasing physical activity in your kids, remember that adults exercise for many reasons, including to optimize health and fitness, lose weight, get stronger, compete, or feel better overall. Many parents enroll their children in various physical activity programs to optimize these types of health benefits. But kids may be motivated to participate in physical activity programs for different reasons (such as to have fun or to hang out with friends). You can guide and oversee your child's activity program to help him reach the goals you had in mind, but it's important to respect your child's motivators. Parents should strive to not put so much pressure on a child to achieve a particular outcome that the activities lose their allure and are no longer fun for the child.

> ### Five Everyday Ways for Families to Increase Physical Activity
>
> - Play a round of Simon Says or tag with your kids. They'll love it, and you'll both be sure to get your heart pumping.
> - Play with your kids in child-driven and child-directed activities 30 minutes a day.
> - During commercials, have the whole family do sit-ups in front of the TV. See how many you can do in total by the end of the show. Next week, try to do a few more. Continue to build up the number you can do.
> - Take a family walk after dinner. During each walk, try to cover the same ground in less time. The next week, add some distance.
> - Walk the kids to school. Not only is it a great opportunity for physical activity and modeling a commitment to a healthy lifestyle, but it also gives you a few minutes of uninterrupted time together.

# Counterstrategies

While this chapter has offered several general recommendations to increase physical activity in kids, the following are a few pointed suggestions to not only get your kids moving but also help a lot more of the kids in your community at the same time.

## Restore Play

You can help restore play in your child's day by not only making changes at home but also advocating for your child in the community. For example, start by finding out what opportunities your child has for free play and physical activity during the school day. Does he have recess? Engage your PTA and school board. Given the compelling evidence that play improves academic success, ask if they'll consider reinstituting recess into every elementary schoolchild's day. The National Association for Sport and Physical Education advises that recess should be provided at least once per day for at least 20 minutes.[16] As a parent, you can advocate that your child's school includes opportunities for physical activity. For the younger kids, opportunities for free play could be one of your considerations when seeking out a preschool.

It's also important to take a look at your own home life. Is every minute of your child's day scheduled or do your kids have a little downtime each day for child-centered, child-led, and child-driven play? Do you sometimes stop what you're doing to play with your kids or at least observe them play? If you're like most parents these days, an honest answer to these questions might be an impetus to conscientiously provide opportunities for your kids to play. The following are a few recommendations from the AAP to help you get started:[6]

- Encourage your kids to spend a little bit of screen-free time each day to be creative and decompress in child-driven free play.

- Set limits to screen time and passive entertainment. The AAP recommends that each child spend fewer than two hours each day with electronic media.
- Remember that active child-centered play is a great way to help kids be fit and healthy.
- Spend a little bit of time each day in unscheduled spontaneous play with your children.
- Talk to your child's pediatrician if your child shows signs of significant stress, anxiety, or depression.
- Advocate for "safe spaces" for kids to play. This can include a school, library, community center, or even a gym or fitness facility.

## Lead by Example

Every step you take, your kids are watching you. One of the most effective ways to get your kids moving is for them to see you be physically active every day. More than that, you can be an agent for change by actively promoting kids' fitness. You could do this in many ways—two of which include coaching your child's team and mobilizing your community through efforts such as starting a Walk to School campaign in your neighborhood. The sidebar "Counterstrategies in Action: Real-Life Successes" offers a few other real-life examples of now-parents committed to a physically active lifestyle thanks to the actions of their own parents.

### Coach a Team

The influence of a youth athletic coach extends far beyond honing a skill, promoting fitness, and making exercise fun. Coaches can shape a child's attitudes, values, and self-esteem. Coaches can ignite passion. You don't have to be an exceptional athlete to be a great coach. You don't even have to play a sport. For example, Girls on the Run, a national program that uses running to teach 9- to 11-year old girls confidence and healthy lifestyles, offers opportunities throughout the country. Coaches are selected based on their passion and commitment to the kids, not how fast they can run a mile. Whether it's your child's Little League team, a national organization, or a school program, parent coaches who have made a personal commitment to make a difference are in high demand.

### Mobilize Your Community

Everyone knows that childhood obesity and physical inactivity are problems. But what are communities doing about them? As a parent, you're ideally positioned to become a voice of change. The following can help you with this endeavor:

- Attend school board and PTA meetings to advocate for increased time and resources for recess and physical education courses and healthier food choices in district schools.
- Join organizations such as Action for Healthy Kids, a national initiative to improve nutrition and physical education in schools. This initiative is

## Counterstrategies in Action: Real-Life Successes

Our experiences as kids shape the priorities and expectations we have for own children. The following are a few examples of parents today who were profoundly influenced by the philosophies and foresight of their parents. As a result, these parents got hooked on physical activity and have passed it on to their own kids.

- "In seventh grade, I hit puberty and switched schools. It was a very hard time for me, and I gained weight. My dad enrolled me in a weight training class at the YMCA and also had a friend sign up with me. In this class, we had a person from the YMCA show us how to do each machine, and he set up our seats and weight. He talked to us about repetition and when to move the weight up and good form while lifting. We were then given a sheet that had all of our information, and we were able to come whenever we wanted (with a parent). This was wonderful for my self-esteem, plus I was gaining knowledge. I never felt uncomfortable in the gym because I knew how to use all of the equipment. I remember in college, no girl would lift weights because they didn't know how. I was so proud of myself that I was comfortable in the weight room, but I also knew how to use the machines properly."

  —Bridget

- "When I was 17, my mom and I, with dirt plastered on our faces and 35-pound packs strapped to our backs, trekked out of the Grand Canyon after a three-day intensive hike to the base of the canyon and back out. After a childhood of being overweight and with a mom who always struggled with her weight and sticking with an exercise program, this physical challenge pushed both of us way outside our comfort zones and proved that if you set a goal and stick to the plan, you really can achieve anything. That experience was a major turning point in my life."

  —Natalie

supported by such organizations as the American Academy of Pediatrics, the National School Board Association, the U.S. Department of Health and Human Services, and the American Federation of Teachers.

- Join a school health advisory committee. These committees advise school administrators and the school board on various health-related topics, including overall health, physical activity, nutrition, tobacco prevention, and sex education. Committee members make recommendations regarding the number of hours in the school day that should be devoted to health and physical education and appropriate changes to improve the nutritional quality of foods offered in the school. As an active committee member, you would be well positioned to make change happen.
- Adopt the walk-to-school initiative in your neighborhood. Check out http://www.walktoschool-usa.org for a step-by-step guide to get started.

- "My family was always big into sports. My dad was a college athlete, and my mom was convinced that team sports would help us build life skills. They didn't care what sports we chose or whether we played on an official team or [a] pickup [team], but they always went out of their way to help make it fun for us. My dad coached my Little League team, and my mom tirelessly shuttled the four of us kids around for practices and games. Looking back, they must have been exhausted, but they really did instill in us a love of sports and exercise."

  —Bob

- "I hated that I always dreaded doing that damn mile in gym class once a year, so when I saw an article in some teen magazine about how you could "run 30 minutes in 30 days," I tore it out and convinced my sister to do it with me. ... My mom started running with us after that and, as is her usual style, soon surpassed us by starting to train for marathons. Both my brothers started running after that too. ... [My brother] still runs races with my mom occasionally. I think my mom's persistent love of running has kept me motivated to either keep going or restart running when I have been away from it for a while. ... She always talks about her runs to me—a little friendly reminder on an almost daily basis for me to stay active. ... Growing up with three siblings, it was special to have some alone time together, and if I went to work out with my mom or on a walk or run together, we were able to spend some extra time together in a setting that was conducive to having uninterrupted conversations. When my mom comes to visit me, we go running together to get time alone to catch up."

  —Amber

# Developmental Considerations

As you get your kids up and moving, it's best to set expectations and develop strategies that coincide with their developmental stages (Figure 9-2).

## Infant (0–1 years)

A baby can begin to engage in physical activities at about one month of age, with multiple short bouts of "tummy time" each day. Tummy time is when a baby is placed on his stomach while awake and closely monitored. Tummy time challenges an infant to learn to develop upper-body strength as he tries to push up. Once an infant learns to roll, he can be allowed to practice his new skill in a safe and baby-proofed environment. Outdoor free play and exploration under close adult supervision provide an infant with cognitive stimulation as

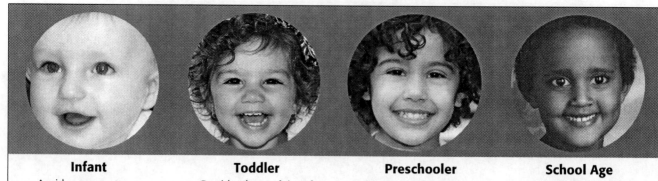

| Infant | Toddler | Preschooler | School Age |
|---|---|---|---|
| • Avoid exposure to electronic media (such as TV, cell phones, etc.).<br>• Aim for a total of one hour of "tummy time" throughout the day.<br>• Create safe spaces for exploration and play. | • Provide plenty of time for free play.<br>• Introduce your child to the fun and beauty of the outdoors and nature in your own yard and at parks and playgrounds.<br>• Introduce sports equipment for exploration. | • Encourage at least 30 minutes of free play every day.<br>• Increase opportunities for daily physical activity. Encourage walking, running, tumbling, and climbing.<br>• Introduce the idea of sports, with an emphasis on fun. | • Continue to introduce sports. Choose those with flexible rules, short instruction time, and fun aspects.<br>• Continue to encourage free play.<br>• Restrict screen time to fewer than two hours per day. |

Figure 9-2. Developmental considerations

well as a fun experience. The AAP recommends that children younger than two not be exposed to any television or electronic media.

## Toddler (1–3 years)

Toddlerhood and learning to walk open up all kinds of opportunities for kids to be active. Running around outdoors, learning to kick a ball and swing a bat, and being allowed to spend playdates with other kids engaged in free play indoors and outdoors in parks and playgrounds are some examples.

## Preschooler (3–5 years)

A preschooler loves to play! The goals at this age are to create ample opportunities for fun free play, exploration, and experimentation while also being careful to provide adequate supervision and a safe environment. Running, swimming, tumbling, throwing, and catching are especially fun for preschool children who are just starting to learn many of these skills. A preschooler can also go for family walks and be encouraged to take extra steps in the day, such as taking the stairs instead of the elevator. Preschoolers should watch fewer than two hours of television each day.

## School Age (5–10 years)

As children enter elementary school, they begin to develop the physical, emotional, and cognitive maturity to play sports. They can physically master the skills, emotionally engage in competition, and cognitively understand the rules. For best results, organized sports should have flexible rules and short instruction, allow for free time during practice, and emphasize fun rather than serious competition. Children who can follow directions and are developmentally ready for sports would also do fine with a resistance training program. Like preschoolers, school-aged children should watch fewer than two hours of television each day.

# Chapter Summary

Are you ready to get your family moving? The following summarizes the major points from this chapter, but don't feel constricted. Really, it's just simply about getting back to moving our bodies—one step at a time:

- Allow for child-directed, child-driven free play at least 30 minutes most days. Make finding time for this free play a priority when you contemplate what after-school activities and programs your children will do.
- Remember, the most important component to any exercise program for kids is the fun factor.
- Limit screen time to fewer than two hours per day for kids older than two. Avoid TV and screen time for infants and toddlers zero to two.
- Advocate for regular physical education and recess in your child's school.
- Once your child is developmentally ready, introduce your child to sports, but be careful not to push too hard.
- Increase opportunities for everyday physical activity in your home and as a family.
- Come up with a sample "schedule" of how your kid might meet the physical activity guidelines without making exercise a drag.
- Lead by example. Commit to increase your everyday physical activity and be active about one hour on most, if not all, days of the week.
- Encourage activities most appropriate for your child's developmental stage.
- Mobilize your community for the sake of all kids.

# Recipes: Healthy Snacks After Serious Physical Activity

## Homemade Trail Mix Granola Bars

1 1/2 cups rolled oats
1 1/2 cups crispy brown rice cereal
1 cup brown rice syrup
1/4 cup brown sugar
1 cup whole or slivered almonds
1 cup raisins
1/2 cup of chocolate chips
1 tablespoon ground cinnamon
1 teaspoon salt
2 tablespoons of butter, melted and cooled
2 tablespoons of flaxseed meal or flaxseeds (optional)

Preheat oven to 375 degrees. Mix all ingredients together in a mixing bowl. Spray a 9x13 pan with nonstick cooking spray. Pour mixture into the baking pan and press down. Bake in oven for 25 minutes. Cool to room temperature before cutting into bars.

### Five-Layer Bean Dip With Fresh Vegetables and Baked Pita Chips

2 15-ounce cans of black beans
6 tomatoes, seeded and chopped
2 ripe avocados
1/2 cup of fresh cilantro, chopped
2 bunches of green onion, chopped
1/2 cup of shredded cheddar cheese
1 1/2 cups of Greek yogurt
Juice of 1 lime
1/4 medium white onion, finely chopped

Place beans, including the water from the can, into a small pot over medium heat. Bring to boil and then remove from heat. Using a fork or potato masher, mash the beans in the pot and then place in an 8x8 baking dish. To make the guacamole, spoon the avocado into a bowl. Mix in the chopped white onion and lime juice and sprinkle with salt and pepper. Mash the avocado with the onion and lime mixture. Then, add 1/4 cup of Greek yogurt to the avocado mixture and mix well. Spread the guacamole on top of the bean layer. Next, layer the chopped tomatoes on top of the guacamole. On top of the tomatoes, spread the remainder of the Greek yogurt evenly. Sprinkle the cheddar cheese on top of the yogurt and then the chopped cilantro and green onion.

Serve with fresh carrots, bell peppers, celery, cucumbers, or baked pita chips.

### Whole Grain Waffle Apple Peanut Butter Sandwiches

4 frozen whole grain waffles, defrosted
8 tablespoons of peanut butter
2 apples

Toast waffles until golden brown. Cut each apple in half, remove the core, and cut apples into thin slices. Once waffles are toasted, cut each in half. Place 1 tablespoon of peanut butter on each waffle half. Place apple slices evenly among the waffle halves and top with remaining waffle half.

## References

1. Rideout, V.J., U.G. Foehr, and D.F. Roberts. (2010). Generation M2: Media in the Lives of 8- to 18-Year-Olds. Menlo Park, CA: Henry J. Kaiser Family Foundation. Available at http://www.kff.org/entmedia/upload/8010.pdf.

2. Eaton, D.K., L. Kann, S. Kinchen, S. Shanklin, J. Ross, J. Hawkins, W.A. Harris, R. Lowry, T. McManus, D. Chyen, C. Lim, L. Whittle, N.D. Brener, and H. Wechsler. (2010). Youth risk behavior surveillance—United States, 2009. *MMWR Surveill Summ. 59*(5): p. 1-142.

3. Biddiss, E., and J. Irwin. (2010). Active video games to promote physical activity in children and youth: A systematic review. *Arch Pediatr Adolesc Med. 164*(7): p. 664-72.

4. Floriani, V., and C. Kennedy. (2008). Promotion of physical activity in children. *Curr Opin Pediatr. 20*(1): p. 90-5.

5. Miller, E., and J. Almon. (2009). *Crisis in Kindergarten: Why Children Need to Play in School*. New York: Alliance for Childhood.

6. Ginsburg, K.R. (2007). The importance of play in promoting healthy child development and maintaining strong parent-child bonds. *Pediatrics. 119*(1): p. 182-91.

7. Diamond, A., W.S. Barnett, J. Thomas, and S. Munro. (2007). Preschool program improves cognitive control. *Science. 318*(5855): p. 1387-8.

8. Barros, R.M., E.J. Silver, and R.E. Stein. (2009). School recess and group classroom behavior. *Pediatrics. 123*(2): p. 431-6.

9. Tofler, I.R., and G.J. Butterbaugh. (2005). Developmental overview of child and youth sports for the twenty-first century. *Clin Sports Med. 24*(4): p. vii-viii, 783-804.

10. *Physical Activity Guidelines for Americans.* (2008). Washington, DC: Department of Health and Human Services.

11. Benjamin, H.J., and K.M. Glow. (2003). Strength training for children and adolescents: What can physicians recommend? *Phys Sportsmed. 31*(9): p. 19-26.

12. Guy, J.A., and L.J. Micheli. (2001). Strength training for children and adolescents. *J Am Acad Orthop Surg. 9*(1): p. 29-36.

13. Faigenbaum, A.D., W.L. Westcott, R.L. Loud, and C. Long. (1999). The effects of different resistance training protocols on muscular strength and endurance development in children. *Pediatrics. 104*(1): p. e5.

14. Faigenbaum, A.D., and L.J. Micheli. (1998). Youth resistance training. *Sports Medicine Bulletin. 32*(2): p. 28.

15. Atlantis, E., E.H. Barnes, and M.A. Singh. (2006). Efficacy of exercise for treating overweight in children and adolescents: A systematic review. *Int J Obes (Lond). 30*(7): p. 1027-40.

16. *Recess in Elementary Schools: A Position Paper of the Council on Physical Education for Children.* (2001). Reston, VA: National Association for Sports and Physical Education.

17. Zabinski, M.F., B.E. Saelens, R.I. Stein, H.A. Hayden-Wade, and D.E. Wilfley. (2003). Overweight children's barriers to and support for physical activity. *Obes Res. 11*(2): p. 238-46.

# THE OVERLOOKED MISTAKES

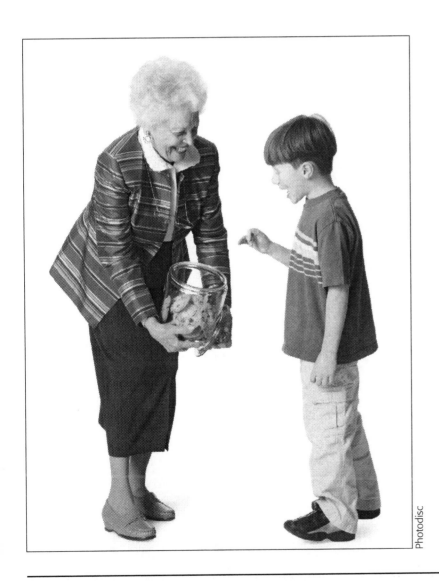

Photodisc

**Part Four**

# 10

# Mistake #10— Remaining Speechless at Doctor's Visits

*"If the doctors of today do not become the nutritionists of tomorrow, then the nutritionists of today will become the doctors of tomorrow."*
—Rockefeller Institute of Medicine Research

Hailey is a very picky one-year-old. When she was born, she was average weight, but now her weight gain has slowed considerably and she's in the eighth percentile. Her mom is worried that she doesn't eat very much and she's rarely hungry. She's also concerned that Hailey might be at risk for nutritional deficiencies due to the limited variety of foods in her diet. Hailey's mom has brought this up with Hailey's doctor, who says that he isn't too concerned, but he still keeps asking Hailey and her parents to come back every four weeks to do "weight checks." He also did a blood test, but Hailey's mom isn't sure what the test was for or what exactly the results were.

Michael is Hailey's seven-year-old brother. He has the opposite problem. At his last physical exam, the doctor told Michael and his parents that Michael weighs too much for his height and that he needs to eat less and exercise more. The doctor ordered a bunch of blood tests to make sure Michael doesn't have any early signs of obesity-related diseases. They all came back normal.

Hailey and Michael's mom isn't quite sure how she ended up with an underweight kid and an overweight kid or what she should do to make sure that each gets just the right amount and type of food. She describes herself as very sensitive and can't help but get defensive when the doctor continues to question her on how and what she's feeding her kids. Although she wants what's best for her kids, she's not quite sure what to make of the doctor's advice.

# The Parent-Pediatrician Partnership

These days, with childhood obesity, physical inactivity, and very poor overall eating habits widespread throughout the United States and the world, pediatricians have become even more diligent in assessing a child's weight and nutrition and activity habits. While this overall is a trend in the right direction, it also opens up a sensitive area for many families. After all, feeding a child is one of the most important and treasured roles a parent plays. When a parent senses criticism or judgment of parenting skills from an outside observer who's not present at the home on a day-to-day basis and doesn't truly understand the challenges a parent faces, it's natural for the parent to feel slighted and defensive. But if parents and pediatricians form a strong partnership, they're a potent force in the effort to improve a child's nutrition, activity, and weight.

While this is the ideal scenario, on many occasions—especially in the case of a child who's under- or overweight—parents' and pediatricians' intentions may collide, leaving a parent feeling defensive and undermined, while the doctor feels like his efforts are in vain and that it's unlikely that changes will be made at home. In this situation, chances are pretty low that much will come from a discussion about weight, nutrition, and physical activity at a routine physical exam. The parent is unlikely to ask many questions, and the doctor is unlikely to spend much time exploring potential solutions.

One of the most important steps you can take to build a solid and healthy partnership with your child's doctor is to *not* remain speechless at doctor's visits. In other words, take the opportunity during physical exams and well-child checks to engage your child's doctor in your pursuit to optimize your child's health. One way to do this is to be familiar with the lingo, motivations, and constraints your child's doctor faces. Then, you can take the conversation to the next level and really get the most from the visit.

# Counterstrategies

To make the most of doctor's visits, a few simple steps are recommended.

### Plan Ahead

Start by planning ahead. First, ask yourself some important questions: Are you already doing everything that you can to optimize your child's health? How well does he really eat? How active is he? Are there any changes you could make to help him to be even healthier? Check out the quick sample quiz in the sidebar "'The Big Five' Scoring Worksheet" to help identify a starting point for how much work really needs to be done.

Then, before taking your child to his doctor's appointment, ask yourself what you hope to get from the visit. With doctors having only a few short minutes to examine your child and provide you with general guidance, your best bet is to walk in the door with a plan of what you'd like to accomplish during the visit. The questions for parents listed in the sidebar "Preparing for Your Child's

Checkup" can help you get started in thinking about what questions you should be able to answer in case your child's pediatrician asks.

## Understand the Pediatrician's Lingo

At each checkup, pediatricians discuss with patients and their families a variety of topics, such as safety, development, nutrition, and physical activity.[1] Many pediatrician recommendations are based on the Bright Futures guidelines, a set of guidelines endorsed by the American Academy of Pediatrics which advise pediatricians of the most important questions to ask and the most relevant information to share during routine physical exams and well-child checks. Among many other aspects of well-child care, the guidelines include recommendations for promoting healthy weight, healthy nutrition, and physical activity.

### *Promoting Healthy Weight*

Every time your child goes to the doctor for a routine checkup, your child's height and weight should be measured. From this, your child's doctor will calculate BMI (body mass index). (See the sidebar "Understanding BMI.") This number is plotted on a gender-specific growth chart. If your child has a BMI that's less than 5 percent for age, then your child is underweight. (See the sidebar "What to Do About Underweight Kids?" for a discussion of care for an underweight child.) If it's from 5 to 84 percent, your child is at a healthy weight. If it's 85 to 94 percent, your child is overweight. If it's greater than 95 percent, your child is considered "obese." Pediatricians understand that no parent wants to be told that their child is "obese." While pediatricians characterize BMI greater than 95 percent as obese, a sensitive pediatrician is most likely to share that a child with a BMI greater than 95 percent is at an "unhealthy weight," rather than using the term "obese." (See the sidebar "The Problem With Childhood Obesity" for a detailed discussion of the health consequences of carrying too much weight.)

Even if your child is at a healthy weight, your pediatrician should still talk about weight and the importance of maintaining a healthy weight. The AAP recommends promotion of the 5-2-1-0 campaign to promote a healthy weight:

**5** servings of fruits and vegetables per day

**2** hours or fewer of screen time per day (including television, computer, video games, cell phone games, etc.)

**1** hour of physical activity each day

**0** servings of sugar-sweetened beverages per day

### *Promoting Healthy Nutrition*

The Bright Futures guidelines advise pediatricians to discuss nutrition at every checkup. The nutritional advice you can expect to hear from your pediatrician will likely include the following themes:

- *Nutrition for appropriate growth.* The goal is to consume adequate calories and nutrients for optimal growth but not overfeed and contribute to obesity.

# "The Big Five"—Scoring Worksheet

Some habits contribute more than others to excess weight. Complete this brief scoring sheet on behalf of your child. Keep in mind that all children should have good nutrition and physical activity habits, regardless of whether they are overweight.

## 1. Sweetened beverages

Sweetened beverages include fruit juices (whole juice or from concentrate), fruit drinks and punches, regular-calorie soft drinks, sports drink (e.g., Gatorade®), energy drinks, regular sweetened iced tea, and chocolate or other flavored milk. One serving of a sweetened beverage is 12 oz.

How many servings of sweetened beverages does your child consume in a typical day? (Round up any half servings to the next whole number of servings.)

A.   One or no servings = 0
B.   Two servings = 5
C.   Three servings = 10
D.   Four servings = 15
E.   Five or more servings = 20

*Record your child's score here:* _____

## 2. Fast food (excluding sweetened beverages)

Traditional fast food (e.g., burgers [with any type of meat], hot dogs, French fries, chicken nuggets, onion rings)

In a typical week, how often does your child eat traditional fast food?

A.   One time or less = 0
B.   Two times = 5
C.   Three times = 10
D.   Four times = 15
E.   Five or more times = 20

*Record your child's score here:* _____

## 3. Family meals

Eating dinner while being supervised by at least one parent is protective against obesity.

How often does your child eat dinner with at least one parent during a typical week?

A.   One time or less = 20
B.   Two or three times = 10
C.   Four or five times = 5
D.   Six or seven times = 0

*Record your child's score here:* _____

### 4. Media time

Media time is defined as the amount of time your child spends watching television, using a computer (apart from homework), playing video games, or listening to a music device while sitting or lying still.

In a typical day, how much total media time does your child have?

A. Less than one hour = 0
B. One or two hours = 5
C. Two to three hours = 10
D. Three to four hours = 15
E. More than four hours = 20

*Record your child's score here:* _____

### 5. Habitual physical activity

Regular physical activity is protective against obesity. This can include most sports as long as your child is out of breath at least once while playing (softball and bowling do not usually count). It can also include walking, riding a bike, skateboarding, etc., regardless of whether your child is out of breath. Gym class does not count.

In a typical week, on how many days does your child participate in physical activity (sports to the point of being out of breath) or walking, riding a bike, etc., for at least 30 minutes total per day?

A. Zero or one day = 20
B. Two or three days = 10
C. Four or five days = 5
D. Six or seven days = 0

*Record your child's score here:* _____

*Total score:* _____

**To calculate your child's total score, add up the scores above, and then subtract that number from 100. For example, if the sum of the scores above is 60, your child's score would be: 100–60=40.**

### Scoring guide:

*80 to 100 points.* Excellent. Although there is always room for improvement, it's obvious that your child is practicing habits that will help him or her achieve or maintain a healthy weight.

*60 to 80 points.* Good. Your child has many good habits, but there is still significant room for improvement.

*40 to 60 points.* Fair. To achieve or maintain a healthy weight, there are many healthy behaviors your child needs to adopt.

*Less than 40 points.* Poor. Your child is at high risk of becoming obese or remaining obese. You should speak to your doctor about helping your child achieve a healthy weight.

## Preparing for Your Child's Checkup

While you consider what questions you'd like to ask your pediatrician, it's also worth being prepared to answer questions your pediatrician may ask you. The following are a few questions your pediatrician may ask at your child's next routine checkup.

### Eliciting Concerns

- What concerns do you have about your child in general?
- What concerns do you have about your child's eating habits, activity level, and weight—if any?

### Understanding Lifestyle Habits

- How frequently does your family eat meals together?
- What types of fruits and vegetables does your child eat each day?
- About how many servings of fruits and vegetables does your child eat?
- How many minutes of physical activity does your child get on most days?
- How much time does your child spend in front of a screen (TV, computer, phone, tablet, video games, etc.)?
- Does your child have a television in the bedroom?
- Does your family watch television during mealtimes?
- How often does your child eat fast food or at a restaurant? What does your child typically order?
- How many times per day does your child drink soda, sports drinks, or powdered drinks?
- How often does your child eat breakfast?
- How many hours does your child sleep each night? Does your child have any difficulty falling or staying asleep?

- *Nutrition and development of feeding and eating skills.* The pediatrician should help you understand your child's developmental stage and how well he should be able to feed himself and make food choices.
- *Healthy feeding and eating habits.* The pediatrician should help you create an environment in which children learn to consume all the essential nutrients their bodies need to grow.
- *Healthy eating relationships.* Parents and pediatricians should work together to promote healthy adult-child feeding relationships (free of mealtime food battles and coercive practices) as well as a positive relationship between children and food (such as an avoidance of emotional eating).
- *Nutrition for children with special health care needs.* Pediatricians should help parents decide if a child with special needs requires supplements. The doctor should help parents navigate the medical system and access needed specialists, including occupational therapists to help with feeding problems.

## Identifying Strengths

- What habits does your child have that make you proud?
- What healthy foods does your child like most?
- What physical activities does your child enjoy?

## Setting Goals

- What behaviors would you like to change most?
- What behaviors does your child want to change most?
- What barriers get in the way of making these changes?
- On a scale of 0 to 10—with 10 being very important—how important is it for you to make this behavioral change?
- On a scale of 0 to 10—with 10 being very confident—assuming you decided to makes this change, how confident are you that you could succeed?
- Why did you not choose a lower number? Why did you not choose a higher number?
- What would it take you to move to a higher number?
- How are you feeling about making a change?
- What might be a good first step for you and your child?

## Following Up

- When is a good time to follow up on these goals?

Any parent that suspects a child may have a nutritional disorder should be able to count on the pediatrician to help evaluate and treat the child for potential problems, such as food allergies and lactose or gluten intolerance.

*Promoting Physical Activity*

With the epidemic of inactivity and the low quantity and quality of physical activity in most schools, the encouragement of regular physical activity is a major priority for most pediatricians at checkup visits. The AAP advises that all children get at least 60 minutes of activity each day. Many pediatricians also emphasize that children under two shouldn't watch any television and those older than two should spend two hours or fewer each day on screen time. Along these lines, most pediatricians feel strongly that children shouldn't have a television in their rooms. During your visit, your pediatrician may describe why physical activity is important and offer contact information for community resources that provide quality physical activity opportunities.

## Understanding BMI

Body mass index (BMI) is a measure of your child's height and weight. The formula for BMI is weight (in kilograms) divided by height (in centimeters) squared. It's used as a way of estimating a person's body fat. But it's not a perfect measure for everyone. BMI may overestimate fat in muscular individuals, such as a football player who's "overweight" but not "overfat," and may underestimate fat in others with normal weight but a high percentage of body fat compared with muscle. Still, it offers a pretty good idea of whether to be concerned about your child's weight.

In adults, BMI ranges are set: any adult with a BMI greater than 25 is considered overweight and those with BMI over 30 are considered "obese." Because children are continually growing and experience spurts at certain ages (for example, a typical child will have a decrease in BMI around four years and then progressively increase throughout childhood), BMI is plotted on an age- and gender-appropriate growth chart. From there, you can determine a child's BMI percentile.

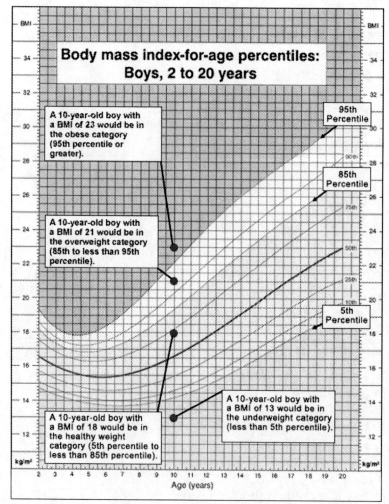

A 10-year-old boy with a BMI of 23 would be in the obese category (95th percentile or greater).

A 10-year-old boy with a BMI of 21 would be in the overweight category (85th to less than 95th percentile).

A 10-year-old boy with a BMI of 18 would be in the healthy weight category (5th percentile to less than 85th percentile).

A 10-year-old boy with a BMI of 13 would be in the underweight category (less than 5th percentile).

For example, let's look at Dave, a 10-year-old male. He's 4'10" and 110 pounds. His BMI is 23, which puts him in the 96th percentile. That means he weighs more than 96 percent of children based on 1976 norms. (The BMI percentiles are based on the distribution of children's weights in 1976. These days, a lot more than 5 percent of kids have a BMI greater than 95 percent.) He would be considered "obese."

Because his weight is in the high risk category, Dave and his parents need to make urgent lifestyle changes. Dave, his parents, and his doctor could work together to develop strategies for Dave to achieve a healthier weight. It's also important to continue to monitor his BMI over time to make sure he's getting closer to his goal. (First goal: get in the yellow zone. Second goal: get in the green zone and maintain green zone throughout childhood, thus entering adulthood at a healthy weight.) To reach his goals, Dave doesn't necessarily need to lost weight. If he maintains his current weight, as he grows, his BMI will progressively decrease and his percentile rank on the BMI chart will continue to fall until he's below 85 percent.

*Source*: Division of Nutrition, Physical Activity and Obesity, National Center for Chronic Disease Prevention and Health Promotion (http://apps.nccd.cdc.gov/dnpabmi/Calculator.aspx)

## Ask All the Right Questions

The following are a few questions you might consider asking your pediatrician, along with some background information that might help you to best use the information.

### *What's My Child's BMI and What Does It Mean?*

BMI helps to characterize your child's weight status. Your child's pediatrician should plot BMI at every well-child visit, show you the growth chart, and explain to you what your child's number means. (Refer to the sidebar "Understanding BMI" for a sample BMI chart and description of how to interpret it.)

### *If My Child Is Overweight or Obese, What Physical Exams and Laboratory Measures—If Any—Will Be Ordered to Rule Out Any Underlying Illness or Early Complications From Being Overweight?*

At a minimum, the physical exam should include pulse, blood pressure, and a search for signs commonly associated with excess weight, including a large liver and skin darkening behind the neck. If your child is classified as "obese" based on BMI, the doctor may also order labs to check for high cholesterol, type 2 diabetes, or kidney damage, which could result from long-standing high blood pressure or diabetes.

### *Can We Brainstorm Potential Strategies to Help Improve My Child's Nutrition and Fitness?*

Even if your child is at a perfect weight, chances are pretty good he has some less-than-ideal nutrition or physical activity behaviors. Challenge your child's pediatrician to actively engage you in coming up with a doable plan to help optimize your child's health.

### *What's Our Ultimate Goal?*

Refuse to leave the visit until your child, you, and the pediatrician have collectively come up with a SMART (specific, measurable, achievable, results-driven, and time-bound) goal that will help your child be healthier. Have a plan for monitoring the goal and following up with your doctor.

### *What Innovative Strategies Have Worked for Other Patients and Families Struggling With Weight/Picky Eating/Refusal to Exercise?*

Your pediatrician has the advantage of seeing many patients with similar struggles. Ask what has worked for others. This will not only help you come up with your own best plan, but it also reminds the doctor to keep tabs on what works and what doesn't and to continue to hone his skills to provide even better, more effective coaching to patients.

## What to Do About Underweight Kids?

With all the talk of childhood obesity, kids on the other end of the growth chart—those with weight or BMI less than the 5 percent for gender and age—are rarely discussed in the media or mass public health campaigns. Kids with low weight for height—known as "failure to thrive" in young children and "underweight" in older kids—are at risk for a variety of medical and nutritional challenges.

While much of the research on the long-term complications of failure to thrive is incomplete and somewhat contradictory, concern for possible negative effects on intellect, learning, and behavior drives many pediatricians to aggressively treat undernutrition—usually in the form of pushing high-calorie foods and nutritional supplements, such as PediaSure® or Boost®, or, in extreme cases, a feeding tube. While well meaning, pediatrician efforts to quickly reverse failure to thrive can sometimes contribute to increased stress in families struggling to get their child to eat more and gain weight. Many times, parents become defensive or overwhelmed when they perceive that a doctor is questioning their parenting skills or ability to fulfill one of their most fundamental responsibilities of parenthood—ensuring adequate nutrition for a child to grow.

While inadequate food intake is usually the reason for the low weight, it's rarely due to poor parenting and neglect. Common reasons a child doesn't eat enough include food insecurity (not having enough food to eat as a result of poverty), well-meaning but ultimately unhelpful food restrictions (such as putting a young child on the same low-calorie, low-fat "diet" the rest of the family may be on), breastfeeding challenges, and picky eating, which can often be due to feeding aversions or difficulty coordinating feeding. When a child

*What Are the Latest Evidence-Based Recommendations for Optimal Children's Nutrition, Obesity, and Eating Disorder Prevention and Management for Someone My Child's Age?*

When you throw out the term *evidence based*, you're asking your doctor to share with you what really works based on available research and studies—not based on opinion. If your doctor isn't familiar with the latest research and findings, ask him if he can help you find that information.

*When Can We Schedule a Follow-Up Appointment to Assess Our Progress?*

If your child is either underweight or overweight, regular follow-up is important to monitor progress and provide adjustments to the treatment plan—as needed. The expert guidelines for the treatment of childhood obesity recommend that pediatricians schedule follow-up visits every one to three months to track weight and progress on goals.[2]

*What Resources Are Available to Help Us in This Community?*

While so much effort is spent on discussing individual lifestyle habits, the reality is that multiple factors come into play in the development and ultimate correction

has failure to thrive, the parents and pediatrician are allies in the joint effort to get to the root of the mealtime struggles and figure out how to get the family the support and possible interventions they may need (such as from an occupational therapist to help a child with challenges eating certain textures or types of foods) to ensure the child's adequate growth.

An underlying medical condition is responsible for about 10 percent of infants and young children with failure to thrive. These problems usually lead to either malabsorption of consumed foods (such as with cystic fibrosis and celiac disease or food protein intolerance) or increased metabolism (such as with many metabolic disorders and genetic syndromes). If a pediatrician suspects this may be the cause, he will refer the family to the appropriate specialists for further evaluation and intervention.

Low weight in school-aged children can be due to genetic factors and a possible predisposition to be small or, especially in preadolescent and adolescent girls (but certainly not limited to them), a restriction of calories. This can happen on the part of the child in response to perceived increased weight. Or it can occur accidentally in some cases, such as in very active children who don't eat enough to support physical demands. If a child restricts food and is losing weight instead of gaining or if a child is engaging in unhealthy amounts of exercise, the child's parents and pediatrician should work closely together to evaluate the situation and help the child receive the services and knowledge necessary to maintain a healthy weight and eliminate disordered thinking—if present. Management of a full-blown eating disorder, such as anorexia, bulimia, or binge eating, is usually outside the scope of a general pediatrician, although that doctor should facilitate a referral to the appropriate professionals and continue to monitor to help the child change course.

of weight issues and poor lifestyle habits. Communities generally contain many assets and opportunities for healthy activity and nutrition. Pediatricians are often familiar with programs available nearby, and if you ask, your child's pediatrician may be able to provide you with a large range of potential programs and opportunities for your child to eat better and exercise more.

## Take It Outside the Office

Even the most motivated children, families, doctors, and communities are up against powerful barriers when trying to commit to healthy lifestyle changes and promote health. In one study, pediatricians counted fast-food availability, soft drink availability, school food environment, and school physical activity environment among the most powerful impediments.[3] Parents commonly list lack of time, lack of support from community and pediatrician, difficulty changing kids' nutrition and activity preferences, and cost as barriers to adopting healthier lifestyles.[3]

Parents inclined toward advocacy might consider engaging in efforts to improve the nutrition and fitness environment for children in the community and begin to overcome barriers. You could start by exploring your community's strengths and needs. What's already under way regarding obesity prevention? What school and

## The Problem With Childhood Obesity

It's no secret that the United States faces an epidemic of childhood obesity. Obesity prevalence among children has increased from 5 percent in the 1960s to about 17 percent currently. Another nearly 20 percent of children are overweight.[6] Black girls (24 percent), Mexican American boys (22 percent), and children from lower-income communities with little access to healthy foods and physical activity opportunities suffer the highest rates.[6] While genes and environment contribute to obesity risk, the increasing prevalence of childhood obesity has occurred too rapidly to be explained by a genetic shift.[2] Changes in the way we live—from how we get to work and school to what we eat for snacks and meals—are responsible for the rapid and alarming widening of our waistlines from infancy to old age. With many children now on the same medications as their grandparents, childhood obesity experts speculate that this may be the first generation with a shorter life span than their parents.

The effects of childhood obesity extend far beyond aesthetics. Obese children suffer alarming social consequences from their weight. They're more frequently bullied, do worse in school, and are often socially marginalized by their peers. And childhood obesity left ignored can progress to serious complications in adolescence and adulthood—and sometimes even sooner. Childhood obesity negatively affects nearly every organ of the body, causing complications as varied as asthma and sleep apnea to gallstones, liver dysfunction, bone fractures, and infertility in girls.[2] In fact, many complications of obesity that are common in adults—such as type 2 diabetes, high blood pressure, and abnormal cholesterol—are present in obese children.[7] If current trends continue, one study predicted that the average boy born in the year 2000 has a 33 percent chance of developing diabetes in his lifetime, while the average girl has a 39 percent chance.[8]

Being an obese kid is tough. While it's not "easy" to attain a healthier weight, with the right tools and support, children are more successful than their adult counterparts. A change in lifestyle habits is what caused the obesity epidemic, and a change in lifestyle is the solution. Childhood obesity results from an imbalance between energy intake and energy expenditure. By improving nutrition habits and increasing physical activity, many children can avert the harmful consequences of obesity to achieve and maintain a healthy weight. Without a partnership with the pediatrician, parents may not even realize if their child is or isn't at a healthy weight, whether there any signs of obesity-associated disease, and what resources are available to help families adopt healthier lifestyles.

community policies interfere with supporting optimal nutrition and opportunities for activity? Consider engaging your child's pediatrician in this conversation.

The sidebar "Counterstrategies in Action: Engaging With the Community to Optimize Children's Health" highlights ways a few parents have made a positive health difference in their communities.

# Developmental Considerations

The Bright Futures guidelines task pediatricians with sharing large amounts of information on weight management, nutrition, and physical activity with parents. The recommendations are based on a child's age and developmental stage. The weight, nutrition, and physical activity guidance that pediatricians should share with their patients' families is highlighted the following sections. The hope is that if you go to your child's checkups already armed with this information, you'll have more time with the doctor to ask specific questions and raise concerns (Figure 10-1).

## Infant (0–1 years)

Infancy is an important period of time in establishing a healthy growth trajectory and the promotion of developmental milestones, such as feeding oneself and learning to walk.

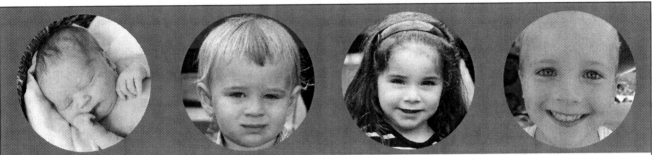

### Infant

- Monitor weight gain in the first weeks and months of life to ensure adequate but not excessive growth.
- Discuss with the pediatrician strategies for introducing solids.
- Ask whether your infant needs an iron and/or vitamin D supplement.
- Discuss with the pediatrician any eating concerns or challenges.
- Facilitate motor development and physical activity with tummy time and opportunities to move around freely.

### Toddler

- Begin to monitor BMI starting at two years of age. Be sure to find out what BMI means and where your child falls.
- Talk with the pediatrician about how to best facilitate your child's development when it comes to self-feeding and food choices.
- Expose your child to developmentally appropriate physical activities to keep his body moving and help him hone his new-found skills.

### Preschooler

- When discussing a child's weight, be sensitive to the child's experiences and thoughts.
- Encourage your child to share his food likes and dislikes with the doctor.
- As your child develops more advanced motor skills, give him opportunities to use these skills, such as with bike riding, exposure to the water and swimming (closely supervised), and introduction to simpler sports, such as T-ball and soccer.

### School Age

- Be on the lookout for potential physical or emotional consequences of overweight or perceived overweight. Discuss any concerns with the pediatrician.
- Encourage your child to take an increasingly active role in making nutrition choices and sharing requested information with the doctor at checkups.
- Assess for potential nutritional inadequacies or deficiencies (such as calcium, vitamin D, or iron).
- Advance from activities that focus on fundamental skills to those that require increasing strategy and teamwork.

Figure 10-1. Developmental considerations

## Counterstrategies in Action: Engaging With the Community to Optimize Children's Health

- For the past 20 years, volunteer parents and grandparents of children at Oak Meadow Elementary School in San Antonio, Texas, have maintained the "Garden Angel" program. The parents and grandparents, together with the kids, plant, care for, harvest, and eat a wide variety of fruits and vegetables. This parent-school partnership gives children the powerful experience of eating what they grow—a surefire way to get a child to be willing to try (and love) a variety of vegetables.

- While Oak Meadow Elementary has been at it for 20 years, a new movement for school garden "learning laboratories" is underway in the United States. In fact, organizations such as the American Heart Association (AHA) are taking an active role in helping communities build gardens through programs like AHA's Teaching Gardens. As stated by Kelly Hurter, a mother of two boys, a runner, and the North Carolina AHA Development Director who helped develop the Hope Valley Elementary School garden in Durham, North Carolina: "In today's world, many children don't really know where fruits and vegetables come from. They think they come from the grocery store…. We realized the importance of teaching children how simple gardening is and that it's easy to eat healthy."

- At Maybury Elementary School in Detroit, Michigan, parents organized a "walking school bus." The parents first received pedestrian safety training and then coordinated morning walking pickups. The school helped to arrange for extra crossing guards at busy intersections on the walking route. The program continues to grow and has well over 50 students who regularly walk to school.

- Molly Barker is a mom, four-time Ironman triathlete, and social worker who, during a run one day, pondered the struggles of girls during middle childhood. During that run, she developed a vision for a program that would use physical activity to help girls build self-esteem and confidence. From there, she developed a 24-lesson program called "Girls on the Run." She piloted her program with 13 girls. It grew to 26, then 75. Now it is a 501(c)(3) with over 170 programs across the United States and Canada.

- Once a high-powered attorney in New York City, Bettina Elias Siegel chose to stay home with her first child. It turns out that decision was career-changing. Siegel joined a writing workshop for stay-at-home moms and unexpectedly discovered a new passion for writing. This interest, combined with a passion for food, inspired her to start a mommy blog on "kids and food, in school and out" named "The Lunch Tray," which was voted one of the top 25 "foodie mom" blogs by the Circle of Moms online community (www.circleofmoms.com). Highly involved in her local community as a member of the Houston Independent School District's Food Services Parent Advisory Committee and chair of the food/nutrition subcommittee of the School Health Advisory Council, Siegel also authors the blog "The Spork Report" which keeps local parents up to date on the school district's food news.

*Weight Management*

In the first two to six weeks of a child's life, he does little more than eat, sleep, cry, and grow. It's normal for a newborn to lose up to 10 percent of his birth weight in the first week of life, but he should gain back to birth weight by two weeks. From there, he grows rapidly, gaining about two pounds per month. Most babies will double their birth weight by their four-month checkup. A baby who loses more than 10 percent of birth weight in the first week of life will likely be closely followed by his pediatrician until he regains birth weight.

While a chubby baby is often considered a healthy baby, a growing body of research suggests that obesity can begin in infancy and too rapid weight gain in the first year can set the stage for long-standing struggles with overweight and obesity.[4–5] Typically, breastfed babies gain more than formula-fed babies in the first six months, but then formula-fed infants tend to gain more rapidly during the rest of the first year. BMI isn't calculated for children younger than two years old because length (with the baby lying down) is measured instead of height (with the child standing up). Instead, an infant's weight-for-length can be recorded to assess growth. By their first birthday, most babies will have tripled their birth weight and increased their length by 50 percent. Exclusive breastfeeding and avoidance of overfeeding in formula-fed infants can help to assure adequate but not excessive growth.

*Nutrition*

Most pediatricians encourage mothers to breastfeed due to the large body of evidence that it benefits the health and well-being of both mother and baby. Formula-fed infants should receive formula that's fortified with iron. Infants who show signs of milk intolerance, such as loose stools, excessive spitting up, or vomiting, may need elemental formulas (transitioning from milk to soy formula doesn't seem to help symptoms). If you have concerns that your child may have a milk-protein allergy, you should discuss the best alternatives for your child with your child's pediatrician. Spitting up is extremely common in infancy and could result from drinking too fast, inadequate burping, or improper feeding (bottle propped, bottle not adequately tipped, shaking formula too much before feeding). If your child still spits up frequently despite all your efforts, it's worth discussing with your pediatrician.

In the first several months of life, breastfed infants will eat about every 2 to 3 hours, for a total of 8 to 12 feeds in a 24-hour period. As they grow older, they'll eat less frequently but take more volume with each feed. Because formula isn't digested as rapidly as breast milk, formula-fed newborns tend to need to eat every three to four hours instead of every two to three. To avoid overfeeding, the AAP recommends offering your baby two ounces of formula every two to three hours in the first week of life. If your baby still seems hungry, then offer more until he shows signs that he's full. Signs of hunger include hand-to-mouth movements, lip smacking, smiling, cooing, and gazing at the feeding parent. Crying is a late sign. For optimal development and attachment, parents should aim to feed a newborn as soon as he shows signs of hunger. (Later in the first year, when an infant is more secure in his trust, a parent can wait longer for feedings.) Satiety cues include turning away from the nipple, falling asleep, spitting up milk or refusing the nipple, becoming fussy during feeding, slowing the pace of eating, or stopping sucking. The average newborn needs about 20 ounces of formula per day, with a range of 16 to 24 ounces. As he grows older, he'll need larger volumes less frequently. At 4 months, the average infant consumes about 31 ounces per day, with a range of 26 to 36 ounces, although his intake may fluctuate from day to day. More importantly, babies should never be put to bed with a bottle, as it contributes to cavities as well as overfeeding.

Parents should introduce solid foods around four to six months of age, when most infants are developmentally ready to expand their diet. The AAP recommends that exclusively breastfeeding moms wait to the six months mark to optimize the benefits of breastfeeding. Signs that an infant is ready to start solids include increased demand for breastfeeding that continues for a few days, ability to sit with arm support, good head and neck control, ability to indicate desire for food by opening his mouth and leaning forward, ability to indicate disinterest by leaning back and turning away, and loss of the extrusion reflex (in which the infant thrusts out his tongue when given food). It's well established that introducing solids earlier than four months contributes to childhood obesity.

It doesn't really matter what solid foods are given first. While parents have historically been advised to start with rice cereal and to hold off on meat until seven or eight months, most babies may actually be better off with iron-containing vegetables or meat to help reduce the risk of iron-deficiency anemia, the most common nutritional deficiency in infancy and toddlerhood. Historically, pediatricians have recommended that vegetables be introduced before fruits for fear that a child exposed to the sweet taste of fruits will subsequently reject the bitter taste of vegetables. While intuitively it makes sense, no evidence exists to support this belief. Luckily, most infants are open to trying (and liking) a wide variety of foods.

Parents should begin solids with single-ingredient foods at two- to seven-day intervals, so if a food allergy does develop, it will be possible to tell which food is the culprit. (See the sidebar "Does My Baby Have a Food Allergy?") After the baby has accepted the new foods, he should eat solids about two or three times per day. Remember to let him control how much he eats. By the end of the first year, an infant should have been exposed to fruits, vegetables, whole grains, and lean meats. Fruit juice should be limited to no more than four ounces per day, and ideally, an infant won't be exposed to such nutrient-poor foods as sodas, chips, sweetened drinks, and French fries. Parents should also make an effort to establish regular meal and snack times to avoid grazing, which can contribute to being overweight or underweight.

The AAP recommends that pediatricians consider iron and vitamin $B_{12}$ supplements for certain high-risk infants and vitamin D for all infants. Exclusively breastfed, premature, and babies on iron-free formula (not recommended) are at highest risk of deficiency, which is associated with lower IQ. Breastfed infants also are at risk for vitamin D deficiency, and those breastfed infants with vegan mothers are at risk for vitamin $B_{12}$ deficiency. Parents should discuss the need for supplements with their child's doctor.

## Does My Baby Have a Food Allergy?

A food allergy or *hypersensitivity reaction* occurs when a protein or another component of a food causes the same problem every time the child is exposed to that particular food. It's relatively uncommon, occurring in 2 to 8 percent of infants and children younger than three years old. Common symptoms of food allergy include vomiting, cramps, diarrhea, eczema, hives, and, in severe cases, anaphylaxis (throat swelling and difficulty breathing). The most common allergy-causing foods in kids include milk, eggs, peanuts, soy, and wheat. Tree nuts, shellfish, and fish are common causes in older kids and adults.

It used to be that pediatricians advised avoiding highly allergic foods until at least one year of age, whenever possible. However, more recent research says that you're actually better off introducing highly allergic foods earlier to decrease risk of later food allergy.[9–10] The following is a summary of the latest recommendations when it comes to food allergy prevention:

- Maternal dietary restrictions during pregnancy and lactation probably don't decrease the risk of food allergies, with the possible exception of eczema, which may be lessened with avoidance of highly allergic foods, such as those mentioned earlier.
- Exclusive breastfeeding for at least three months decreases the risk of wheezing in early childhood. Breastfeeding for at least four months decreases the risk of cow milk allergy and eczema in the first two years of life.
- No benefit exists to delaying the introduction of highly allergic foods. Thus, such foods as fish, eggs, and foods containing peanuts may be introduced at four to six months when other first foods are introduced (but not whole peanuts since they are a choking hazard). In fact, introducing these foods prior to the first birthday may lead to a decreased risk of food allergy later.
- Soy-based infant formula doesn't prevent or treat cow milk allergy.

Up to 25 percent of infants have some type of feeding problem (the number jumps to 80 percent in children with developmental disability).[1] Whether it's refusing food; difficulty transitioning to textured food; gagging, choking, or vomiting with feeding; inadequate food volume; picky eating; prolonged feeding time (more than 30 minutes); or other problems, your child's pediatrician should be a ready source of information and referrals to best evaluate and manage the challenge. While parents often blame themselves for these feeding problems, the difficulties most often are related to a problem with a child's ability to coordinate feeding.

### Physical Activity

The importance of physical activity begins in infancy. An infant starts with involuntary reflexes, which give way to coordinated movements. The timeline for motor skill development varies somewhat from child to child, but the progression is usually the same: roll over (about 4 months), sit up (about 6 months), crawl (about 9 months), pull-to-stand (about 9 months), and walk (about 12 months). Parents can facilitate their child's development of these skills by providing physical stimulation. This includes "tummy time"; such games as pat-a-cake, peek-a-boo, and "How big is baby?"; and the opportunity to move around freely. Shorts bursts of time with toys, such as a jumperoo, also offer an infant an opportunity to be active. Sedentary activities, such as television and other media, aren't educational or helpful for children at this age despite the gimmicks intended to entice parents to make purchases to help "educate" babies.

## Toddler (1–3 years)

With growing independence and ability to communicate, toddlers are able to exert more control over their food and activity choices. When healthy habits are fostered, a child can develop long-lasting lifestyle preferences for healthy foods and physical activity. However, if the opportunity is missed, the opposite can happen and a child can get into a fast-food, video-game rut.

*Weight Management*

Toddlerhood offers an opportunity to set the stage for lifelong healthy habits that help to protect against excessive weight gain (or loss). Children should be encouraged to self-regulate caloric intake and use internal cues of hunger and fullness to guide intake. If overweight/obesity or underweight is detected at this age, the pediatrician and parent should proceed carefully in addressing weight. In the case of overweight, attempting to restrict food intake or limit access to food can be counterproductive and override a child's ability to use hunger to guide intake. Some pediatricians may counsel a parent to restrict young children's access to certain foods in an attempt to slow weight gain. If this is done, it's important that it doesn't interfere with a child's ability to respond to cues of hunger and that it's done thoughtfully so as to avoid excess restriction (see Chapter 4). If a pediatrician is concerned about a child's weight, he'll often ask questions about portion sizes, types of foods served, and how often the child eats.

*Nutrition*

After a child's first birthday, the rapid weight gain of infancy begins to slow, leading to a notable decrease in appetite and food intake. To supply the body with needed calories, the toddler tends to eat foods with higher caloric density. After the age of one, most children will eat the same foods that adults eat, although parents should watch out for choking hazards, such as peanuts, gum, popcorn, chips, hot dogs or sausages, carrot sticks, whole grapes, hard candy, large pieces of fruits and vegetables, and tough meat. Because toddlers are able to eat many of the same foods that the older family members eat, it's especially important to offer a healthy, varied, and portion-controlled diet. But remember, picky eating is especially common in this age group. If you stay the course and consistently expose your kids to a variety of new and familiar foods, this pickiness will resolve by the time a child begins kindergarten. As your toddler develops and perfects self-feeding skills, he should be encouraged to use a spoon; transition from bottle to sippy cup to small cup; and, counterintuitively, "play with his food" as a form of food exploration, which will help him be more accepting of the food in the future.

*Physical Activity*

Being physically active is second nature to rambunctious toddlers. Not only is it an excellent outlet for excess energy and an opportunity to expend calories, but it also helps to facilitate motor skill development. Most children develop motor skills from walking to marching, galloping, hopping, running, navigating obstacles, and skipping. Giving a child the opportunity to play outside and walk, run, climb, and explore the outdoors allows him to practice his motor skills and enjoy moving his body. Simple games and dancing are also great opportunities to be active in a safe and supervised environment.

## Preschooler (3–5 years)

Much of the advice for toddlers also applies to preschool-aged children.

*Weight Management*

Refer to the previous section for a discussion of weight management in toddlers, which also applies to preschoolers. Furthermore, if fostered, preschoolers have an ability to choose a healthy diet and control portions based on their hunger. However, if unhealthy foods are easily accessible or children are taught to ignore their signs of hunger and eat even when they aren't hungry, they'll quickly lose this innate ability.

*Nutrition*

See the section on toddlers for a discussion about nutrition for them. These principles also apply to preschoolers. In addition, parents have an opportunity to take advantage of a preschool child's newfound willingness to try new foods after getting over the neophobia and pickiness of toddlerhood.

*Physical Activity*

The physical activity principles described for toddlers also apply to preschoolers. After toddlerhood, preschoolers develop more advanced activity skills, and they begin to improve eye-hand and eye-foot coordination, balance, and depth perception.

## School Age (5–10 years)

Because peer influence, the school environment, and the surrounding community play an increasingly important role in a child's eating and activity behaviors, parents and pediatricians should aim to understand the environment the child engages with each day and identify areas of concern or opportunities for advocacy to help improve the situation.

*Weight Management*

Middle childhood is a period of slow, steady physical growth. As with younger children, a pediatrician should continue to plot BMI and identify weight concerns early.

*Nutrition*

A school-aged child needs three meals and two to three healthy snacks each day. Calcium should be aggressively incorporated into the school-aged child's diet because the majority of kids this age are calcium deficient. (Kids need about three to four servings of calcium-rich foods each day [800 to 1,300 milligrams a day]. Calcium-rich foods include cheese, yogurt, milk, sardines, leafy green vegetables, such as spinach and kale, soybeans, and fortified and enriched cereals and grains.) Parents should encourage school-aged children to play an increasingly active role in helping with food planning and preparation.

*Physical Activity*

The school-age years are when a child is developmentally ready to begin to master athletic skills. The five- to six-year-old perfects the fundamental skills of running, galloping, jumping, hopping, skipping, throwing, catching, and kicking. The best activities at this age are ones that emphasize fun and develop motor skills; require little instruction; and are repetitive and don't require complex motor and cognitive skills. These are considered "fundamental" skills. Great examples include running, swimming, tumbling, and throwing and catching a ball. At the age of seven to nine, a child develops "fundamental transitional" skills, such as throwing for distance or accuracy. A child at this age is ready to begin sports, such as baseball or soccer, but emphasis should still be on having fun rather than competition. Around the age of 10, a child moves into a "transitional complex" phase of motor development in which he learns to play more complicated sports, such as basketball, in which strategy and teamwork are especially important.

# Chapter Summary

Parents and pediatricians are natural allies in the pursuit to raise healthy, active, well-adjusted children. When both work together to foster a strong partnership, a child benefits immensely, especially when that child has weight, nutrition, or activity challenges. One way to nurture this relationship is to take an active role in doctor's visits and ask all the right questions to get the answers you need to help your child thrive.

The following recap highlights the major points of this chapter:
- Rely on your child's pediatrician as an ally in your effort to help your child optimize health, including growth, nutrition, and physical activity. If you're unhappy with the care that your child is receiving, look for another doctor who's a better match.

- Ask the pediatrician what your child's BMI is and what it means.
- Be willing to work with your child and the pediatrician to help your child achieve or maintain a healthy weight.
- Make sure to discuss your child's nutrition and physical activity habits at each checkup.
- Ask yourself some important questions: How healthy of an environment does your child live in? What changes should be made? How can the pediatrician be of the most help?
- Plan ahead for doctor's visits. Write your questions down.
- Be transparent when expressing your concerns and reactions to information that the pediatrician shares.
- Get involved in advocacy efforts in your community.
- Understand your child's developmental stage and what tasks he should be able to accomplish. Challenge him to meet these milestones. If he can't, talk with your child's pediatrician.
- Don't remain speechless at doctor's visits. Ask for help and support when you need it. And don't be afraid to ask for clarification if you don't fully understand what the doctor says or recommends.

# Recipes: Living the MyPlate Life

Putting together a meal that meets the USDA MyPlate recommendations can be intimidating. But take these basic recipes and spice it up with the marinades in Chapter 8 and you'll have endless combinations for a balanced and healthy meal!

## PROTEIN

### Simple Baked Chicken Breast

Preheat oven to 350 degrees. Place chicken breasts on a baking sheet. Drizzle with olive oil, salt, and pepper. Bake in oven for 30 to 45 minutes or until thoroughly cooked.

*Tip:* Make extra chicken and use in sandwiches, tacos, and wraps for the rest of the week.

### Perfect Steamed Fish

Preheat oven to 350 degrees. Tear a piece of foil approximately 3 times the size of the fish filet. Place the 4-ounce filet in the center of the foil. Bring up all sides of the foil perpendicular to the fish (as if creating 4 walls). Place 2 tablespoons of liquid of your choice (e.g., water, lemon juice, orange juice, soy sauce) on top of the fish. Bring two opposite sides of the foil together in the middle and roll down until it meets the fish. Roll the remaining sides of the foil into the center, which creates a package where the fish in completely enclosed.

Place on a baking sheet and bake for 20 to 25 minutes.

*Tip:* Add julienned vegetables on top of fish before cooking for an easy and quick meal.

## Flavorful Tofu

Using the extra firm variety of tofu, cut the tofu into 1/2-inch slabs. Marinate the tofu in any spice mixture or sauce overnight so the tofu absorbs the flavor. Place 2 tablespoons of olive oil in a pan over medium heat. Panfry the tofu on each side for 6 to 7 minutes.

*Tip:* Try marinating with BBQ sauce for a healthier alternative in sandwiches.

## VEGGIES—EASY COOKED VEGETABLES

### Smashed Cauliflower and Potatoes

1 head of cauliflower, trimmed and cut into small florets
1 medium-sized potato, washed and cut into 1/2-inch cubes
1/4 cup yogurt
Salt and pepper

Place cauliflower and potatoes into a pot. Add water until the vegetables are completely submerged in the water. Bring the pot to a boil and then reduce to medium heat and cook for 20 to 30 minutes. Once the vegetables are tender, remove from heat and mash with a potato masher or fork. Add 1/4 cup of yogurt, 1 teaspoon of salt, and pepper.

### Roasted Garlicky and Cheesy Broccoli

1 head of broccoli, trimmed and cut into florets
3 cloves of garlic, cut into thin slices
1/4 cup shredded Parmesan cheese
Olive oil
Salt and pepper

Preheat oven to 375 degrees. Toss the broccoli florets with 3 tablespoons of olive oil, garlic, salt, and pepper. Spread broccoli in an even layer on a baking sheet. Bake in oven for 20 minutes. Remove from oven and sprinkle cheese on broccoli before serving.

## VEGGIES—QUICK AND FRESH SALADS

### Cucumber and Carrot Sesame Salad

2 medium-sized carrots
1 large cucumber
1 to 2 stalks of green onions
1 tablespoon of sesame seeds
2 tablespoons of vinegar or juice of one lime

Peel carrots. Slice carrots in half lengthwise and then lay carrots flat and cut into thin slices across. Put into large bowl. Next, cut cucumber in half lengthwise. Using a spoon, scrape out the seeds and then place cucumber flat and cut into thin slices across. Place cucumber into bowl with carrots and add green onions and sesame seeds. Mix in vinegar or lime juice and stir. Add salt and pepper.

## Corn and Black Bean Salad

2 cups of cooked brown rice

1 package of frozen corn, defrosted

1 can of black beans, drained

1 medium cucumber

1 red bell pepper

1/2 cup of cilantro (or green onions)

Juice from one lime

Slice in half lengthwise. Scoop seeds out with a spoon. Lay flat and cut cucumber across into thin slices. Cut red bell pepper in half and remove seeds. Dice into small pieces. Place cucumber and red bell pepper in a mixing bowl. Add corn and beans and then cilantro and lime. Salt and pepper as needed.

## CARBS

## Basic Quinoa

1 cup of dry quinoa

2 cups of water

Bring water to boil in a pot. Add quinoa and lower heat to low-medium. Cover and let cook for 20 minutes.

## Basic Whole Wheat Couscous

1 cup of dry couscous

1 1/2 cups of water

Bring water to boil in pot. Add couscous, cover pot, and turn off heat. Let stand for 10 minutes and then use fork to fluff couscous.

## Basic Barley

1 cup of barley

2 cups of water

Bring water to boil in pot. Add barley and lower heat to low-medium. Cover and let cook for 30 minutes. Drain excess water from barley.

*Tips:*

- Add any of these grains to a salad for a heartier meal.
- Substitute water for chicken or vegetable broth for a tastier grain!

## References

1. Hagan, J.F., J.S. Shaw, and P.M. Duncan. (2008). *Bright Futures: Guidelines for Health Supervision of Infants, Children, and Adolescents* (3rd ed.). Washington, DC: American Academy of Pediatrics.

2. Barlow, S.E. (2007). Expert committee recommendations regarding the prevention, assessment, and treatment of child and adolescent overweight and obesity: Summary report. *Pediatrics. 120*(Suppl 4): p. S164-92.

3. Perrin, E.M., K.B. Flower, J. Garrett, and A.S. Ammerman. (2005). Preventing and treating obesity: Pediatricians' self-efficacy, barriers, resources, and advocacy. *Ambul Pediatr. 5*(3): p. 150-6.

4. Ong, K.K., and R.J. Loos. (2006). Rapid infancy weight gain and subsequent obesity: Systematic reviews and hopeful suggestions. *Acta Paediatr. 95*(8): p. 904-8.

5. Taveras, E.M., M.W. Gillman, K. Kleinman, J.W. Rich-Edwards, and S.L. Rifas-Shiman. (2010). Racial/ethnic differences in early-life risk factors for childhood obesity. *Pediatrics. 125*(4): p. 686-95.

6. Ogden, C.L., M.D. Carroll, B.K. Kit, and K.M. Flegal. (2012). Prevalence of obesity and trends in body mass index among US children and adolescents, 1999-2010. *JAMA. 307*(5): p. 483-90.

7. Weiss, R., J. Dziura, T.S. Burgert, W.V. Tamborlane, S.E. Taksali, C.W. Yeckel, K.Allen, M. Lopes, M. Savoye, J. Morrison, R.S. Sherwin, and S. Caprio. (2004). Obesity and the metabolic syndrome in children and adolescents. *N Engl J Med. 350*(23): p. 2362-74.

8. Narayan, K.M., J.P. Boyle, T.J. Thompson, S.W. Sorensen, and D.F. Williamson. (2003). Lifetime risk for diabetes mellitus in the United States. *JAMA. 290*(14): p. 1884-90.

9. Nwaru, B.I., M. Erkkola, S. Ahonen, M. Kaila, A.-M. Haapala, C. Kronberg-Kippilä, R. Salmelin, R. Veijola, J. Ilonen, O. Simell, M. Knip, and S.M. Virtanen. (2010). Age at the introduction of solid foods during the first year and allergic sensitization at age 5 years. *Pediatrics. 125*(1): p. 50-9.

10. Greer, F.R., S.H. Sicherer, and A.W. Burks. (2008). Effects of early nutritional interventions on the development of atopic disease in infants and children: The role of maternal dietary restriction, breastfeeding, timing of introduction of complementary foods, and hydrolyzed formulas. *Pediatrics. 121*(1): p. 183-91.

## Resource

Hagan, J.F., J.S. Shaw, and P.M. Duncan. (2008). *Bright Futures: Guidelines for Health Supervision of Infants, Children, and Adolescents* (3rd ed.). Washington, DC: American Academy of Pediatrics.

# 11

# Mistake #11— Mishandling Grandparent Sabotage

*"Grandmas are moms with lots of frosting."*
—Author unknown

Marion and Anneliese adore their grandma Gail, whom they call GG. She spoils them with love and affection, toys, and lots and lots of food. In fact, Marion and Anneliese's mom swears that all meals together with Grandma end with ice cream. If Anneliese is sad, GG helps heal her pain with a visit to the neighborhood chocolate shop. The children look forward to splurges galore at GG's house. As with many grandparents, food is how GG expresses her love. And efforts to control GG's behavior are more futile than trying to rationalize with a three-year-old. While it may be easier to "let bygones be bygones," grandparent sabotage can wreak havoc on parents' other nutrition successes. But how do you speak up without offending and annoying Grandma and Grandpa who, as we all recognize, are mighty and powerful influences?

## The Science Behind "Grandparent Sabotage"

Grandparents are profoundly important in the lives of children. With both parents working in many families, grandparents now living longer and often into a grandchild's adult years, divorce rates hovering around 50 percent, and the increasing number of environmental and family stressors, grandparents help to provide stability, support, and child care to young families. Not to mention the simple fact that grandparents by the very nature of their title have "been there, done that." They've raised a few kids in their day, and most of their kids probably turned out all right. In most cases, it would be a mistake to shun the help of a loving grandparent. At the same time, without some structure, nudging, and general "guidelines" for when the kids are with their grandparents, you might find that an influential, firm-minded grandparent could swiftly and completely sabotage your hard-won successes.

For example, take results from a study of 12,000 preschoolers living in the United Kingdom. Those kids who between the ages of nine months and three years were cared for by a grandparent—full time or part time—were more likely to be overweight than the kids cared for primarily by a parent or those who attended formal daycare. These results held even after controlling for mom's prepregnancy weight, ethnicity, number of children living in the house, whether the mother smoked during the pregnancy, the mother's age at the time of birth of the first-born child, the child's birth weight, breastfeeding, and timing of introducing solids.[1] Something about the grandparent-grandchild relationship contributes to kids eating more calories and consequently gaining too much weight. We're left to speculate what that "something" is because very little published research has explored this phenomenon. But the parents interviewed for this book have a few good guesses.

## The Reality Behind Grandparent Sabotage

The following are just a sampling of responses from a survey asking parents how they think their kids likely eat when they're with their grandparents. While a few said that the grandparents are very health conscious or that they typically follow the recommendations of the parents, most of the feedback fell along the lines of the following:

> *"Grandparents feed the kids whatever they want! Usually unhealthy snacks!"*
>
> —Jenelle, mother of eight-year-old
> Avery and six-year-old Morgan

> *"For almost every visit, my mother brings doughnut holes. She is known as 'Doughnut Hole' Grandma!"*
>
> —Barbara, mother of 12-year-old Zac
> and 10-year-old Samantha

> *"My in-laws follow all the rules. My parents love to break them all."*
>
> —Jen, mother of two-year-old
> Joseph

> *"The kids spend time with their grandma quite a bit and she does not listen to my food recommendations. She says, 'I'm Grandma. I can give them whatever I want.'"*
>
> —Anonymous

If parents and grandparents are on the same page with approaches to taking care of the kids, then you don't have too much to worry about and visits will go well. However, when parents and grandparents disagree, major conflicts can ensue. Add to that a child who's very adept at pushing the boundaries and discovering weak spots (i.e., a loving grandparent who just can't say "No" to an adorable, begging child) and you've got a situation in need of intervention. The impact of grandparent splurges on a child's overall health is amplified when grandparents play a major role in child rearing compared with those who infrequently drop by for a short visit. While parents who struggle with highly influential, independent-minded, very-involved grandparents may be eager for tools to help manage these relationships, even parents with the most supportive and obliging parents will benefit from the strategies described in this chapter.

## An Approach to Partnering With Grandparents

While you may occasionally have disagreements, parents and grandparents are typically on the same page with their overall goals for the children. They want to raise well-balanced, polite, fun-loving, and healthy kids. It's just that they often take very different approaches. Before engaging in the next big heated debate over this, consider sitting down with your child's grandparents to share your concerns and explore how to best resolve differences. (See the sidebar "Five Ways Grandparents Can Help Raise Healthier Kids" for the grandparent equivalent of the following advice, which you may consider sharing with your parents and in-laws.)

- *Identify your motivations.* First, explain to your parents or in-laws your major motivations and goals. For example, share with the grandparents that your goal is to raise physically active children who are familiar with a wide variety of healthy foods, who use hunger to guide their intake, and who have a healthy relationship with food.
- *Share a few basic and simple "guidelines."* Share with the grandparents the major principles you would like to follow to meet your goals. For example, you could describe how you try to avoid using food as a reward; don't require "cleaning the plate"; rarely store unhealthy foods in the home (although they're not off limits); and limit TV and other electronic media to two hours or fewer per day.
- *Serve as a role model.* Let the grandparents watch you follow your guidelines and witness how your child's overall nutrition and fitness status transforms. (Remember, it takes consistent application and time for the transformation to occur so the grandparents may also witness some of the bumps along the way.)
- *Communicate.* Keep the dialogue open. Encourage your parents and in-laws to explore and share their concerns with you.

Say you had this conversation and the grandparents are still engaging in all kinds of behaviors that seem to slowly sabotage your efforts. In that case, you might have to move to Plan B, which includes a few carefully planned strategies to influence your parents to come around to your way of raising the kids.

## An Approach to Influencing Adults

In the late 1950s, social psychologists Raven and French described a theory of "interpersonal influence and social power" that relied on six power strategies to influence others: informational power, expert power, referent power,

## Five Ways Grandparents Can Help Raise Healthier Kids

The strong bond grandparent and grandchild share provides grandparents an incredible opportunity to help parents raise healthier, more active children. While grandparents may have an entirely different philosophy than the parents on the best way to make this happen, if both work together, the children's health (as well as everyone's overall sanity) will benefit.

To deal with conflicting approaches to childrearing, grandparents might consider following these approaches:

- *Identify your motivations.* Grandparents should self-reflect and ask themselves what's their philosophy on what it means to be a grandparent and in what kind of environment a child should be raised for optimal health and well-being.

- *Communicate with the parents.* A lot of parent-grandparent strife occurs when expectations differ, conflicts are ignored, and parents and grandparents don't talk to each other about their concerns.

- *Follow a few basic and simple "guidelines."* Parents may suggest a few ideas of how to approach helping a child develop the healthiest eating and activity habits as possible. While the parent shouldn't be overbearing in the rules, try your best to follow the few guidelines the parents believe are most important.

- *Serve as a role model.* The grandkids are watching you. Take this opportunity to serve as a positive role model by choosing to eat a healthy, balanced diet and trying to fit in regular physical activity every day.

- *Check yourself.* It's easy to fall into the grandparent role of child-spoiler and rule-breaker. If you notice that you've gotten a bit too lenient with the grandkids, check yourself. Remember your promises to the parents and touch base with them to see if there are any hard feelings. When conflicts do arise, the American Association for Retired Persons (AARP) offers the following suggestions:
  - ✓ Let the parents be the parents.
  - ✓ Accept new parenting methods.
  - ✓ Give advice only when asked.
  - ✓ Respect children and grandchildren.
  - ✓ Use love, not gifts, to win affection.
  - ✓ Set boundaries for grandchildren.
  - ✓ Discuss disagreements with children when grandchildren aren't present.
  - ✓ Work out hard feelings when conflicts arise.

legitimate power, reward power, and coercive power (described in more detail in subsequent sections).[2] Over the years, these methods have been tweaked and updated by other authors, but for the most part, the strategies still offer an approach you can use to influence interactions with your parents, in-laws, and other well-meaning adults who may unknowingly interfere with your best-laid child-rearing plans. (After all, it's not always just the grandparents. See the sidebar "It's Not Just the Grandparents" for more on this subject.)

## Common Gripes and How to Overcome Them

The following are a few examples of the strategies and how you could use them to transform your parents from antagonists to fierce allies in your pursuit to raise healthier children. The strategies will also help you minimize conflicts along the way.

*Grandparents Who, No Matter What You Request, Give In to the Child's Begging for the "Same Old, Same Old" Foods (Such as Macaroni and Cheese, Cheese Pizza, Peanut Butter and Jelly, or Chicken Nuggets)*

In this situation, it's easier for grandparents to serve the "tried and true" (which also tends to be very easy to prepare), and as an added bonus, the kids are thrilled. As far as they're concerned, it's a win-win. The grandparents are happy; the kids are happy. So, what's the big deal? When you insist that a grandparent do more work to prepare a wholesome meal *and* put up with the kids groaning that they don't want to eat that anyway, you put the grandparents in an unpleasant situation. Unless they're 100 percent on board with you that it's important for children to be offered a healthy meal, then it's not worthwhile to hope they're going to comply with your requests. Your best bet is to use your *informational power.*

Do this by explaining your rationale for why you'd like your child to have a more balanced meal. And make it easy on them. For example, explain how you try to include a protein, fruit, vegetable, and high-quality carbohydrate at every meal. Then, tell your mother or mother-in-law not to fret, the kids can still have the cheese pizza, but would Grandma be willing to also offer some carrot sticks and apple slices—two easy-to-prepare sides you're sure the kids will like?

If you've already tried this strategy and it's failed, then take it to the next step. How important is it to you that your parents give your kids healthy meals? Your answer to this question might depend on how often your parents are responsible for providing meals, how strict you are with your children's food offerings (including in response to a child's food allergies or sensitivities), and how likely it is that this conflict will lead to longer-term hard feelings and ill will. If you still feel very strongly, then you may need to consider another approach.

*Grandparents Who Offer Lots of Sweets—for Snacks, as Rewards, to Heal Pain, or Just for the Fun of It*

Grandparents know that candy and sugar aren't healthy foods. The most likely reasons that they're constantly allowing your kids all this junk food include

## It's Not Just the Grandparents

While grandparents may be the most notorious for their disregard for your eating rules, they're not the only ones exposing your kids to less-than-desirable eating habits. A study of 300 families with school-aged kids set out to understand what factors are most associated with increased time spent in fast-food and full-service restaurants. Along with parenting style, parental work patterns, importance to parents of family meals, and time spent traveling, kids who spent more time with their fathers were more likely to eat out at fast-food and full-service restaurants. (However, those fathers who think of dinner as an important family ritual ate out less frequently.)[3] Turns out you might need to take a second glance at how dad is feeding the kids too.

Kids also spend a large amount of time in either child care or preschool. Whether their exposure to these settings affects weight or overall health depends in large part on the individual characteristics of the day care or school, including the philosophy of the director as well as political and financial constraints when it comes to funding snacks and meals.

As peer influence becomes more important as children age, the beliefs and actions of your child's friends as well as those children's parents may also influence your child's eating attitudes and behaviors. For example, one mom shared how the brown rice and broccoli that her daughter normally loves was swiftly rejected when a cousin got to eat chicken nuggets during a playdate.

Ultimately, you can't possibly go out and protect your child from all potentially "harmful" influencers. You wouldn't want to anyway because highly controlling and restrictive parents tend to have children who rebel against their best wishes anyway. However, you can be aware of the major influencers in your child's life and take extra care to consistently apply your own family's nutritional philosophy. This will help your child want to eat the healthy food, even when you're not there looking over his shoulder.

wanting to win over the love and admiration of your kids and perhaps satisfy their own sweet tooth. You've likely tried using your informational power but to no avail. Not exposing your kids to endless amounts of sugar, especially in a way that contributes to emotional eating down the line (especially when desserts are used as rewards and for comfort), is extremely important to you; thus, you want to find some way to get your parents to stop this habit.

In many cases the next best strategy after using information is *expert power*. The main difference between these two strategies is that with informational power, the grandparents understand the reason why they're making a change. With expert power, they do it just because someone with more know-how tells them they should. To make this one work, you need to get some supporting documentation from a well-respected expert to back you up. If your child's pediatrician is on board with your efforts, you could bring the grandparents along for a checkup. To maximize the chances that this will work, talk with the pediatrician ahead of time. Many parents report some success with this technique.

This is just one example: Maria's eight-year-old obese daughter Ariel is "Grandpa's girl." The grandparents watch Ariel after school five days per week. Despite repeated requests from Maria that he stops, Grandpa continues to sneak Ariel candy on a daily basis. Whether the candy helped create it or is a result of it, you can tell that Grandpa and Ariel have a strong relationship. In fact, when Ariel had to get shots at the doctor's office, she cried for Grandpa. This situation is a perfect example of how a grandparent can sabotage a parent's efforts to optimize a child's health. At the pediatrician's urging, on the next visit, Grandpa came with Maria for Ariel's appointment. The pediatrician offered alternatives to candy and a few suggestions of ways that Grandpa and Ariel could spend quality time together sans candy. When Ariel was in the playroom at the office, the pediatrician explained to her grandpa why it's so important to help Ariel achieve a healthy weight to avoid the childhood onset of adult health problems, such as high blood pressure, high cholesterol, and diabetes. Grandpa took this to heart and said he'd remove the candy from his house.

*Grandparents Who Plop the Kids in Front of the Television for Unlimited TV Viewing (and Possibly With Little Supervision)*

Grandparents are known for their leniency when it comes to TV time. You might have already tried everything. You explained how too much TV time negatively affects language development, how TV advertisements for all that sugar cereal and junk food make the kids beg for the junk, how zombies in front of the TV interfere with normal playtime and physical activity. But still, every time you walk in the door when the grandparents are babysitting, you see them all engrossed with some TV program. (Information did not work.) You may have explained how the American Academy of Pediatrics says kids younger than two should have no TV exposure and that kids older than two should get two hours max. But still, you come home to the TV on as background noise. (Experts ignored.) Just like with your children, you may have to be a little bit less obvious in your demands. (Remember when your kids ignored requests to "Eat your vegetables!" but then when you made the vegetables easily accessible and made them taste good, the kids were somehow more willing to give them a try?) Just like you turn to your kids' healthy-eating peers to inspire some vegetable intake, for the particularly stubborn grandparent who simply ignores your requests, you may consider turning to other grandparents who *don't* let the kids play video games for hours on end or spend the entire evening together on the computer. Capitalize on the other grandparents' *referent power*. To make this one work, try the following actions:

- Identify a good friend of your parents who engages in some healthy activity with their grandkids that you wish your parents would do with yours. (For example, does she take the kids to the pool, plan an art class, or regularly take them to visit a museum?)

- Make arrangements to see that friend. Whether you help coordinate them taking all of the grandkids out together or you help set up a time for them to get coffee, conversations will inevitably come to the grandkids. This offers a great time for your parent to pick up on some of the fun activities that the other grandparent-grandchild duo do together.
- Follow up. After the outing, ask your parent how it went. What did they do? What kind of things does the friend like to do with her grandkids? This helps to remind your parent of potential ideas she might have picked up to get your kids off the couch and doing more.

Just as peer influence is powerful in influencing kids, it's equally powerful for the older generation.

*Grandparents Who Eat a Generally Unbalanced and Unhealthy Diet and, By Default, Offer the Same Generally Unbalanced and Unhealthy Meals to Your Kids*

The chances of getting a grandparent who has less-than-ideal eating habits to provide your child with only the healthiest and most balanced meals are low. These eating habits have been ingrained into the grandparent's way of life, and as everyone knows, eating habits are very difficult to change, especially when the person has no interest in doing so. In these situations, it may be that your best chance to ensure that your child eats a healthy, balanced diet when your parents are in charge is to use your *legitimate power*. This is when you say "I'm the mom, and when you're at my house, I need you to follow the guidelines and rules I have set for my kids."

Kids are very place specific. You can minimize mealtime food fights and struggles if you implement and enforce consistent rules in your home. For example, you may require that everyone sit together to eat dinner as a family. That no one has to clean his plate. That dessert isn't used as a reward for eating vegetables. By being very clear and consistent with your mealtime expectations, mealtimes will be more enjoyable for everyone, including your kids and the grandparents. You might just find that your parents don't mind reinforcing your rules because they see the problems and struggles that ensue when using various forms of negotiation, power plays, and coercion. Of course, in order for grandparents to voluntarily go along with this plan, you've got to also make it easy for them to follow your guidelines. In addition to making your goals and expectations explicit, you also can increase your chances of success by making it very easy on your parents. Have easy-to-make healthy meals and snacks on hand when they're scheduled to watch your kids.

Increase the likelihood that this whole idea will work by allowing Grandma to practice her "legitimate power" to have her own rules when taking care of the kids at her house. The kids may learn that different rules apply at Grandma's, but at least that won't interfere with the work you're trying to accomplish at home. (This strategy may not work so well if it turns out that your kids spend more or equal amount of time at Grandma's than at home.)

*Grandparents Who Follow the Same-Old Routines and Are Resistant to Make Changes in Their Approach to Interacting With the Grandkids*

Everyone is motivated to some extent by rewards. While you can't guarantee that the behavior will keep happening once the rewards stop, you can set the stage to use rewards to build long-term habits. Think about what motivates your parents the most when it comes to the grandkids. A lot of the time, it's the kids' love and affection. Other times, it may just be a little bit of appreciation and gratitude. Give some sincere consideration to what truly makes your parents happy and then use your *rewards power* when your parents do something with the kids that you'd like to reinforce. For example:

- If Grandma takes the kids to play at the park, thank her with a framed photograph of the kids swinging, riding a bike, or playing on the playground equipment.

- If Grandpa decides to take the kids to Subway for lunch or dinner (and while there buys them healthy meals), commend him for such a healthy lunch idea and buy him a gift card for Subway so he can take the kids back again.

- If your mother-in-law goes outside her comfort zone to prepare a truly gourmet (and also very healthy) dinner, take the extra effort to help the kids write a thank-you note to thank her for such a wonderful meal.

*Grandparents Who Will Do Whatever They Want—Regardless of What You Ask*

In this case, you've already tried every other possible method to get your parents to listen—to no avail. Sometimes, a behavior may be so important to you that you require compliance. And if the request isn't followed, then you may need to use punishments to force the desired behavior. It goes without saying that this strategy should be used only as a last resort for the most serious issues because you're very likely to create familial discord, hard feelings, and a motivation on the grandparents' side to hide facts and information. But when it comes down to it, this is a useful strategy. If your parents refuse to do X, you may have to use this *coercive power*, which may mean hiring a babysitter who will follow your requests, cutting off opportunities for a period of time, or taking away certain "privileges." (See the sidebar "GG Speaks.")

# Other Counterstrategies

You *can* undo grandparent sabotage. You and your parents want what's best for your kids—you may just take different approaches to getting there. Increase the chances that your influence strategies will work with some of these supporting counterstrategies.

## Make It Easy on Them—Provide a Few Snacks and Samples

You can increase the odds your parents will provide your children with healthy snacks and take them to engage in fun physical activities if you make it easy on them. Have snack ideas and adventure itineraries readily accessible so they can choose to follow your lead if they feel so inclined.

## GG Speaks

The content of this book is based on the latest research, anecdotes from parents, and, in some cases (including this chapter), personal experiences. GG is a real-life character. This strong-willed, highly influential, and difficult-to-persuade grandma—who also happens to be my mom—agreed to share her unedited viewpoint on the matter.

Dr. Nat describes me and, interestingly, many of my "grandparent" peers with the candor and straight talk characteristic of hers. Reading this chapter brought up poignant and sobering memories about the challenges of communicating child-rearing expectations with my parents and in-laws, all of whom were card-carrying members of the "traditional generation." For them, loyalty to the past accompanied by an unquestioning belief in "the way we were raised" yielded predictable and nonnegotiable habits and practices—many of which I questioned and resisted as a young parent. Understanding why we do what we do when it comes to feeding our grandchildren—in terms of nourishing the body and nurturing the spirit—and how we choose to act on those values is at the heart of the message behind "grandparent sabotage."

Yes, I'm motivated by feelings, aspirations, and hopes that my grandchildren enjoy a happy and healthy life—as *children* and as *adults*. Blessed with four of them ranging in age from infancy to adolescence, I sometimes behave in ways that are inconsistent or misaligned with my stated values. I imagine that makes me "human." More importantly, like many caring adults, I believe my day-to-day actions are guided by a thoughtful desire to make a difference in their lives and to leave a legacy of "gifts" that bring them happiness and a solid foundation for a healthy and happy future. This is when I realize how important it is to nurture the relationship with their parents by respecting and honoring their rules, speaking truthfully to

## Reinforce Healthy Eating Habits in Kids so They'll Not Want a Lot of Junk

You've got to meet your parents halfway. If you're going to request that they create an optimally healthy environment for your kids, you've got to do the same. Make sure that you have a healthy home environment and that you "train" your kids so they actually like and request the healthy stuff.

me when my behavior falls into the sphere of "grandparent sabotage," and regrouping to do better next time. Clearly, the challenge remains because my generation and that of my children have cultivated different assumptions and habits about food and the emotional ties associated with eating. We grew up at different times, survived and thrived under different circumstances, and learned to parent by watching and experiencing our own parents.

With that said, it seems to me, as one who's "strong-willed, highly influential, and difficult to persuade," that investing in the longer-term vision of a healthy, nutritionally balanced, active, and happy grandchild is well worth the ups and downs of a conscientious and sometimes challenging effort to support his parents. We're dedicated to the same outcome: healthy, nutritionally balanced, active, and fulfilled adults. What makes this easier to accomplish is articulating an explicit and shared commitment. This happens because together we talk and agree on several important things, including clear expectations, a time and a place to share our views and the promise of being heard (in other words, having some influence with each other), the will and commensurate skill to follow through on expectations, and accountability.

This last one is critical to the immediate and long-term success of our partnership. Acknowledgement and expression of genuine gratitude go a long way to reinforce and sustain commitment. At the same time, feedback and honest conversation when behavior doesn't align with what we promised to do are equally important in refocusing and revitalizing our shared expectations. I don't claim that this approach is easy, but I know it's effective.

So, thanks, Dr. Nat, for the thoughtful chapter and informative "wake-up call."

—GG

## Expect Some Spoiling Is Going On

If grandparents were given a job description, they would demand that spoiling be a part of it. Many grandparents take great pleasure and joy from spoiling their grandkids. Expect that some spoiling is going on—and choose your battles wisely.

### Do Not Forbid Ice Cream and Potato Chips

The more you forbid your kids from eating the "junk" food, the more enticing it becomes not only to the kids but also to the grandparents, who can offer it up when you're not around. Make this stuff an occasional occurrence in your house so you can lessen some of the allure of binging on these foods when you're not looking.

### Make It Up With Physical Activity

Kids love to run around, be active, and play about as much as they love to go out for ice cream and pick up an occasional fast-food dinner. If you're concerned that the calorie intake is excessive when spending time with your parents, then rather than forcing the kids or parents to cut out all junk food, you can support them in creating opportunities to be active and subsequently burn off energy and a lot of those extra calories.

### Try to "Go With the Flow" as Much as Possible

Ultimately, you can do what's best for your kids and your parents with minimal conflict and distress if you continue to be flexible and understanding but also clear and encouraging in your approach to create a healthy environment for your kids when they're being cared for by their grandparents.

The sidebar "Counterstrategies in Action: Grandparents as Allies" highlights effective approaches some parents have taken when working together with their parents, in-laws, and other influential adults.

# Developmental Considerations

The grandparent-grandchild bond begins in infancy and grows with the child. From the newborn baby nestled in the nape of Grandma's neck and the rambunctious toddler playing T-ball with Grandpa to the school-aged child learning to read and the awkward adolescent trying to manage his growing need for independence, grandparents play a tremendous role in the growth and development of their grandchildren. To harness grandparents' potential as powerful allies in not only optimizing your child's physical health but also his intellectual, social, and emotional health, help your parents tailor their activities to the child's age and developmental stage (Figure 11-1).

### Infant (0–1 years)

The coddling, holding, and adoration that a grandparent provides a newborn baby helps to build the baby's confidence and trust in the world. It's impossible to spoil a newborn. The joy and gift of helping care for a new baby is many grandmothers' dream. In the second half of the first year, the infant begins to form strong attachments to primary caretakers, which may include a grandparent, especially if he or she is a primary caretaker. Habits that start this early tend to last. Encourage your parents to take the baby for long walks, read together, and play music. These are interactive activities that stimulate a child's rapidly growing brain.

## Counterstrategies in Action: Grandparents as Allies

A child benefits tremendously when parents and grandparents take a team approach to parenting. The following are a few examples of this chapter's counterstrategies in action.

- *Make it easy.* Nina figured out an easy way to get her mother and mother-in-law on board with feeding her daughter Nora healthy foods. On Monday through Thursday, Nora's grandmas share caretaker responsibilities. And when Nora is dropped off, she comes fully equipped with daytime meals and snacks. Her mom says: "They feed her what I leave for her, which is all healthy. They respect that because I have made it clear how important it is to me that she eats well."

- *Reinforce healthy habits.* Tali, mother of six-year-old Averie, four-year-old Sami, and two-year-old Bennett, shares her philosophy on reinforcing healthy habits at home and also giving grandparents the opportunity to set their own guidelines: "Our children spend time with their grandparents frequently. Although we'd love for the grandparents to follow all of our rules, we think it's equally important for our children to learn that different homes have different rules. Therefore, we do not impose our rules on our grandparents or family members (unless they're regarding safety) if our children are at their houses. If they are in our home, they follow our rules."

- *Expect spoiling.* As the mother of a toddler, Shannon understands that some spoiling is going on at Grandma's—and she's okay with that. In fact, she agrees "that's what they're here for—to spoil!" (This is especially applicable for grandparents who only get to see the grandkids on occasion.)

- *Don't restrict the unhealthy food.* Katie, mother of two toddlers, takes a laid-back but still authoritative approach to teaching her kids about healthy eating—whether they eat at home or at their grandparents' homes. "We really try to eat mostly healthy and teach about eating sweets in moderation," she says. With that, Katie and her husband are pretty laid back and flexible (without many requests or restrictions) when they drop the kids off with their grandpas two days per week. And it seems to be working. Katie describes her kids as fantastic eaters who will try anything once and don't go overboard when given "sometimes" foods.

- *Make it up with physical activity.* Grandparents keeping the kids busy and away from sitting comatose in front the television all afternoon goes a long way in helping kids to get healthy! Not only are the kids moving their bodies and bonding with their grandparents, but they're also not mindlessly eating and loading up on calorie-rich, nutrient-poor foods. Sam, mom of six-year-old twins Nick and Bella, doesn't worry so much about the grandparents sometimes giving the kids not-so-healthy foods because most of the time, the kids and their grandparents are running around and playing outside together. Jessica has made it very easy for the grandparents to promote physical activity with her kids: "My mom watches my daughter one day a week—and I found a dance class for her at the park district that falls on that same day. It's good for my daughter—and it gives my mom a little break!"

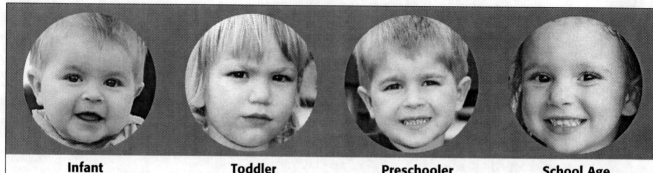

| Infant | Toddler | Preschooler | School Age |
|---|---|---|---|
| • Let grandparents spoil a newborn.<br>• Encourage grandparents to take a new baby for walks, to read together, and play music together. | • Encourage firm limit setting.<br>• Work with grandparents as a team.<br>• Encourage grandparents to experiment with healthy variations of favorite foods. | • Encourage grandparents to play and explore with the grandchild.<br>• Continue to encourage grandparents to experiment with healthy foods and activities. | • Encourage grandparents to expose the child to intellectually stimulating bonding experiences.<br>• Set the stage for grandparents and kids to cook together. |

Figure 11-1. Developmental considerations

### Toddler (1–3 years)

Toddlerhood may be a particularly trying time for the parent-grandparent relationship because this is the age when kids tend to be the most picky, particular, and vulnerable to developing undesirable behaviors in response to spoiling (and it turns out that this may be the time when grandparents love to spoil the most). Without firm limits and a team approach to dealing with a toddler, major family strife can occur. Although grandparents may be tempted to give in to the toddler's constant requests for the same foods, they could experiment with healthy variations of favorites. (See this chapter's recipes for some ideas).

### Preschooler (3–5 years)

As toddlers become preschoolers, they're more interested in trying new foods and activities and thus will be more flexible with a grandparent trying out healthier eating and activity approaches. A great complement to a preschooler's high energy and short attention span are short adventures, such as taking the dog for a walk or going to the park or playground.

### School Age (5–10 years)

A school-aged child is inquisitive and interested in trying out new experiences. A venture to a museum, aquarium, or a long hike in a local preserve or state or national forest offers an opportunity for grandparent-grandchild bonding as well as ample opportunities for physical activity, conversation, and intellectual stimulation. A school-age child may also be excited to learn to cook healthy and delicious foods with a grandparent.

# Chapter Summary

While no foolproof way exists to get grandparents on board in your effort to shape your child's eating and activity habits, the goal is that some of these strategies may be directly applicable to your situation and make it a little bit easier to get the all-important grandparents on your team. The following are crucial points from this chapter:

- Always try to show your appreciation and gratitude to grandparents, especially when they go out of their way to help out or go along with your requests.
- Share your concerns in a transparent and open manner.
- Make it easy for the grandparents to follow your "guidelines."
- Explain the rationale for why you do what you do.
- Choose your battles wisely.
- Enlist the help of others who grandparents respect and trust.
- You set the "rules" at your house, but consider letting Grandma "set the rules" at her house.
- Reinforce healthy eating habits in your kids so they actually want the healthy stuff.
- Tolerate some spoiling.
- Create opportunities for kids and their grandparents to be healthy and active together.

# Recipes: Foods Kids Can Make With Their Grandparents

## Homemade Whole Wheat Rosemary Pizza

2 cups whole wheat flour

2 cups of bread flour

2 teaspoons of salt

2 tablespoons of fresh rosemary, finely chopped

1 3/4 cups of water, slightly warmer than room temperature

3 tablespoons of olive oil

1 package of rapidly rising yeast

Lots of your favorite vegetables

Place warm water into a bowl and sprinkle in yeast. Let sit for 4 to 5 minutes and then mix in the olive oil. Add the flours, salt, and rosemary and mix with a wooden spoon. Knead by hand for approximately 10 minutes, ensuring the dough comes together. Place in a large bowl and cover with a kitchen towel. Let rise for 1 1/2 to 2 hours and watch the dough grow!

After the dough has risen, punch it down in the bowl. Makes dough for 6 individual pizzas. Roll dough out on a well-floured surface. Top with your favorite toppings. Bake in oven at 450 degrees for 12 to 15 minutes.

## Fruity Tropical Creamsicles

2 cups of plain nonfat yogurt
1/2 cup of pineapple chunks
1 banana
1 orange, peeled and cut in half
1/2 cup of mango chunks
1/2 cup of strawberries
1/4 cup honey
Small paper cups
Popsicle sticks

Place all ingredients into a blender and blend until smooth. Pour into paper cups and place a popsicle stick in the middle. Freeze overnight. To serve, peel the paper cups off of the popsicles and enjoy!

## Coconutty Blueberry Granola

3 cups rolled oats
1 cup pecans, chopped
1 cup cashews, chopped
1 1/2 cups dried blueberries
1 1/2 cups shredded coconut
1 teaspoon salt
1 tablespoon ground cinnamon
1 tablespoon vanilla extract
1/2 cup brown sugar
3 tablespoons butter, melted
3 tablespoons brown rice syrup or honey

Preheat oven to 325 degrees. Mix all ingredients together in a large mixing bowl. Pour evenly onto a baking sheet. Bake for 20 minutes and then remove from oven and stir. Place back into oven and cook for another 15 minutes. Remove from oven and stir. Let cool to room temperature. Serve with milk or yogurt.

## References

1.  Pearce, A., L. Li, J. Abbas, B. Ferguson, H. Graham, and C. Law. (2010). Is childcare associated with the risk of overweight and obesity in the early years? Findings from the UK Millennium Cohort Study. *Int J Obes (Lond). 34*(7): p. 1160-8.

2.  Raven, B. (2008). Bases of power and the power/interaction model of interpersonal influence. *Analyses of Social Issues and Public Policy. 8*(1): p. 1-22.

3.  McIntosh, A., K.S. Kubena, G. Tolle, W. Dean, M.-J. Kim, J.-S. Jan, and J. Anding. (2011). Determinants of children's use of and time spent in fast-food and full-service restaurants. *J Nutr Educ Behav. 43*(3): p. 142-9.

# 12

# Mistake #12— Missing Opportunities

*If I had my child to raise over again,*
*I'd finger paint more, and point the finger less.*
*I'd do less correcting and more connecting.*
*I'd take my eyes off my watch and watch with my eyes.*
*I would care to know less and know to care more.*
*I'd take more hikes and fly more kites.*
*I'd stop playing serious and seriously play.*
*I'd run through more fields and gaze at more stars.*
*I'd do more hugging and less tugging.*
*I would be firm less often and affirm much more.*
*I'd build self-esteem first, and the house later.*
*I'd teach less about the love of power,*
*And more about the power of love.*

—If I Had My Child To Raise Over
Again*, Diana Loomans © 2012,
www.dianaloomans.com

When today's adults look back at their childhood, they may remember playing ball, climbing trees, and generally causing mischief outside with friends until their mom called them in for dinner. Now, you could drive through comfortable suburban neighborhoods on a sunny and cool fall day and not find a kid in sight. But, of course, the drive-through line at any given fast-food place will be packed. And if you listen carefully, you may hear the noise of a blaring TV through open windows. What happened?

Kids these days spend more time in front of electronic media, such as the TV, computer screen, and phone, than they spend in school. Even our

*Reprinted with permission

youngest children are bombarded with appealing advertising to buy more and eat more. Of course, a life of inactivity and wasted time isn't true for all kids. "The generation of 'solution-focused,' 'results-driven,' thrusting adults has created a performance-measured world where children can't 'just play'—they must have 'structured activities' ... where they cannot just daydream and fantasize ... where even fetuses in utero must have their potential maximized, ..." researcher Philip Darbyshire points out in an article on the death of childhood.[1] Society pressures parents to push their kids even harder at even younger ages in the pursuit of the perfect child with the perfect level of measured success. As any parent quickly recognizes, childhood today is different from how it was 20 or 30 years ago. But it doesn't have to be worse.

Just as childhood should be fun, parenting is also supposed to be fun—despite its accompanying demands, stresses, mistakes, and disappointments. Parents have an incredible opportunity to teach their children about the wonders and amazement that the world has to offer. While this role extends far beyond shaping kids' health habits, you can make eating healthy and being physically active fun and exciting. Seize these opportunities to teach your kids a little bit about the world and spend quality time together while also fostering lifelong healthy habits and attitudes.

Plant a small garden and teach your children how to use what you grow to make delicious recipes. Take the children to a farmers' market and let them pick out a new vegetable or fruit to try at home. Go on a pretend "trip around the world" by learning about various countries and then prepare traditional meals from some of those countries. Once per month, make dinner a festive celebration by having the kids decorate and be responsible for serving the hors d'oeuvres of their choice.

However you decide to do it and whatever approach you take, consider evaluating your priorities, goals, and commitments to your children. You may reach the conclusion that it's really not all that important if they eat a vegetable at every meal; clean their plate of all the food you offer; or sometimes splurge on ice cream, cookies, or junk food. But it's important that they regularly be offered fresh and wholesome foods and have fruits and vegetables readily accessible should they choose to eat them; that they learn to let their bodies tell them when they're hungry and when they're full; that they learn how to critically evaluate and be skeptical of marketing gimmicks and ads that try to persuade them; that they have frequent opportunities to move their bodies, run around, and just play; that at each step of the way, they have a loving adult at their side to teach them what it means and what it looks like to be healthy, have a healthy relationship with food, and still have a bit of fun along the way.

The purpose of this book was to provide you with tools, examples, and ideas to help you in your pursuit to get your children to eat healthier and be more physically active. One of the major objectives of the book was to emphasize that it's not so much about what your child eats but more about your approach—the consistent, persistent, and predictable decisions you make each day that shows them what healthy looks like—the choices that give your kids a fun, stimulating, and full childhood. The goal is that one day, when you least expect it, you find that your picky, don't-give-me-that-green-thing, hate-to-play-outside child has suddenly grown up into a healthy, active, well-adjusted young adult. And then you may look back and be glad you didn't insist "Eat your vegetables!" or fall for some of the other mistakes that parents unwittingly make.

Hopefully, this book helped you minimize the mealtime food battles and take a more relaxed approach to feeding your kids. To tie it all together, this final chapter's recap highlights the book's major themes.

# The 10 "Power Ps"

We're not talking crispy green vegetables here. These 10 "Power Ps" offer a recap of the major tenets of this book and comprise final advice for parents who feel they've tried everything—to no avail:

- *Packaging.* Borrow the tricks of the multi-billion-dollar food industry and creatively package and "brand" healthy foods. An appealingly decorated or snazzy-named snack can transform a rejected food into a food a picky child will at least try. As one Cornell study showed, a quick name change from drab "peas" to snazzy "power peas" doubled children's pea consumption.[2]

- *Parenting.* Taking an authoritative parenting approach in which you set boundaries and guidelines for your children but they're given the freedom to make choices within those guidelines helps you to raise the most well-adjusted and overall healthy children. Put this to practice at mealtimes, when you determine what types of foods are prepared and the children decide what and how much to eat.

- *Psychology.* Always remember that your kids have minds of their own (as if you could forget!) and they'll resist overt coercion. A power struggle with a strong-willed child is an unpleasant experience to be avoided whenever possible. You're better off creating situations in which your child is given the opportunity to choose between equally healthy options. You get what you want (after all, you're the one who decided his choice options) and your child gets what he wants (the opportunity to exert a little control).

- *Physiology.* The human body needs certain vitamins and nutrients for optimal health and well-being, while other foodstuffs are needed only in small amounts (or occasionally not at all). Take advantage of opportunities to teach your children what's healthy for their growing bodies and why you keep reminding them to drink three glasses of milk per day or ask them to consider giving the iron-rich, dark green veggies a try.

- *Practice.* Unfortunately, these strategies won't turn your picky eater into an adventurous food connoisseur overnight. And you may not intuitively be inclined to ignore the fact that your two-year-old blatantly refuses to eat anything you have put on his plate, although that's what this book recommends. In order for these strategies to work, you've got to practice using them—day in and day out.

- *Persistence.* Despite urges to give in to the unnerving whining, begging, pleading, and screaming, to get the results you want (active and healthy children), you have to be persistent and consistent. As operant conditioning shows us, not reinforcing the negative behavior will extinguish it.

- *Peers.* Never underestimate the power of peer influence for your kids and for you. Your child's friends can make or break your efforts to get him to eat healthier. At the same time, teams of parents working together to make lasting changes in their kids are most likely to be successful in their efforts (and may even encourage each other to step up their own nutrition and exercise plans).

- *Price.* When the frustration overwhelms and the desire to just give in and forget about it increases, remember the high price of being overweight on a child's health and well being. Also, remember that even if your child isn't even close to being one of the 30 percent of children who are already overweight, he's got a decent chance of being overweight in the future if he doesn't adopt healthy nutrition and activity habits in childhood. (Two-thirds of adults are overweight or obese.)

- *Payback.* The strategies and tips recommended in this book require persistence and patience, but ultimately, if applied consistently and effectively, they'll give you the payback you envision—well-rounded, healthy, active children with a firm grasp of how to take care of their bodies.

- *Pep talk.* You're not in this alone. Generations of parents have struggled to figure out the best way to feed their children. Hopefully, this book helped you reexamine your beliefs about how to raise healthy eaters. But don't go it alone. Open the conversation with your friends. Together, you can encourage, strategize, and rejuvenate to end the food fight once and for all.

# Recipes: A Multicultural Extravaganza

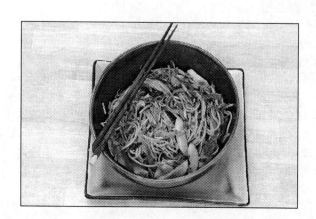

### Whole Wheat Chow Mein

1 pack of whole wheat spaghetti, cooked

3 cups of chopped assorted vegetables (mushrooms, spinach, peppers, carrots, snap peas)

1 1/2 cups of meat, sliced thin (chicken, pork, beef or tofu)

1 medium onion, sliced

3 to 4 cloves of garlic, finely chopped

1-inch piece of fresh ginger, finely chopped

1 cup of green onions, chopped

1/4 cup of soy sauce

1 tablespoon of honey

Place 2 tablespoons of olive oil in a pan over medium heat. Place onions, ginger, and garlic in pan and cook for 3 to 4 minutes, stirring occasionally. Add sliced meat to pan and cook for 6 to 7 minutes or until meat is almost cooked. Add vegetables to pan and then soy sauce and honey and cook for 2 minutes. Lastly, add cooked noodles to pan and mix all ingredients well. Cook for another 2 to 3 minutes and then serve.

## Baked Egg Rolls

8 egg roll wrappers

2 carrots, peeled and grated

1/2 head of green cabbage

1 9-ounce bag of baby spinach

3 tablespoons of soy sauce

1/2 inch piece of fresh ginger

Olive oil

To prepare vegetables: Wash and dry all vegetables. Chop cabbage into thin slices and place into a mixing bowl. Peel and grate the carrots and place into mixing bowl. Using the fine grating holes, grate the ginger and mix in with vegetables. Place 2 tablespoons of olive oil in a pan over medium heat. Pour vegetables from mixing bowl into pan and cook until cabbage is soft, approximately 10 minutes. Add spinach to pan and stir. Once spinach has wilted, add the soy sauce, stir, and remove from heat and let cool.

To prepare egg rolls: Preheat oven to 375 degrees. If egg roll wrappers are square, arrange so it's a diamond shape in front of you. Dip your index finger in water and paint the perimeter of the wrapper with water. Place 3 tablespoons of cooled vegetable filling in the center of the wrapper but favoring the half of the wrapper closest to you. Fold in the left and right corners of the wrapper toward the filling. Then, fold the corner of the wrapper closest to you toward the filling. Next, roll the covered filling toward the last corner and place on a baking sheet. With a pastry brush (or your index finger), lightly brush a thin layer of olive oil on both sides of the egg roll. Bake in the oven for approximately 15 minutes or until brown and crispy.

## Parmesan Crusted Baked Pasta

1 pack of whole wheat short pasta (penne, rigatoni, macaroni), cooked

3 cups of chopped assorted vegetables

1 jar of tomato or marinara sauce

1/2 cup of grated parmesan or mozzarella

Cook pasta as instructed on label. Place 2 tablespoons of olive oil in a pan over medium heat. Place vegetables in pan and cook for 3 to 4 minutes, until vegetables are tender. Pour vegetables into large mixing bowl. Add tomato/ marinara sauce. Add cooked pasta and stir. Pour contents of bowl into a large baking casserole tray.

Preheat oven to 375 degrees. Place dish into oven and cook for 30 minutes. Remove dish from oven and sprinkle cheese on top. Return dish to oven and cook another 15 minutes, until cheese is melted.

### Curry Salmon Tomato Kabobs and Vegetable Biryani

*Curry Salmon Tomato Kabobs*

1 pound of salmon filets, cut into 1-inch cubes
1 cup of plain nonfat yogurt
2 tablespoons of curry powder
1 pint of cherry tomatoes
Wooden skewers

*Vegetable Biryani*

2 cups of brown rice, cooked
2 cups of chopped vegetables (zucchini, broccoli, cauliflower)
1 medium onion, chopped
1 teaspoon of ground cumin
1 teaspoon of ground cinnamon
1 teaspoon of ground cardamom
2 garlic cloves, finely chopped
1/2 inch of fresh ginger, grated (or 1 teaspoon of ginger powder)
1 teaspoon of chili powder (optional)
1/2 cup fresh cilantro, chopped
Olive oil

To prepare salmon: Mix salmon cubes with yogurt and curry powder in a mixing bowl. Let sit in refrigerator for 30 minutes.

Remove salmon from refrigerator and place approximately 4 to 5 pieces of salmon on skewer, alternating with cherry tomatoes. Preheat oven to 375 degrees. Place skewers on baking sheet, approximately 2 inches apart. Bake for 20 to 25 minutes, until salmon is well done.

To prepare biryani: Wash and dry all vegetables. Place 2 tablespoons of olive oil in pan over medium heat. Place onions and spices in pan and sauté for 2 minutes. Add chopped vegetables and cook for 3 to 4 minutes. Add rice and stir.

Place skewers over rice, sprinkle with chopped cilantro, and serve. If serving younger children, remove salmon and tomatoes from skewer before serving.

### Moroccan Chicken With Raisin Couscous

6 bone-in chicken thighs
1 medium onion, chopped
2 garlic cloves, finely chopped
1 lemon, cut into 1/4-inch slices
1/2 cup of green olives, pitted and halved

1 teaspoon of ground cardamom

2 teaspoons of cinnamon

2 teaspoons of ground coriander

2 cups of chicken or vegetable broth

Salt and pepper

Olive oil

*Raisin Couscous*

1 1/2 cups of dry couscous

1 3/4 cups of water

1/2 cup of raisins

1/2 cup of fresh parsley, chopped

To prepare chicken: Heat a wide bottomed pot over medium heat. Place 3 tablespoons of olive oil in pot. Sprinkle the chicken with salt and pepper. Place the chicken skin-side down in the pot and cook for 6 minutes. Flip chicken over and cook for another 5 minutes. Remove chicken from pot and set aside.

Place onions, garlic, and spices in same pot and cook for approximately 5 minutes, stirring occasionally. Add lemon slices and cook for another 2 to 3 minutes. Return chicken to the pot in an even layer. Add olives and then broth to the pot. Bring to gentle boil and then turn heat to low. Let simmer for 25 minutes.

To prepare couscous: Bring water to a boil in a pot with a fitted lid. Once water is boiling, add dry couscous and raisins to pot, cover with the lid, and turn off the heat. Let sit for approximately 10 minutes and then remove lid and fluff couscous with a fork.

Serve chicken on top of raisin couscous and top with chopped parsley.

## Grilled Chicken Tacos With Pico de Gallo and Elote (Mexican Corn on the Cob)

2 Simple Baked Chicken Breasts—Mexican inspired (see Simple Baked Chicken Breast recipe in Chapter 10 and Mexican Spice Marinade recipe in Chapter 8)

8 corn tortillas

*Pico de Gallo*

1/4 medium onion, finely chopped

4 tomatoes, chopped

1 large cucumber, seeded and chopped

1/2 cup fresh cilantro, chopped

Juice of one lime

Salt and pepper

*Elote*

4 fresh ears of corn, husks removed

3 tablespoons of Greek yogurt

1 tablespoon of mayonnaise

1/4 cup grated parmesan

1 teaspoon of cayenne pepper (optional)

1 lime, quartered

To prepare the elote: Bring a large pot of water to boil. Place corn into boiling water and cook for approximately 5 minutes. Remove corn from water and turn off stove. Place a pan over medium heat. Once the pan is hot, place corn on pan for 3 to 4 minutes on each side or until kernels are slightly charred. In a small bowl, mix the Greek yogurt, mayonnaise, and cayenne pepper (if using) together. Remove the corn from the pan and let cool slightly. Spread 1 tablespoon of yogurt mixture on each ear of corn and then sprinkle with 1 tablespoon of grated parmesan. Serve with lime wedges.

To prepare the pico de gallo: Mix the chopped tomatoes, onion, cucumber, and cilantro in a bowl. Add the juice of one lime. Sprinkle 1 teaspoon of salt and pepper.

Assemble tacos by heating the corn tortillas in a pan or in the oven. Chop the chicken breasts into 1/4-inch cubes. Place a small amount of chicken in the middle of the tortilla and top with pico de gallo. Serve tacos with elote on the side.

## References

1.  Darbyshire, P. (2007). 'Childhood': Are reports of its death greatly exagerrated? *Journal of Child Health Care.* *11*(2): p. 85-97.

2.  Cuellar, S. (2009). Names turn preschoolers into vegetable lovers. *The Mindless Eater.* Available at http://foodpsychology.cornell.edu/pdf/newsletters/Newsletter_Spring_09.pdf.

# Cooking Basics

This appendix provides the tips and tools you need to best prepare delicious recipes. The information is adapted from *Cooking Basics* prepared by Janie Burney, Ph.D., RD for the University of Tennessee Extension[1].

Topics include:

- Kitchen equipment
- Measuring
- Measurement equivalents
- Recipe preparation steps
- Cooking terms
- Ingredient substitutions
- Healthy cooking tips
- Cooking with herbs, spices, and seasonings
- Seasoning your food with less salt
- Food yields
- Putting out a cooking fire

**Appendix**

# Kitchen Equipment

| Kitchen Equipment | Substitute Items |
| --- | --- |
| Measuring cup | Marked jar or baby bottle |
| Strainer | Pan with a lid or cover |
| Cookie sheet | Cake pan, pizza pan |
| Rolling pin | Smooth bottle or glass |
| Potato masher | Forks |
| Measuring spoons | Regular teaspoon and/or tablespoon |
| Vegetable peeler | Sharp knife |
| Mixing bowls | Kettle, pan, or storage containers |
| Cutting board | Sturdy plate |
| Pie pan | Flat cake pan |
| Round cake pan | Square or oblong pan |
| Biscuit/cookie cutters | Lids, rims of jars, rims of cans, glasses |
| Ladle for serving soup | Cup with handle |
| Pancake turner | Two knives, fork |
| Cooling rack | Oven rack |
| Rotary beater | Fork |
| Wire whisk | Two forks or jar with tight lid |
| Pot holder | Folded towel |
| Pastry blender | Two knives |
| Grater | Sharp knife |

# Measuring

*Note*: Do not measure any ingredients over the mixing bowl.

### Measuring Liquid Ingredients

- Use a liquid measuring cup to measure water, oil, fluid milk, juices, and syrup.
- Measure liquids in marked, clear containers.
- Set measuring cup on a flat surface. Check at eye level to make sure the correct amount is measured.

### Measuring Dry Ingredients

- Measure dry ingredients in containers that allow you to level off the ingredients across the top edge.
- Use a dry measuring cup to measure ingredients like flour, sugar, cornmeal, dry milk, and solid shortening.
- Sift or fluff dry ingredients, like flour, with a fork before measuring.
- Spoon dry ingredients into dry measuring cup. Level off ingredients with the flat edge of a knife.

## Measurement Equivalents

| | | |
|---|---|---|
| 3 teaspoons | = | 1 tablespoon |
| 4 tablespoons | = | 1/4 cup |
| 5 1/3 tablespoons | = | 1/3 cup |
| 8 tablespoons | = | 1/2 cup |
| 10 2/3 tablespoons | = | 2/3 cup |
| 12 tablespoons | = | 3/4 cup |
| 16 tablespoons | = | 1 cup |
| 2 tablespoons | = | 1 fluid ounce |
| 1 cup | = | 8 fluid ounces |
| 1 cup | = | 1/2 pint |
| 2 cups | = | 1 pint |
| 4 cups | = | 1 quart |
| 4 quarts | = | 1 gallon |

### Abbreviations

| | | |
|---|---|---|
| Tbsp. | = | Tablespoon |
| Tsp. | = | Teaspoon |
| Oz. | = | Ounce |

## Recipe Preparation Steps

1. Read the recipe to make sure you have all the food and equipment you need. Be sure you have enough time to prepare the recipe.
2. Clear and clean a work area.
3. Set out all ingredients needed.
4. When necessary, preheat the oven, then grease and flour pans.
5. Prepare the recipe.

## Cooking Terms

*Boil*: To heat liquid until bubbles break the surface, or to cook in boiling water.

*Broil*: To use direct heat to cook.

*Coat*: To cover entire surface with a mixture, such as flour or bread crumbs.

*Core*: To remove the core/seeds of a fruit using a sharp knife.

*Cream*: To stir one or more foods until they are soft.

*Crisp-tender*: Describes the "doneness" of vegetables when they are cooked until only tender and remain slightly crisp in texture.

*Cut in*: To mix fat into dry ingredients using a pastry blender, fork, or two knives, with as little blending as possible until the fat is in small pieces.

*Dice*: To cut into small, square-shaped pieces.

*Drain*: To put food and liquid into a strainer (or colander), or to pour liquid out of a pot by keeping the lid slightly away from the edge of the pan and pouring away from you.

*Flute*: To pinch the edge of dough, such as on a pie crust.

*Fork-tender*: Describes the "doneness" of a food when a fork can easily penetrate the food.

*Knead*: To mix by "pushing" and folding.

*Marinate*: To soak in a seasoned liquid to increase flavor and tenderness.

*Mince*: To cut or chop food into small pieces.

*Mix*: To combine ingredients using a fork or spoon.

*Oil*: To apply a thin layer of vegetable oil on a dish or pan. Vegetable spray may be used instead.

*Sauté*: To cook in a small amount of fat or water.

*Scald*: To heat milk until bubbles appear (bubbles should not be "breaking" on the surface).

*Shred*: To rub foods against a grater to divide into small pieces.

*Simmer*: To cook at a temperature that is just below the boiling point. Bubbles form slowly but do not reach the surface.

*Steam*: To cover over boiling water.

*Stir-fry*: A method of cooking in which vegetables are fried quickly to a crisp-tender state while stirring constantly.

*Stock*: Water in which vegetable(s) or meat has been cooked. Stock liquid should be stored in the refrigerator.

# Ingredient Substitutions

| Ingredient | Amount | Substitutions |
|---|---|---|
| Baking powder | 1 teaspoon | 1/4 teaspoon baking soda plus 5/8 teaspoon cream of tartar, or 1/4 teaspoon baking soda plus 1/2 cup sour milk or buttermilk (if using sour milk or buttermilk, decrease liquid called for in recipe by 1/2 cup) |
| Beef or chicken broth | 1 (14 1/2 ounce) can | 2 teaspoons instant beef or chicken bouillon granules with water to equal amount of broth specified |
| Bouillon cube | 1 | 1 tablespoon soy sauce |
| Dry bread crumbs | 1/4 cup | 1/4 cup cracker crumbs, cornmeal, rolled oats, or crushed bran cereal, or 1 cup soft bread crumbs |
| Butter, margarine, shortening, oil | 1 cup | 1/2 cup applesauce or prune puree plus 1/2 cup of butter, margarine, shortening, or oil |
| Corn syrup | 1 cup | 1 cup sugar plus 1/4 cup liquid (use the type of liquid that is called for in the recipe) |
| Cornstarch | 1 tablespoon | 2 tablespoons all-purpose flour, or 2 tablespoons quick-cooking tapioca |
| Cream | 1/4 cup | 1/4 cup fat-free half and half or evaporated skim milk |
| Egg (cake batter only) | 1 | 2 tablespoons mayonnaise |
| Flour, all-purpose | 1 tablespoon | 1/2 tablespoon cornstarch or quick-cooking tapioca (for thickening) |
| Flour, all-purpose | 1 cup sifted | 1 cup plus 2 tablespoons sifted cake flour or 1 cup unsifted all-purpose flour minus 2 tablespoons |
| Flour, cake | 1 cup sifted | 1 cup minus 2 tablespoons sifted all-purpose flour |
| Garlic | 1 clove, small | 1/8 teaspoon garlic powder |
| Gelatin, flavored | 3 ounce package | 1 tablespoon plain gelatin plus 2 cups fruit juice (prepared with water) |
| Herbs, fresh | 1 tablespoon | 1 teaspoon dried herbs |
| Honey | 1 cup | 1 1/2 cups sugar plus 1/4 cup liquid (use liquid called for in recipe) |
| Lemon | 1 medium | 2–3 tablespoons juice and 1–2 teaspoons rind |
| Lemon juice | 1 teaspoon | 1/2 teaspoon vinegar (for use as acid source in cooking only) |
| Milk, buttermilk | 1 cup | 1 cup yogurt |
| Milk, whole | 1 cup | 1/2 cup evaporated milk plus 1/2 cup water, low-fat milk, or skim milk |
| Milk, skim | 1 cup | 5 tablespoons nonfat dry milk and 1 cup water |
| Onion, fresh | 1 small | 1 tablespoon dry minced onion, rehydrated |
| Prepared mustard | 1 tablespoon | 1 teaspoon dried mustard |
| Parsley, dried | 1 teaspoon | 3 teaspoons chopped fresh parsley |
| Shortening, melted | 1 cup | 1 cup vegetable oil |
| Sour cream | 1 cup | 1 cup yogurt |
| Sugar, white | 1 cup | 1 cup corn syrup minus 1/4 cup liquid in recipe, or 1 cup brown sugar (firmly packed), or 1 cup honey (reduce liquid in recipe by 1/4 cup), or 1 3/4 cup confectioners' (powdered) sugar (packed) |
| Tomato juice | 1 cup | 1/2 cup tomato sauce plus 1/2 cup water |
| Tomato sauce | 1 (15 ounce can) | 1 (6 ounce can) tomato paste and 1 cup water |
| Tomatoes, canned | 1 (16 ounce can) | 3 fresh medium tomatoes, cut up |

# Healthy Cooking Tips

### Ways to Increase Fiber

- Choose whole grains instead of refined products. For example, use whole wheat flour, brown rice, oatmeal, whole cornmeal, and barley.
- Whole wheat flour can usually be substituted for up to 1/2 of the white flour in recipes. For example, if a recipe calls for 2 cups of flour, try 1 cup of white and 1 cup of whole wheat flour.
- Add grated or mashed vegetables or fruit to sauces or baked goods. For example, you can add grated carrots to spaghetti sauce and meat loaf.

### Ways to Decrease Sugar

- Try using 1/4 to 1/3 less sugar in baked foods and desserts (do not do this if sugar in the recipe has already been reduced). For example, if a fruit pie recipe calls for 1 cup of sugar, use 2/3 or 3/4 cup sugar. This works best with quick breads, cookies, pie fillings, custard, puddings, and fruit crisps. It may not work for some cakes. Do not decrease the small amount of sugar in plain yeast breads because it provides food for the yeast and helps the bread to rise.
- You do not have to add sugar when canning or freezing fruits. Or, you can buy unsweetened frozen fruit or fruit canned in its own juice or water.
- Increase the amount of cinnamon, vanilla, or nutmeg in a recipe to make it seem sweeter.

# Cooking With Herbs, Spices, and Seasonings*

Herbs and spices can add flavor and variety to your food. Use a little at first, then add more when you are sure you like the flavor. To substitute dry herbs for fresh, use 1/4 teaspoon powder or 1 teaspoon crushed for 1 tablespoon fresh chopped herbs. Some herbs and spices are expensive. You might want to buy only a few of the less expensive herbs and spices you will use.

Herbs and spices lose flavor and can spoil if kept in the cupboard longer than a year. If you use herbs and spices slowly, buy small containers, or store them in the freezer.

*Adapted from Wisconsin Nutrition Education Program. (1996). Cooking with herbs and spices. In: *Creative Cooking*, University of Wisconsin-Extension.

| Herbs, Spices, and Seasonings | Uses |
|---|---|
| Allspice (a mixture of cinnamon, nutmeg, and cloves) | Fruit desserts, pumpkin pie, apple cider, cakes, cookies, chicken, beef, and fish dishes |
| Basil | Tomato and egg dishes, stews, soups, and salads |
| Bay leaves | Tomato dishes, fish and meat dishes |
| Celery seed | Juices, soups, salads, vegetables, pot roasts, poultry, rolls, and biscuits |
| Chili powder | Chili, bean, and rice dishes |
| Chives | Potato dishes, soups, dips, and sauces |
| Cilantro (coriander leaves) | Latin American, Indian, and Chinese dishes, salsa, stir-fries, legume or rice salads, hot cooked rice, grilled chicken or fish, or a dish of ripe tomatoes; use fresh if possible |
| Cinnamon | French toast, fruit and fruit salads, sweet potatoes, pumpkin and squash, puddings and apple desserts, ham or pork chops |
| Cloves | Whole cloves on ham or pork roast; ground cloves to season pear or apple desserts, beets, beans, tomatoes, squash, and sweet potatoes |
| Coriander seed | Middle Eastern dishes, spice cakes and cookies, soups, roast pork, and salad dressing |
| Cumin | Mexican, Middle Eastern, and Indian dishes; beef and lamb, dry bean dishes, marinades, chili and tomato sauces; ingredient in curry powder |
| Dillweed | Tuna or salmon salad, potato salad, pickles, dips, and sauces |
| Garlic | Mexican, Italian, and Asian dishes and in salad dressings; can be used fresh or dried, minced or powder |
| Ginger (fresh) | Asian dishes, marinades for chicken or fish, fruit salad, dressings |
| Ginger (ground) | Gingerbread, spice cake, pumpkin pie, poultry or meat, soups, stews, stuffing, squash, sweet potatoes |
| Ground peppers: black, cayenne, and white pepper | Meats, casseroles, vegetables, and soups |
| Italian seasoning (a mixture of marjoram, oregano, basil, and rosemary) | Italian dishes such as spaghetti |
| Marjoram | Egg and cheese dishes, meats, fish, poultry, and vegetables |
| Mint | Fruit salads and fruit soups, melon, berries, cold fruit beverages, cooked carrots or peas, chilled yogurt soup, lamb, tabbouleh |
| Mustard | Sauces for meat and fish, in marinades, salad dressings, chutneys, pickles, and relishes |
| Nutmeg | Cooked fruits, pies and desserts, baked items, spinach, sweet potatoes, eggnog, and French toast |
| Onion | Any dish where onion flavor is desired; can be used fresh or dried (minced or powder) |
| Oregano | Italian dishes, chili, omelets, beef stew, meat loaf, pork, and vegetables such as broccoli or tomatoes |
| Parsley | Meat, soup, or vegetable dishes; adds color |
| Paprika | Stew, chicken, fish, potatoes, rice, and hard-boiled eggs |
| Rosemary | Egg dishes, meats, fish, soups and stews, and vegetables |
| Thyme | Fish, poultry, or meats, in soups or stews, vegetable salads |

# Seasoning Your Food With Less Salt*

Try using herbs and spices to season your food. You may find that you can cut down the amount of salt you use.

Some seasonings contain salt and/or sodium. Use the following sparingly: garlic salt, celery salt, seasoned salt, soy sauce, onion salt, monosodium glutamate (MSG).

Many seasoning mixtures contain a lot of salt—read the label!

# Food Yields

| Food | Amount | Yield |
|------|--------|-------|
| Apples | 1 pound | = 3 medium = 3 cups slices |
| Bananas | 1 pound | = 3–4 medium = 1 1/2 cups mashed = 2 cups sliced |
| Beans (dry) | 1 pound | = 2–2 1/2 cups (dry) = 6 cups cooked |
| Bread crumbs | 4 slices bread | = 2 cups fresh crumbs = 1 1/3 cups dry crumbs |
| Butter, margarine, shortening | 1 pound | = 2 cups |
| Cabbage | 1 pound | = 6 cups shredded = 2–3 cups cooked |
| Carrots | 1 pound | = 3 cups sliced = 1 1/2 cups shredded |
| Cheese | 4 ounces | = 1–1 1/3 cups shredded |
| Coffee | 1 pound | = 40–50 cups brewed |
| Eggs (medium) | 1 dozen | = 2 cups |
| Egg whites (large) | 8 eggs | = 1 cup |
| Flour, all-purpose | 1 pound | = 4 cups sifted |
| Flour, whole wheat | 1 pound | = 3 1/2–3 3/4 |
| Graham crackers | 12 squares | = 1 cup crumbs |
| Ground meat (beef, turkey, pork) | 1 pound | = 2 cups ground |
| Lemons | 1 lemon | = 2–4 tablespoons juice |
| Macaroni, spaghetti | 1 pound | = 5 cups (dry) = 8–10 cups cooked |
| Milk, evaporated | 6 ounce can | = 1 1/2 cups reconstituted |
| Oatmeal | 1/2 cup (dry) | = 1 cup cooked |
| Onions | 1 pound | = 3 large |
| Oranges | 1 orange | = 6 tablespoons juice |
| Potatoes | 1 pound | = 3 medium = 3 1/2 cups sliced = 2 cups mashed |
| Raisins | 1 pound | = 1 3/4–3 cups |
| Rice, white or brown | 1 pound | = 2 1/2 cups (dry) = 7 1/2 cups cooked |
| Sugar, white-granulated | 1 pound | = 2 cups |
| Sugar, brown | 1 pound | = 2 1/4 cup (firmly packed) |

*Source*: Brody, J. (1990). *Jane Brody's Good Food Gourmet*. New York: W.W. Norton & Co. Inc.

*Adapted from Wisconsin Nutrition Education Program. (1996). Cooking with herbs and spices. In: *Creative Cooking*, University of Wisconsin-Extension.

# Putting Out a Cooking Fire

1. Turn the stove or oven off immediately.
2. Use a fire extinguisher to put out a fire. If you do not have a fire extinguisher, cover the pan with a lid or other non-flammable object to suffocate the fire. If covering the pan is not possible, pour salt or baking soda on the fire.
3. If the fire does not go out immediately, call the fire department.

*Tips*:

- Don't throw water on grease fires.
- The best way to put out a fire is with a fire extinguisher. Many buildings, such as apartment buildings, must have fire extinguishers in the hall or other areas close to each unit. If there is a fire extinguisher where you live, know where it is located and how to use it.

## Reference

1. University of Tennessee Extension Expanded Food and Nutrition Education Program (2002). *Eat Smart: Get Your Family to the Table—Cooking Basics*. Available at https://utextension.tennessee.edu/publications/Documents/SP732.pdf.

# About the Authors

**Natalie Digate Muth**, MD, MPH, RD, is a pediatrician, registered dietitian, and mother of two. She completed her pediatrics training at Mattel Children's Hospital UCLA, where she was in the Community Health and Advocacy Training program. She's a spokesperson for the American Council on Exercise and has been widely featured as a health and nutrition expert in the media, including *ABC World News Now*, *San Diego Living*, *Health* magazine, and *The New York Times*.

**Mary Saph Tanaka**, MD, MS, developed her love for cooking at a young age, with fond memories of planting and cooking vegetables from the garden with her mother. She regularly utilizes locally grown ingredients and her knowledge of nutrition and herbs to prepare nutritious meals for family and friends. She completed her pediatric training at Mattel Children's Hospital UCLA as part of the Community Health and Advocacy Training program.